# CRASH COURSE

*Third Edition*

# Ophthalmology
# Dermatology
# ENT

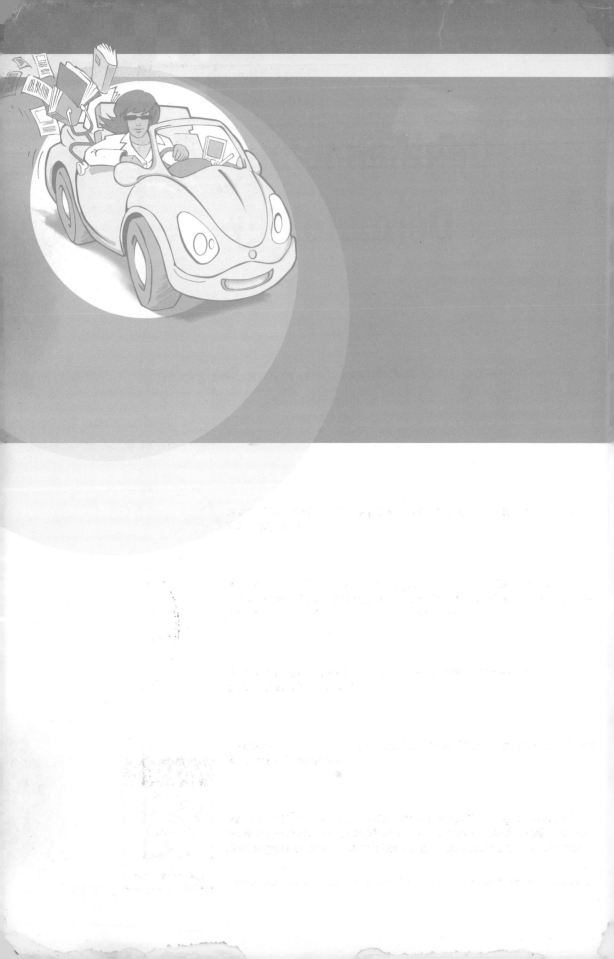

# CRASH COURSE

# Ophthalmology
# Dermatology
# ENT

Series editor
**Daniel Horton-Szar**
BSc(Hons) MBBS(Hons) MRCGP

Northgate Medical Practice,
Canterbury,
Kent, UK

## Seau-Tak Cheung
BMedSci(Hons) MBChB MRCP
Locum Dermatology Consultant, Heart of England Foundation NHS Trust,
Birmingham, UK

## Niaz Islam
BSc(Hons) MBBS FRCOphth
Consultant Ophthalmic Surgeon, Queen's Hospital, Romford, Essex,
and Locum Consultant and Medical Education Fellow, Moorfields Eye
Hospital NHS Foundation Trust, London, UK

## David Keegan
PhD FRCSI(Oph) FRCOphth
Consultant Ophthalmic Surgeon, Mater Misericordiae University
Hospital, Dublin, Ireland

## John McGuinness
FDS RCS FRCS(Oto/HNS)
Specialist Registrar in ENT Head and Neck Surgery, The Royal Marsden
Hospital, London, UK

## Nicholas G Strouthidis
MD MRCOphth
Specialist Registrar, Glaucoma Research Unit, Moorfields Eye Hospital
NHS Foundation Trust, London, UK, and Post-Doctoral Scientist, Optic Nerve
Head Research Laboratory, Devers Eye Institute, Portland, Oregon, USA

MOSBY

ELSEVIER

Edinburgh • London • New York • Oxford • Philadelphia • St Louis • Sydney • Toronto 2009

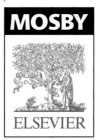

| | |
|---|---|
| Commissioning Editor: | Alison Taylor |
| Development Editor: | Siân Jarman |
| Project Manager: | Gail Wright |
| Designer: | Sarah Russell |
| Cover Designer: | Stewart Larking |
| Illustration Manager: | Bruce Hogarth |

First published 2009
Reprinted 2010

ISBN: 978-0-7234-3369-9

**British Library Cataloguing in Publication Data**
A catalogue record for this book is available from the British Library

**Library of Congress Cataloging in Publication Data**
A catalog record for this book is available from the Library of Congress

**Notice**

Knowledge and best practice in this field are constantly changing. As new research and experience broaden our knowledge, changes in practice, treatment and drug therapy may become necessary or appropriate. Readers are advised to check the most current information provided (i) on procedures featured or (ii) by the manufacturer of each product to be administered, to verify the recommended dose or formula, the method and duration of administration, and contraindications. It is the responsibility of the practitioner, relying on their own experience and knowledge of the patient, to make diagnoses, to determine dosages and the best treatment for each individual patient, and to take all appropriate safety precautions. To the fullest extent of the law, neither the Publisher nor the Authors assumes any liability for any injury and/or damage to persons or property arising out or related to any use of the material contained in this book.

The purpose of the ophthalmology section is to present an up-to-date, systemic and practical overview for undergraduate medical students. A good teacher explains, but a great teacher inspires. We hope our readers are inspired!

**Niaz Islam**

More than a decade has now passed since work began on the *Crash Course* series. Medicine never stands still, and the work of keeping this series relevant for today's students is an ongoing process. As the series keeps up to date with the latest medical research and developments in pharmacology and current best practice, this title builds upon the success of the preceding books.

As always, we listen to feedback from the thousands of students who use *Crash Course* and have made further improvements to the layout and structure of the books.

Despite the ongoing revisions and improvements, we hold fast to the principles on which we first developed the series: *Crash Course* will always bring you all the information you need to revise in compact, manageable volumes that integrate pathology and therapeutics with best clinical practice. The books still maintain the balance between clarity and conciseness, and provide sufficient depth for those aiming at distinction.

I wish you all the best for your future careers!

**Dr Dan Horton-Szar**
**Series Editor**

# Contributors and Acknowledgements

**Gus Gazzard** MA MD FRCOphth
Consultant Ophthalmic Surgeon,
King's College Hospital,
London, UK
*Chapter 9*. Glaucoma

**Rajni Jain** MBBS FRCOphth
Consultant Ophthalmic Surgeon,
The Western Eye Hospital,
London, UK
*Chapter 7*. Adnexal (eyelids, lacrimal system and orbit) and
*Chapter 12*. Strabismus and paediatrics

## Ophthalmology

I would like to acknowledge the following ophthalmic consultant surgeons: Miss Narciss Okhravi and Professor Sue Lightman (Moorfields Eye Hospital) and Mr Andrew Coombes and Mr Mark Westcott (Royal London Hospital) for their kind help and support throughout my medical retina/medical educational teaching fellowship.

**Niaz Islam**

# Contents

# Contents

# Glossary

**Anisocoria**  A difference in size between the two pupils. Occurs in 20% of UK population.

**Chemosis**  Conjunctival oedema.

**Cotton wool spot**  A white fluffy lesion due to a superficial retinal infarction.

**Crowding phenomenon**  Individual letters can be read better than a whole line; most commonly seen in amblyopic patients.

**Diplopia**  Double vision.

**Ectopia lentis**  Dislocated lens.

**Flare**  Increased protein in the anterior chamber fluid, permitting visualization of the slit-lamp beam.

**Floaters**  Visual perception of dots or spots which may seem to 'swim' or shift location when the position of gaze is shifted.

**Fovea**  An area of the retina corresponding to central vision, located temporal and slightly inferior to the centre of the optic disc.

**Hard exudates**  Deep retinal lipid, often glistening yellow in appearance.

**Hypemetropia (long sighted)**  The eye is too short or the refractive power too weak to bring objects at distance or near into clear focus (without the use of accommodation).

**Hyphaema**  Blood in the anterior chamber.

**Hypopyon**  Layer of white blood cells inferiorly in the anterior chamber.

**Keratic precipitates**  Lymphocytic cellular aggregates that form on the corneal endothelium, often inferiorly, in a base-down triangular pattern.

**Leukocoria**  A grossly visible white pupil.

**Macula**  An area four disc diameters in size centred at the posterior part of the retina.

**Meibomianitis**  Inflamed, inspissated oil glands along the eyelid margins, reflecting inflammation of the meibomian glands.

**Miosis**  Constriction of the pupil.

**Mydriasis**  Dilatation of the pupil.

**Myopia (short sighted)**  The eye is too long or the refractive power too great to bring objects at a distance clearly into focus.

**Nystagmus**  Rhythmic oscillations or tremors of the eyes that occur independently of normal movements.

**Optic neuritis**  Inflammation of the optic nerve.

**Papilloedema**  Optic disc swelling produced by increased intracranial pressure.

**Peripapillary**  Surrounding the optic disc.

**Peripheral iridectomy**  Removal of a portion of the peripheral iris.

**Photophobia**  Ocular pain on exposure to light.

**Photopsia**  Flashes of light; most commonly indicative of retinal traction.

**Posterior synechiae**  Adhesions between the iris and the anterior lens capsule.

**Proptosis**  Protrusion of the globe from the bony orbit.

**Ptosis**  Drooping of the upper eyelid.

**Punctum**  The opening of the tear drainage system in the eyelid margin.

**Retinitis**  Retinal inflammation.

**Rhegmatogenous retinal detachment**  Detachment of the retina as a result of a retinal tear or hole.

**Scleritis**  Inflammation of the sclera (white coat of the eye).

**Scotoma**  An area in the visual field with a loss of sensitivity.

**Strabismus**  Ocular misalignment.

**Trabeculectomy**  Surgery to improve aqueous outflow and reduce intraocular pressure in glaucoma patients.

- Gritti... conjun...
- Itching
- Sharp pain, if exp... may suggest a co... corneal abrasic... accompanying s...
- Pain exacerbat... – is usually a fe...
- A dull, boring a... in anterior scl... look similar... patients wil'... severe enc... they may

# The red, painful eye

## Objectives

You should be able to:

- Take an 'ophthalmic' history of red eye.
- Identify salient features in the history pointing to a particular cause of red eye.
- Differentiate between sight threatening and non-sight threatening causes of red eye.
- Understand the anatomical location of each pathological cause of red eye.
- Appreciate how to elicit the necessary physical signs.
- Understand which investigations may be performed to help establish the diagnosis.

Red eye is among the commonest ophthalmic presentations to general practitioners, accident and emergency departments and high street opticians. It is usually accompanied by some degree of pain/discomfort, ranging from the mild (e.g. blepharitis and conjunctivitis) to the severe (e.g. scleritis, iritis and primary angle closure).

The red, painful eye usually suggests a disorder in the anterior segment – i.e. the front parts of the eye (conjunctiva, sclera/episclera, cornea, iris and lens).

- A white, painful eye is more unusual and usually suggests pathology at the back of the eye (posterior scleritis, optic or retrobulbar neuritis). However, in these conditions, other symptoms will predominate – in particular visual loss. Orbital pathology may also present with a painless white eye, although symptoms of proptosis, diplopia or visual loss are likely to predominate.
- The most common cause of a red, painless eye is spontaneous subconjunctival haemorrhage (see Fig. 2.3). In this condition blood is seen overlying the white of the eye (sclera) under the conjunctiva. It looks alarming but is of no visual consequence and patients are usually unaware of it until it is pointed out by friends/family. Usually no cause is identified, although it may occur in patients coughing, sneezing or following any other Valsalva manoeuvre, including straining on the toilet, or in patients taking aspirin or warfarin. Usually one

can reassure the patient; if the haemorrhages recurrent one can consider checking the pa blood pressure or clotting.

Always enquire about a history of trauma in cases of bilateral subconjunctival haemorrhages. Base of skull fractures may present with bilateral subconjunctival h in which the posterior limit may not

It is important mild, self-limiting tivitis, and sight- angle closure, iri Differential di

## DIFFERE

### Key symptoms

Pain.
Watery or sticky (discha
Photophobia?
Visual loss or reduced v

**Fig. 1.1** Common differential diagnoses of a red, painful eye

| Differential | Discharge | Vision | Conjunctiva | Pupil | Cornea | Anterior chamber | IOP |
|---|---|---|---|---|---|---|---|
| Subconjunctival haemorrhage | No | Unaffected | Bright red | Normal | Clear | Quiet | Normal |
| Blepharitis | Occasional | Unaffected | Injected vessels | Normal | Clear | Quiet | Normal |
| Conjunctivitis | Yes | Unaffected | Injected vessels and fornices | Normal | Clear | Quiet | Normal |
| Trauma – abrasion/FB | Watering | Depending on severity | Injected vessels | Normal | Abrasion/FB | Quiet | Normal |
| Keratitis | Watering | May be affected | Injected vessels | Normal | White lesions, hazy | Possible cells | Possibly elevated |
| Iritis | No | May be affected | Injected around cornea | Small, fixed, irregular | Keratic precipitates | Cells | Possibly elevated |
| Episcleritis | No | Unaffected | Sectoral deep injection | Normal | Normal | Normal | Normal |
| Scleritis | No | May be affected | Sectoral deep 'brick red' injection | Normal | Normal | Possible cells | Normal |
| Primary angle closure | Watering | Reduced | Entire eye red | Fixed, mid-dilated | Hazy | Shallow, cells | Elevated |

Foreign body: FB; Intraocular pressure: IOP

## HISTORY

### Des_____ of pain

_____tation – suggestive of
_____lepharitis.
_____tic of *allergic* conjunctivitis.
_____erienced after trauma,
_____rneal foreign body or
_____ye watering is usually an
_____mptom.
_____d by bright lights – photophobia
_____eature of anterior uveitis/iritis.
_____che is characteristically described
_____eritis. Episcleritis (Fig. 1.2) can
_____ut the pain is usually milder, and
_____ never volunteer that the pain is
_____ugh to keep them up at night, which
_____ do with scleritis.

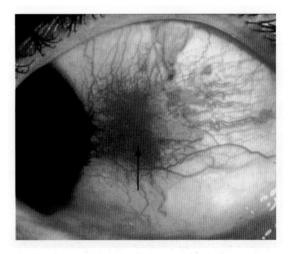

**Fig. 1.2** Episcleritis. A superficial localized red injection between conjunctiva and white sclera.

## Duration of symptoms

- Patients who have experienced trauma whether it be a corneal abrasion, corneal foreign body or a chemical injury will be symptomatic immediately and will present to emergency services accordingly.
- Viral (Fig. 1.3) and bacterial (Fig. 1.4) conjunctivitis may have a period of latency whereby the eye may be mildly irritated for up to 10 days before the redness and discharge develop.
- A red, discharging eye over a period of *months* is unlikely to be bacterial or viral conjunctivitis as these are self-limiting conditions which resolve within 21 days. In these circumstances one should consider the possibility of Chlamydia conjunctivitis, where there is a thick and rope-like mucopurulent discharge. Floppy eyelid syndrome may also present in a similar fashion; such patients have very easily everted upper lids and have the habitus of patients with obstructive sleep apnoea (i.e. obese, short, thick neck, history of snoring). In the younger age group another cause of chronic infective conjunctivitis is molluscum contagiosum; the lesions may be apparent on inspection of the lids.

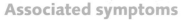

Bringing up the possibility of Chlamydia, a sexually transmitted disease, can be awkward especially as the patient has presented with an eye problem only. Check whether they have heard of Chlamydia and know the implications. Once this has been established, make a direct enquiry regarding the risk of exposure (i.e. take a sexual history). *Remember to ensure the patient's privacy during the consultation!*

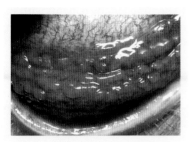

**Fig. 1.3** Viral conjunctivitis. Follicles are visible on the inferior conjunctival surface.

## Associated symptoms

### Watering

- Mild to moderate watering may be seen in blepharitis or conjunctivitis.
- Excessive lacrimation may be seen in corneal abrasions, corneal foreign bodies, subtarsal foreign body (where a foreign body lodges under the top lid and scratches the corneal epithelium with each blink) and trichiasis (where a lash is misdirected onto the globe – this may be particularly uncomfortable if it rubs on the cornea).

### Discharge

- Clear discharge with stickiness of the lids in the morning is common in blepharitis.
- Discharge may be indistinguishable between viral and bacterial conjunctivitis, although in bacterial may be yellow/green compared to yellow/white in viral.
- The discharge in Chlamydia conjunctivitis is thick and accumulates in rope-like strands.
- Gonococcal conjunctival discharge in babies (as ophthalmia neonatorum) is excessive, even 'explosive'.

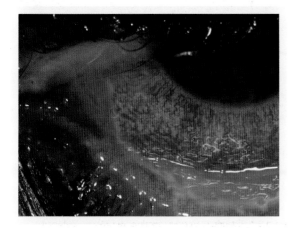

**Fig. 1.4** Bacterial conjunctivitis (yellow/green purulent sticky eye).

## Photophobia

Photophobia is characteristic of anterior uveitis/iritis. However, it may also be a symptom of any condition which causes ciliary muscle spasm, including microbial keratitis, herpetic keratitis, corneal abrasion, recurrent erosion syndrome.

## Visual loss

- Conditions affecting the external lids (blepharitis), the conjunctiva (conjunctivitis) and the episclera (episcleritis) do not usually affect vision, except where the patient is viewing the world through a film of pus or tears (which can of course be wiped away).
- Blurred vision in the context of a red, painful eye will usually suggest either corneal involvement (microbial keratitis, herpetic keratitis, corneal oedema in primary angle closure, large corneal abrasion) or a significant inflammatory component (scleritis or iritis).

## PREVIOUS MEDICAL HISTORY

A number of underlying medical conditions may be associated with red, painful eyes (Fig. 1.5).

A recent history of upper respiratory tract viral illness – cough or sore throat – might be associated with the onset of viral conjunctivitis.

**Fig. 1.5** Common ophthalmic causes of a red eye with an underlying systemic cause.

| Ophthalmic condition | Underlying conditions |
|---|---|
| Scleritis | Rheumatoid arthritis, lupus |
| Iritis | Ankylosing spondylitis, sarcoidosis, juvenile idiopathic arthritis, inflammatory bowel disease, AIDS/HIV-related opportunistic infections, toxoplasmosis (list by no means exhaustive!) |
| Dry eyes | Sjögren's syndrome |
| Thyroid eye disease | Graves' disease |

## PREVIOUS OPHTHALMIC HISTORY

- Ask about recent surgery. Acute iritis, and more seriously endophthalmitis, may occur following cataract surgery. In general endophthalmitis occurs within 10 days of surgery, whereas iritis may occur weeks after the surgery.
- Patients with recurrent erosion syndrome give a classic history. There will be history of traumatic corneal abrasion in the past, which got better. The patient now wakes up with a feeling of the lids sticking together on the side of the previous abrasion and when they open the eyes there is a feeling of 'ripping' or 'tearing'; the symptoms of the original abrasion return.
- Anterior uveitis/iritis and herpes simplex keratitis are recurrent conditions (as is, as the name suggests, recurrent erosion syndrome) and patients may volunteer their diagnosis from the outset.
- Refractive error – primary angle closure is more likely to occur in elderly patients with short, hypermetropic eyes with coexistent cataract.
- Always ask about history of contact lens use. Contact lenses predispose to microbial causes of keratitis, in particular soft lenses. Ask about whether patient sleeps in contact lenses, or swims/showers in them (the latter may point to a diagnosis of acanthamoeba).

Always ask patients about their eye drop history, as patients may develop an allergic conjunctivitis from their drops.

## EXAMINATION

A systematic examination of the anterior segment structures should easily identify the cause of the red, painful eye.

### External lids and adnexae

- Before examining a patient's lids, look at their face. Do they have features of acne rosacea? Is there a vesicular rash over one side of the forehead (herpes zoster ophthalmicus – shingles)?

Do they have features suggestive of thyroid eye disease, such as proptosis?

- Inflammation, redness and swelling of the lids indicate cellulitis, either orbital or pre-septal. As it is the more severe condition, one must exclude features of orbital cellulitis – proptosis, double vision, loss of colour vision, reduced vision, swollen optic disc.
- If you suspect conjunctivitis, palpate the pre-auricular lymph nodes. Tender pre-auricular lymphadenopathy is a feature of viral conjunctivitis.
- Look for signs of herpetic lesions – cold sores or the vesicular lesions of herpes zoster (shingles).
- Examine the lid margin looking for features of blepharitis – crusting of the lashes, telangiectatic vessels at the lid margin, irregular lid margin, meibomian gland orifice capping, inflamed meibomian glands. Also look for other potentially infective lesions – mollusca.

## Internal lids

- Always evert the lids; this way you will be able to identify and remove subtarsal foreign bodies.
- Inspection of the inner aspect of the lids is a reliable way of diagnosing conjunctivitis (look for follicles and papillae).
- Follicles are small and resemble grains of rice, with a surrounding vascular bed. They are characteristic of viral and chlamydial conjunctivitis (where the follicles are much larger).
- Papillae are larger polygonal 'bumps' with a central vascular core. They are non-specific and may be seen in bacterial conjunctivitis, allergic conjunctivitis, foreign bodies (including chronic contact lens wear) and in floppy eyelid syndrome.

## Conjunctiva

- If the conjunctiva is inflamed, injected with follicles +/– tender pre-auricular lymphadenopathy, viral conjunctivitis is likely. Subconjunctival haemorrhages and chemosis ('waterlogged conjunctiva') may also occur in this condition.
- If the conjunctiva is inflamed, injected with subtarsal and bulbar papillae and there is excessive purulent discharge, then bacterial conjunctivitis is likely.

- Acute chemosis and papillae are a feature of allergic/atopic conjunctivitis, as well as chemical conjunctivitis which may be seen following a chemical injury.

Beware the white eye following a chemical injury. Such eyes need to be examined carefully for evidence of conjunctival blood vessel ischaemia. Limbal ischaemia (i.e. absent or constricted vessels at the conjunctival edge by the cornea) are a poor prognostic sign and may result in an opaque cornea.

## Sclera/episclera

- The redness seen in scleritis can be distinguished from episcleritis in a number of ways. In scleritis the redness is sectoral but takes on a brick-like, violet colour with the distension of all the scleral and episcleral vessels which may appear tortuous. This redness is characteristic when viewed in room light. The patient may also report a severe aching pain when the lid is pressed directly over the area of inflammation.
- The injection in episcleritis is also sectoral, but much milder, with a less striking reddish hue. A single drop of phenylephrine 2.5% will allow the episcleral vessels to constrict in episcleritis, making the eye appear more white. This does not happen in scleritis – which may be a useful feature in distinguishing between the two conditions.
- An inflammatory 'nodule' may be present in both episcleritis and scleritis.

## Cornea

Remember to test corneal sensation (which is reduced in herpes simplex keratitis) or the corneal reflex (which tests the integrity of the ophthalmic division of the trigeminal nerve) prior to instilling topical anaesthesia! The results will be meaningless if tested afterwards.

The instillation of topical fluorescein and illumination with cobalt blue light is useful in detected corneal epithelial pathology:

- Corneal abrasions.
- Dendritic ulcers – ulcers with tree-like branches, characteristic of herpes simplex.
- Dry eye – characterized by punctate ('spotty') fluorescein staining.

Multiple vertical corneal scratches may be caused by a subtarsal foreign body. Remember to ask the patient to look down and then evert the upper lid!

The appearance of whitish/cloudy lesions, called infiltrates, within the anterior corneal stroma is a feature of corneal inflammation – keratitis.

- Where corneal infiltrates with overlying epithelial fluorescein staining occur in the context of contact lens wear, microbial keratitis is the most likely diagnosis. In this circumstance one should treat as such, before microbiological confirmation from corneal scrapes (which takes 48 hours) is received.
- Corneal infiltrates occurring near to the limbus, in patients with lid-margin disease, in particular if associated with rosacea, are likely to be a sign of marginal keratitis. The distinction between these infiltrates, which are sterile, and infective infiltrates is difficult if the patient also wears contact lenses. In this circumstance it may be wiser to treat as microbial keratitis in the first instance, as this is the more serious condition.
- Multiple discoid subepithelial infiltrates without fluorescein staining may occur as a sequelae of adenoviral infection. The patient may initially present with adenoviral conjunctivitis and then re-present complaining of reduced vision secondary to these 'adeno-spots'. The infiltrates do clear eventually without treatment, although topical steroids may speed the process considerably.

Corneal oedema – waterlogging of the cornea – is usually apparent as a hazing and thickening of the cornea. It may be present in a localized form in any form of infective keratitis. A more diffuse, generalized form may occur in acute elevations of intraocular pressure, as may occur in primary angle closure.

Keratic precipitates are small spots or discs of inflammatory material adherent to the endothelium which is the innermost aspect of the cornea – they are usually seen in anterior uveitis.

## Anterior chamber

Full examination of the anterior chamber – the fluid space between the cornea and the iris – is difficult without the use of the slit lamp. There are some features which may be apparent using a pen torch or the direct ophthalmoscope:

- A white fluid level within the eye – a hypopyon. It is caused by the settling of inflammatory cells within the anterior chamber. In the context of contact lens wear and a corneal infiltrate this is pathognomonic of an infective keratitis. If seen within a few days of cataract surgery it should set alarm bells ringing in terms of endophthalmitis, a sight-threatening infection. Hypopyon may also be a feature of severe anterior uveitis, as may occur in Behçet's syndrome (strangely, the drug rifabutin can also cause a hypopyon).
- A red fluid level within the eye – a hyphaema. This is caused by the settling of red blood cells within the anterior chamber. Invariably patients will give a report of trauma or surgery. It is important for such patients to have their intraocular pressures checked.
- Anterior chamber shallowing/flattening. This is a feature of primary angle closure; it can be difficult to appreciate without the use of an angled slit beam, as available with the slit lamp.

Other features detectable using a slit lamp are:

- Cells and flare. These are two characteristic features of anterior uveitis – circulating inflammatory cells (cells) and protein exudate (flare) within the anterior chamber. They can only be seen with a slit lamp. When the cells conglomerate within the anterior chamber they can form 'fibrin', which is evidence of a more severe inflammation.

When examining the anterior chamber for cells and flare using the slit lamp, it is important to remember that the aqueous fluid should be clear – this appears as black on the slit lamp. Cells and flare look rather like the beam of light from a cinema or slide projector, with a milky glow equivalent to flare and the dust particles floating about within the beam equivalent to cells.

- Some forms of anterior uveitis – 'hypertensive uveitis'. Another, rarer form, Posner–Schlossman syndrome, is associated with high IOP, very mild anterior reaction and one or two keratic precipitates. Hypertensive uveitis is a common presenting feature of toxoplasma associated uveitis, so always remember to look in the fundus for evidence of active toxoplasma retinitis. Herpes zoster uveitis is also frequently associated with raised pressure.

## Iris and pupil

Primary angle closure, previously known as angle closure glaucoma, may present with a number of iris/pupil signs:

- Fixed, mid-dilated pupil.
- Anterior iris bowing (iris bombé).
- Peripheral iridocorneal touch, as well as shallowing/narrowing of the anterior chamber.

The cornea may be hazy secondary to oedema and the intraocular pressure is elevated. Cataract may also be a predisposing factor.

Iritis may be associated with:

- Posterior synechiae – these are inflammatory adhesions between the pupillary margin of the iris and the anterior lens capsule. When one attempts to dilate the pupil pharmacologically, the pupil may be so stuck down as to not dilate at all, or it may take on an irregular shape secondary to focal adhesions.
- Iris nodules (especially in sarcoid-related anterior uveitis).

Rubeosis occurs when neovascularization occurs in the iris and iridocorneal angle. It is a feature of ischaemic retinopathies such as proliferative diabetic retinopathy, central retinal vein occlusion and certain forms of uveitis. It may cause rubeotic glaucoma whereby the eye becomes painful and red with reduced vision and raised intraocular pressure (IOP).

## Intraocular pressure

This may be elevated in a number of conditions but is seldom in itself a cause of pain, except when extremely high. Causes include:

- Primary angle closure.
- Rubeosis.

The gold standard method of IOP measurement is applanation tonometry, although it is not generally available outside ophthalmology clinics. A simple, subjective alternative is by digital tonometry – whereby the 'tone' of the globe is assessed by balloting the globe (through the closed eyelid!) alternately with the observer's two index fingers.

## INVESTIGATIONS

In ophthalmology most clinical diagnoses can be made on the basis of history and examination without recourse to specific tests. There are a few important investigations to be aware of when a patient presents with a red eye:

- Conjunctival swabs (viral, bacterial, chlamydial) if an infective conjunctivitis is suspected.
- Corneal scrapes – taken if a contact lens-related ulcer/infiltrate is seen. Specimens are plated on to a microscope slide (for rapid microscopy) and onto blood agar, chocolate agar, Sabouraud agar and brain–heart infusion broth (if fungi suspected), and *E. coli* seeded non-nutrient agar (if acanthamoeba suspected).

Systemic investigations are rarely performed in first presentations of scleritis and iritis. Investigations are performed if the presentation is atypical or if recurrent:

- Iritis screen – chest X-ray (tuberculosis/sarcoid), serum ACE (sarcoid), VDRL (syphilis), HLA B27 (ankylosing spondylitis).
- Scleritis screen – cANCA (Wegener's).

CT is useful in the diagnosis of orbital conditions.
B-scan ultrasonography may be required if a view of the posterior segment is not possible, e.g. because of hyphaema.

A basic understanding of ocular (essentially the 'eyeball') and adnexal (the tissue around the eye, including eyelids and orbit) trauma is essential for all doctors who work in an emergency setting. There may be cross-over with other specialties including neurosurgery (if there is a history of head injury), maxillofacial (if there is an orbital fracture) or plastic surgery (if the injuries involve the rest of the face).

> Never forget the theoretical risk of sympathetic ophthalmia, an inflammatory condition which may cause visual loss in the fellow eye following trauma (sometimes years after the event).

## DIFFERENTIAL DIAGNOSIS

The eye's response to trauma will vary according to the mechanism of the injury (Fig. 2.1). By definition, penetrating trauma (i.e. with a sharp instrument) is more likely to result in laceration of the ocular tissues. Blunt trauma, if mild, may only result in superficial tissue damage and bruising. However, where blunt trauma is more forceful, the forces may be transmitted through the globe, perhaps resulting in bruising of the retina (commotio retinae) or globe rupture. Where the force of blunt trauma is transmitted to the orbit, fracture may occur.

The eye may also be subject to injuries from chemical and thermal agents, which present different challenges from mechanical trauma.

Visual loss following trauma may result from:

- Corneal scarring from corneal laceration or opacity following chemical injury.
- Optic nerve compression from retrobulbar haemorrhage or traumatic neuropathy.
- Severely disordered globe anatomy.
- Retinal detachment/choroidal haemorrhage.

## HISTORY

> It is always good practice to clearly document the history and findings of any patients you see. HOWEVER, it is *absolutely essential* you do so in any trauma cases, particularly if they involve assault. Your notes may end up being scrutinized in a court of law, therefore write clearly and in detail. And remember to include the time and date you saw the patient!

### Exclude significant non-ophthalmic trauma

It is essential that potentially life-threatening injuries should be addressed before referral on to ophthalmology services. Upon presentation to the emergency department, most severe traumatic injuries would be managed according to 'advanced trauma life support' protocols and therefore such serious coexisting injuries would be identified and dealt with appropriately.

**Fig. 2.1** Common presentations following trauma to the globe and to the adnexae

| Mechanism | Site | Traumatic consequence |
|---|---|---|
| Blunt trauma | Ocular | Corneal abrasion, corneal foreign body, hyphaema, traumatic iritis, traumatic mydriasis, iridodialysis, angle recession, cataract, lens subluxation/dislocation, commotio retinae, retinal tear/detachment, vitreous haemorrhage, suprachoroidal haemorrhage, globe rupture, traumatic optic neuropathy |
| | Adnexal | Orbital blow-out fracture, lid ecchymosis, retrobulbar haemorrhage, traumatic optic neuropathy |
| Penetrating trauma | Ocular | Corneal laceration, conjunctival laceration, scleral rupture, retained intraocular foreign body |
| | Adnexal | Lid laceration |
| Burn (chemical, thermal) | Ocular | Conjunctival ischaemia, symblepharon, corneal limbal stem cell failure, corneal opacity |
| | Adnexal | Skin burns |

However, there is a risk in more 'trivial' injuries that only the ophthalmic problem is identified:

- Loss of consciousness or variable level of consciousness may indicate neurological trauma. This would need to be excluded as a priority. Likewise other features of raised intracranial pressure or neurological symptoms following trauma should cause concern, requiring urgent imaging (CT/MRI) and possible referral to neurosurgery.
- Take into consideration the SIZE and DIMENSIONS of any instrument responsible for penetrating injury around the globe. Long screwdrivers, bamboo poles, pencils and paintbrush handles may all be long enough to breach the bony confines of the orbit. If an intracranial penetrating trauma is missed, the patient is at risk of death from intracerebral haemorrhage, encephalitis or meningitis. Any history or sign of CSF rhinorrhoea should immediately raise alarm.
- As routine, any patient with history of penetrating trauma should have their tetanus status assessed, in case a booster is required.

## Nature of injury

Record time of trauma.
  For foreign body trauma, identify:

- *Type of object* – whether metal or vegetative matter; the latter may cause risk of fungal infection. In cases of chemical injury, it is important to know whether acid or alkali was involved; alkali burns may cause more serious damage.

- *Velocity, trajectory, distance.* Metal FBs 'blown' into the eye (Fig. 2.2) will usually just land on the corneal surface. Objects at higher velocity (e.g. from a chisel or an air gun) are more likely to penetrate the globe. The risk of penetration increases as the distance of the object from the globe decreases (i.e. the further the object has to travel, the less damage it is likely to cause).
- *Risk of retention.* The likelihood of a foreign body lodging in the globe or adnexal tissue will vary according to velocity and distance as above. Try to establish whether part of a penetrating object (particularly wooden) may have broken off at the time of injury.

For blunt trauma, consider:

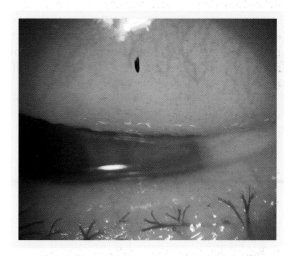

**Fig. 2.2** Subtarsal foreign body.

- *Size of object*. Objects smaller than the orbital rim (e.g. squash ball, 'thumbing' or gouging injury) will transmit forces directly to the globe. The severity of injury increases with force and velocity. Bungee cord (as found on the toggles of children's anoraks) injuries may be particularly vicious, resulting in hyphaema or even globe rupture.

Objects larger than the orbital rim (e.g. fist, tennis ball) will transmit forces to the lids and the bony orbit. So called 'blow-out' fractures occur because the weakest walls of the orbit (floor and medial) are most prone to buckle when the orbital pressure is raised during direct trauma.

## Presenting symptoms

- Red eye – subconjunctival haemorrhage (Fig. 2.3), corneal abrasion, corneal foreign body, penetrating trauma.
- Painful eye – hyphaema (blood in the anterior chamber – Fig. 2.4), traumatic iritis, corneal abrasion, corneal foreign body, penetrating trauma.
- Blurred vision – hyphaema, cataract, vitreous haemorrhage, commotio retinae, retinal detachment, traumatic optic neuropathy.
- Flashing lights and floaters – commotio retinae, vitreous haemorrhage, retinal tear/detachment.
- Double vision – orbital blow-out fracture.
- Pain on eye movement – orbital blow-out fracture.

If you suspect a blow-out, always ask about numbness of the teeth. The infraorbital nerve gives off a sensory branch, the superior alveolar nerve, which supplies the molars. These teeth may become numb if the fracture disturbs the infraorbital nerve.

## EXAMINATION

A systematic examination of the ocular system starting from the lids and working backwards through all of the structures of the eye should easily identify all potential sequelae of trauma.

## Visual acuity

It is absolutely essential that the visual acuity (Snellen) is recorded at first presentation. Some

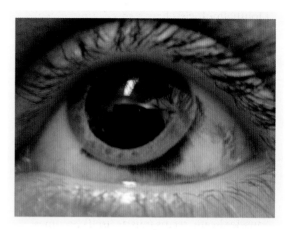

Fig. 2.3 Subconjunctival haemorrhage. Be careful of a base of skull fracture if no posterior limit is visible.

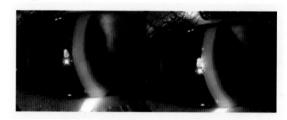

Fig. 2.4 Hyphaema following a football hitting the orbit.

gauge of what the vision was like in the eye prior to injury should be established.

## External eye

### Lids

Likely features include:

- Ecchymoses/bruising.
- Lid lacerations – in general, these should be sutured by an ophthalmologist, particularly if the lid margin is involved. If the canalicular system (the tear drainage system within the medial lid) is suspected to be involved this should be assessed and repaired by an oculoplastic specialist.
- Remember to evert the lids. The inside of the lid and tarsal plate may split following eye lid 'thumbing' – a not uncommon piece of rugby 'skullduggery'.

### Orbit

- Proptosis – forward bulging of the globe. This may be apparent by direct visualization, in particular by looking down on to the eyes from above and behind the patient's head.

Ophthalmologists have a specific instrument, an exophthalmometer, which can measure the degree of proptosis. Proptosis following trauma suggests the presence of blood in the orbit. An acute retrobulbar haemorrhage, where there is rapidly progressing proptosis, diffuse subconjunctival haemorrhage and reducing vision, is a sight-threatening emergency which requires urgent treatment by lateral cantholysis.

- Enopthalmos – this is the reverse of proptosis where the globe is drawn inwards. It is a feature of a blow-out fracture 'with entrapment', in which part of the orbital contents (fat, rectus muscle sheath, rectus muscle itself) becomes caught within the fracture.
- Ocular motility – restriction in up or down gaze is a feature of blow-out fracture with entrapment. The fourth cranial nerve may be particularly susceptible to injury as it emerges from the dorsal surface of the brainstem (i.e. back of the head). Do not forget that sixth nerve palsies may be a non-localizing sign of raised intracranial pressure!
- Palpation – check trigeminal sensation. Look for signs of bony ridges or crepitus (both may be features of orbital fracture).

## Anterior segment

It should be possible to examine the anterior segment using a pen torch and direct visualization. However, for more careful and precise examination, a slit lamp should be used if available.

In an obvious case of globe rupture, the examination should be kept to a minimum. In particular, very little manipulation of the lids or globe should be performed, as this may cause expulsion of ocular contents (vitreous, lens, choroid). A clear shield should be placed over the eye, the patient advised not to blow their nose, and a direct referral to ophthalmology services made.

### Conjunctiva, sclera

- Subconjunctival haemorrhage – this is a common sequela of blunt trauma to the globe. Beware of bilateral subconjunctival haemorrhage

without visible posterior extents. This may be due to skull base fracture.
- Scleral rupture/laceration – beware of any brown or black material on the sclera associated with haemorrhage. This may represent choroidal tissue herniating through disrupted sclera.

## Cornea

- Corneal lacerations may be visible by direct inspection. The anterior chamber will be shallow or flat if there is an aqueous leak. The anterior chamber may be formed if iris tissue plugs the laceration – this may be seen as pigmented tissue on the corneal surface, with the pupil drawn towards the wound.
- Corneal abrasions are best seen with fluorescein and cobalt blue light. Remember, vertical corneal scratches may be secondary to a subtarsal foreign body.
- Corneal foreign body may be visible by direct inspection if large enough, otherwise slit lamp examination will be required.
- Following chemical injury, there may be corneal epithelial disturbance, varying from 'punctate' fluorescein staining, frank epithelial defect (like an abrasion) to corneal opacity (white cornea). A particularly suspicious feature is if there is staining or ischaemia (i.e. absent conjunctival vessels) at the limbus (edge of the cornea).

## Anterior chamber

- Shallow – if a laceration has caused an aqueous leak.
- Deep – if blunt trauma has caused iridocorneal angle recession (long-term risk of developing glaucoma). Anterior chamber will deepen if the lens is avulsed or dislocates.
- Hyphaema – presence of blood in the anterior chamber, with a fluid level/meniscus. A microscopic hyphaema, with circulating red cells in the anterior chamber, may be detectable by slit lamp biomicroscopy.
- Hypopyon – presence of white cells/pus in the anterior chamber with a fluid level/meniscus. This would usually suggest an infection, and would be a late feature of untreated trauma (i.e. corneal foreign body).
- Iritis – cells may be present in the anterior chamber following direct blunt trauma to the globe, a 'traumatic iritis'.

## Iris

- Is there iris tissue outside the globe? This would be a feature of globe rupture/corneal laceration.
- Transillumination defects – a penetrating foreign body may cause a small hole in the iris, visible as a transillumination defect (i.e. one can see the red reflex through the defect). Such injuries may also have a self-sealing corneal perforation, a focal cataract at the site of penetration +/– a retained intraocular foreign body.
- The iris sphincter muscle may rupture following blunt trauma, resulting in a traumatic mydriasis. The pupil is enlarged and poorly reactive to light.

## Relative afferent pupillary defect (RAPD)

This is a poor prognostic sign for visual outcome. It is absolutely essential that the presence or absence of an RAPD is assessed at first presentation. An RAPD following trauma usually indicates a degree of optic nerve compromise:

- Traumatic optic neuropathy – i.e. a contre coup injury transmitting blunt injury force to the optic nerve.
- Optic nerve compression – e.g. by retrobulbar haemorrhage or a piece of bone fragment impinging on the nerve.

Other causes include:

- Macula off retinal detachment.
- Massive choroidal haemorrhage.

## Lens

- Cataract may develop following trauma. A posterior subcapsular cataract may develop some time after blunt trauma. A focal cataract may develop where a foreign body has passed through the lens.
- Remember that the lens is held in place by zonular ligaments which may give out if the force applied is sufficiently high. The lens may stay in place but wobble when the eye moves (phacodynesis), or subluxate (move up or down within the posterior chamber), or fully luxate (dislocate into the vitreous). With sufficient force, the lens may even be expelled out of the eye.

## Posterior segment

Examination of the posterior segment is best performed through a dilated pupil. It may be possible to pick up gross pathology using a direct ophthalmoscope and an undilated pupil, but often more detailed examination will have to be performed by an ophthalmologist.

## Vitreous

- Vitreous haemorrhage should be suspected if there is no red reflex or if there is no view of the fundus with an ophthalmoscope.

## Retina

- Commotio retinae (bruising of the retina) is seen as pale, oedematous patches of retina. The retina may thin out in areas of commotio and the patient is subsequently at risk of retinal detachment.
- Retinal detachment – this frequently occurs in globe ruptures extending posteriorly. Detachments are addressed surgically at a later stage than the primary repair (i.e. putting the outside of the globe back together).
- Suprachoroidal/choroidal haemorrhage – this is seen as an immobile black shadow on fundoscopy. If large, it may have a disastrous prognosis in terms of vision.

## INVESTIGATIONS

- X-rays – facial and orbital views may be useful in detecting orbital fractures; however, orbital CT is the gold standard. It may be possible to detect some radio-opaque (i.e. glass, metal) intraocular foreign bodies using X-ray.

*And REMEMBER – if you suspect an intraocular metal foreign body, don't arrange an MRI!*

In chemical injuries, check the pH of the affected eye(s) using pH paper. Immediately irrigate the eye with normal saline and continue to do so until a pH reading of 7 is detected. Detailed examination of the patient should be withheld until this most important part of the management has been successfully completed.

## Objectives

You should:

- Be able to take a history relevant to visual loss.
- Know the common causes of gradual visual loss.
- Be able to identify which clinical features suggest each cause of gradual visual loss.
- Have a systematic approach to examining the eye with gradual visual loss.

## DIFFERENTIAL DIAGNOSIS

Patients with gradual deterioration of vision usually present for the first time in an optometric practice, on the assumption that the problem will be remedied with the dispensing of glasses. Often the patient will have a refractive error (myopia – short sightedness; hyperopia – long sightedness; astigmatism – 'rugby ball-shaped' cornea; presbyopia – middle age onset poor reading vision), and as such will usually improve with glasses. The vision in two of the commoner presentations in older age, cataract and 'dry' macular degeneration, will also improve, up to a level, with refraction. Often presentation to hospital eye services are made when no improvement can be made on refraction (i.e. glasses do not help).

### Common causes of gradual visual loss

Refractive error.
Cataract.
Posterior capsular opacification (PCO) (post-cataract surgery).
Age-related macular degeneration.
Primary open angle glaucoma (although 'presentation' with visual loss is unusual).

### Rarer causes of gradual visual loss

Extremes of refractive error – keratoconus, myopic degeneration.
Inherited eye disease.
Toxic, drug-related.

## HISTORY

Always establish whether the patient is a driver. If they have significant and irreversible visual loss they may not be eligible (or safe) to drive.

### Duration of symptoms

It can be difficult to get an accurate history of gradual visual loss in terms of time-scale. Patients may attend an optometrist for a routine check-up and be found to have deteriorated since their visit the previous year; in this case the patient will only become aware of the problem when it is pointed out by the optometrist. Detecting gradual monocular (in one eye) visual changes can be particularly difficult as the other (normal) eye will compensate.

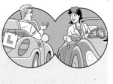

Sometimes a patient presents with sudden visual loss but only a chronic cause is found, e.g. dense cataract. It is helpful to ask whether they became aware of poor vision when they closed the other eye. Be sure to exclude any other causes of sudden visual loss before reassuring the patient as regards their prognosis.

A history of sudden visual loss and presence of a relative afferent pupillary defect (RAPD) is not compatible with a diagnosis of cataract.

If a patient complains of poor vision a few months to years after cataract surgery, ask them if it feels like their cataract has grown back. This suggests that posterior capsular opacification, a thickening of the capsule holding the intraocular lens, has occurred.

## Associated symptoms (Fig. 3.1)

- 'Negative' scotomata occur most commonly following optic nerve disease. The patient is not aware of their central field loss until they try to read.
- By contrast, patients are aware of 'positive' scotomata. Patients with macular degeneration are constantly aware of their central field deficit.
- Visual distortion (metamorphopsia), increase in image size (macropsia) and decrease in image size (micropsia) are reflections of changes in the relative positions of photoreceptors and are a feature of macular disease.

## Family history

Family history is important as it may point to an inherited condition such as retinitis pigmentosa or Stargardt's disease. If a hereditary disorder is suspected, you should always map out a family tree.

## Drug history

Do not forget to take a detailed drug history as some chronic medications may cause poor vision, vigabatrin, tamoxifen and chloroquine being well-known examples. Also, alcohol and tobacco intake may be useful in identifying patients at risk of $B_{12}$ and folate deficiency.

## EXAMINATION

### Visual acuity

- An accurate assessment of visual acuity (VA) (by Snellen or LogMar chart) is essential, if possible with the patient wearing their current spectacles (if any) as this is how they 'see the world'.
- Re-checking visual acuity using a pinhole is essential; an improvement in vision usually points to a condition that may be improved with up-to-date glasses (e.g. cataract or refractive error).

In retinal lesions, particularly macular, visual acuity remains reduced despite using a pinhole.

**Fig. 3.1** Common associated symptoms of gradual visual loss with relevant pathologies

| Symptom | Pathology |
| --- | --- |
| Glare | Cataract |
| Floaters | Vitritis, retinal detachment |
| Night blindness (nyctalopia) | Inherited eye disease, particularly retinitis pigmentosa (RP) |
| Peripheral visual loss ('bumping into things') | Late stage glaucoma, inherited eye disease, e.g. RP |
| Positive central (dark) scotoma | Age-related macular degeneration (ARMD) |
| Visual distortion (metamorphopsia) | Wet ARMD |

## Colour vision

- Usually assessed using Ishihara colour plates.
- Loss of colour vision is an early sign of optic neuritis or neuropathy.

## Visual field

- May be examined by confrontation, or more formally by static automated perimetry.
- Central scotoma is a feature of macular disease.
- An enlarged blind spot is a feature of chronic optic nerve swelling (e.g. benign intracranial hypertension).
- Amsler grid – this is useful for examining the central field in macular disease (see Fig. 10.34).

## Pupils

A relative afferent pupillary defect is a feature of optic nerve compromise, as well as a chronic total retinal detachment.

## Red reflex

Opacities within the red reflex may be observed in cataract. 'Hazy' visual media may be seen in cataract, posterior capsular opacification and corneal scarring or opacity.

## Fundoscopy

Systemic examination of:

### Optic nerve

Optic disc pallor suggests chronic optic neuropathy.
    Optic disc 'cupping' (enlarged optic disc cup with thinning of the neuroretinal rim) is a characteristic feature of glaucomatous optic neuropathy.

### Macula

Drusen (deep yellow flecks) at the macula are a characteristic feature of macular degeneration. As 'dry' macular degeneration progresses, dark pigmentary changes as well as atrophy may be observed at the macula.

## Retinal periphery and vasculature

Peripheral patchy 'bone spicule' pigmentation is a feature of retinitis pigmentosa. The retinal vessels may also be attenuated (the optic disc may also display 'waxy pallor').

## INVESTIGATIONS

These are often not necessary as the diagnosis should normally be apparent from history and examination:

- B-scan ultrasound – may be necessary if fundal examination is precluded by a dense cataract. This is needed to exclude the possibility of a 'sudden' cause for visual loss, given that the cataract is of chronic onset.
- Blood tests – in particular $B_{12}$ and folate; may be useful to rule out nutritional optic neuropathy.
- Electrodiagnostic testing (visual evoked potential, electro-oculogram, electro-retinogram) has two important roles in gradual visual loss:

    — Can identify the location (i.e. rod, cone, macular, optic nerve) of the visual dysfunction
    — Can be used to identify non-organic (i.e. 'functional') visual loss. By the same token it can be used to estimate what the visual acuity should be given the observed integrity of the visual pathway.

ALWAYS consider imaging the brain +/− the orbits by MRI/CT in any cases of unexplained non-functional visual loss.

## Objectives

You should:

- Be able to take a clear history pertaining to sudden visual loss.
- Know the common causes of sudden visual loss.
- Be able to identify risk factors pointing to a particular cause of sudden visual loss.
- Have a systematic approach to examining the eye in all cases of visual loss.

## DIFFERENTIAL DIAGNOSIS

The causes of sudden change in vision may be classified as either painful or painless (Figs 4.1, 4.2).

When confronted with a patient complaining of a sudden change in vision, it is important to remember that *common things are common*. Certain disorders get more common according to the demographics of the patient. Bear this in mind, so you can narrow down your differential even before you take the history.

## Patient demographics

### Age

Some conditions are unlikely under the age of 60, particularly ischaemic optic neuropathy; the arteritic form (i.e. giant cell arteritis) is vanishingly rare in this group. Retino-vascular occlusive conditions (venous and arterial occlusions) are also relatively unusual in a younger age group; if encountered one should suspect an underlying thrombophilic tendency.

### Sex

Benign intracranial hypertension is almost exclusively a condition affecting young (usually overweight) females. Demyelinating optic neuritis is also far more common in young females.

### Race

Always consider the possibility of sickle cell (SC) retinopathy (SC trait) in patients of Afro-Caribbean descent; this may present with a vitreous haemorrhage. Diabetic patients from the Indian subcontinent are prone to more severe retinopathy (both proliferative complications and maculopathy). Some forms of uveitis are more common in certain groups, such as Behçets in Turks/Greeks, toxoplasmosis in South Americans and sarcoidosis in Africans.

## HISTORY

### Duration of symptoms

- Immediate loss of vision – suggests a vascular 'event' (venous or arterial occlusion).
- Progressive loss of field over hours, days – retinal detachment.
- Progressive dimming of vision – optic nerve pathology.
- Transient visual loss, lasting seconds, hours – migraine, giant cell arteritis, benign intracranial hypertension.

### Associated symptoms

- Painful eye – iritis, scleritis, keratitis and primary angle closure (all may have photophobia too!).
- Headache – headache on waking may be a feature of benign intracranial hypertension (as is buzzing in the ear). The headache in temporal arteritis is characteristically centred

**Fig. 4.1** Common causes of painful, sudden visual loss

| Anatomical location | Examples |
| --- | --- |
| Anterior segment | Iritis, scleritis, keratitis, primary angle closure (see Ch. 1) |
| Optic nerve | Optic neuritis (demyelinating) Arteritic ischaemic optic neuropathy (giant cell arteritis) |
| Intracranial | Migraine Benign intracranial hypertension |

**Fig. 4.2** Common causes of painless, sudden loss of vision

| Anatomical location | Examples |
| --- | --- |
| Vitreous | Vitritis, vitreous haemorrhage |
| Retinal – vascular | Branch retinal vein occlusion, central retinal vein occlusion Branch retinal artery occlusion, central retinal artery occlusion |
| Retinal – macula | Exudative (wet) age-related macular degeneration Diabetic maculopathy |
| Retinal | Retinal detachment, retinitis, retinochoroiditis |
| Optic nerve | Non-arteritic ischaemic optic neuropathy Compressive optic neuropathy |
| Intracerebral | Stroke |

on the patient's temple; there may be associated pain in the jaw on chewing ('jaw claudication'). Headache preceded by scintillating lights or 'fortification spectra' is a feature of migraine.
- Photopsia (flashing lights) – this may precede a retinal detachment (or retinal tear). In migraine they are more commonly bilateral; there may be scintillating lights or zig-zag lines.
- Floaters – a sudden increase in floaters may precede retinal detachment. Vitreous haemorrhage and vitritis also present with floaters.
- Loss of colour appreciation – a characteristic feature of demyelinating optic neuritis.
- Distortion of vision ('metamorphopsia') – exudative (wet) macular degeneration.

## Previous ophthalmic history

Certain ophthalmic conditions predispose to particular causes of sudden visual loss:

- Myopia (short sightedness) – the risk of retinal detachment increases with high myopia.
- Hypermetropia (long sightedness) – these patients are more prone to primary angle closure, particularly in combination with dense cataract. Also hypermetropic patients are more likely to have small, crowded optic discs which are more prone to ischaemic optic neuropathy, particularly if the patient is hypertensive.
- Ocular hypertension/glaucoma – predisposes to central retinal vein occlusion.

## Previous medical history

### Hypertension

High blood pressure predisposes patients to venous and arterial occlusions, as well as non-arteritic ischaemic optic neuropathy and stroke.

### Diabetes

It is important to appreciate that poorly controlled diabetics (particularly with coexistent poorly controlled hypertension) are specifically at risk of end-organ damage, whether renal, cardiovascular, neuropathic or retinal. The commonest presentation of sudden visual loss in a diabetic is vitreous haemorrhage in proliferative diabetic retinopathy, although retinal vein occlusions may also present in this way.

### Thyroid/Graves' disease

Visual loss in thyroid eye disease may be caused by three mechanisms: corneal scarring, raised intraocular pressure and compressive optic neuropathy. Of the three, the last presents acutely. It is important that colour vision and visual field are checked in any patient with thyroid eye disease complaining of reduced vision.

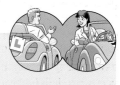

The term 'blind' is a highly emotive label. There are very few conditions which cause 'no perception of light' vision – which may be what the patient understands by blindness. In patients with macular degeneration reassure the patient that they will never be blind, as their peripheral vision will be unaffected by the condition.

## EXAMINATION

### Visual acuity

Snellen chart.

### Colour vision

Ishihara plates.
Reduced in optic nerve pathologies.

### Visual fields

Either to confrontation or by formal perimetry (static or kinetic).

- Homonymous field defects (quadrantinopias, hemianopias) are a feature of stroke.
- Altitudinal defects – are a feature of non-arteritic ischaemic optic neuropathy.
- Central scotomata – optic neuritis, macular degeneration.
- Peripheral field loss – retinal detachment.
- Enlarged blind spots – benign intracranial hypertension.

Amsler grid examination is useful for examining the macular central field and to illicit metamorphopsia.

### Pupils

- An RAPD (relative afferent pupillary defect) is a feature of optic nerve, not macular pathology. It may also be a feature of retinal detachment.
- A fixed mid-dilated pupil is a feature of primary angle closure, whereas a small irregular pupil is a feature of anterior uveitis/iritis.

### Anterior segment examination

As in Chapter 1, slit lamp examination of the anterior chamber will be helpful in identifying iritis, scleritis and primary angle closure.

### Fundoscopy

#### Vitreous

A dense vitreous haemorrhage may preclude a view of the fundus. Inflammatory cells and debris within the vitreous cavity are a feature of vitritis. Pigment cells in the vitreous are strongly suggestive of a retinal break (tear/hole) or detachment.

### Macular pathology

Look for haemorrhages, exudates and oedema which are features of vein occlusion and diabetic maculopathy. Haemorrhages in exudative macular degeneration may present in the pre-retinal zone, within the retina and in the subretinal space. Drusen may also be present.

### Optic nerve pathology

Disc swelling is a feature of most acute optic neuropathies (except retrobulbar neuritis). Disc swelling may also be present in central retinal vein occlusion, posterior scleritis and bilaterally in benign intracranial hypertension.

### Retinal vasculature

Dot, blot haemorrhages and exudates in one sector in the distribution of a vein (which may be seen to be occluded – pale) are features of branch vein occlusion. Central retinal vein occlusions, in contrast, have haemorrhages present in all four quadrants of the retina. In a retinal arterial occlusion, the affected area of retina appears pale yellow owing to retinal oedema; the fovea appears as a cherry red spot.

### Retinal periphery

Retinal detachments appear as mobile retinal 'curtains', billowing with eye movement. They arise from the retinal periphery, where a retinal hole or tear may be observed, and progress towards the posterior pole as fluid collects behind the detaching retina.

## INVESTIGATIONS

### Blood tests

ESR and CRP are usually elevated in giant cell arteritis. It is important to check both in patients over 60 who have any features of temporal arteritis, disc swelling or retinal artery occlusion. They should also be checked in patients over 60 with episodes of transient visual loss or unexplained visual loss.

In cases of retinal vein occlusion, FBC, renal function, lipid screen and glucose should be checked in all cases (as well as blood pressure). In atypical cases (e.g. younger subjects, multiple or recurrent), a thrompophilia screen should be carried out.

## B-scan ultrasonography

Useful in cases of vitreous haemorrhage as it can help exclude a retinal detachment, which would require urgent surgical intervention.

## Fluorescein angiography

This is a particularly useful photographic test which enables the function of the retinal vasculature to be subjectively assessed. It is possible to identify areas of vascular leakage and vascular non-perfusion. It is therefore particularly useful in the diagnosis and in the guiding of the management of exudative vascular conditions (macular degeneration, diabetic retinopathy, vein occlusions, inflammatory vasculopathies) and ischaemic retinopathies (diabetes, vein occlusions).

Fluorescein angiography is one of the most useful diagnostic tools in ophthalmology. However, it is important to remember that it is an invasive test, requiring i.v. injection of 10–20% fluorescein sodium. There is always a small risk of anaphylaxis. The test should therefore really be reserved for cases where the diagnosis is unknown or where the result will affect your management.

## Imaging

CT of the orbits is useful for excluding any compressive orbital or 'intraconal' cause of reduced vision.

MRI of the brain is required to confirm demyelination as a cause of optic neuritis. An MRI of the brain and orbits should be considered in any cases of unexplained reduced vision or field loss.

## Electrodiagnostic testing

In patients with unexplained visual loss, electrodiagnostics may be required to identify a non-organic cause (i.e. malingering).

# Double vision

Double vision (diplopia) can be divided into two categories:

A.   Monocular (one eye) causes.
B.   Binocular (two eyes) causes.

## A.  MONOCULAR DIPLOPIA

### Differential diagnosis

Monocular diplopia is by far the less common presentation of double vision. It is usually caused by some disruption to the ocular media of the affected eye.

- Corneal opacity/scarring/oedema.
- Iris defects – i.e. large iridectomy, post-cataract surgery iris trauma.
- Subluxated natural lens.
- Decentred artificial intraocular lens.
- Uncorrected astigmatism.

### History

In order to establish from the history whether or not the diplopia is monocular or binocular, ask the patient whether the double vision is still present when the unaffected eye is covered. If the diplopia is still present, then the diplopia is truly monocular. The vision should then become single when the affected eye is covered. In binocular diplopia, the double vision only exists when the two eyes are open.

- Establish the refractive status of the patient – when was the last time they went to the optician?
- Have they had any ophthalmic surgery or laser treatment – cataract surgery, corneal surgery, YAG laser peripheral iridotomy? Was cataract surgery complicated, making the intraocular lens more likely to decentre?
- Has there been any direct trauma to the eye which may have caused the natural lens to become unstable in position or to decentre an intraocular lens?
- Does the patient have an underlying medical condition which predisposes them to lens subluxation, such as Marfan's or homocysteinuria?

### Examination

- *Visual acuity.*
- *Refraction* – establish whether the patient is astigmatic.
- *Pinhole.* The use of a pinhole in front of the affected eye should abolish most causes of acquired monocular diplopia.
- *Cover test and ocular motility* (see next section, B. Binocular diplopia). It is important to perform this to document clearly that the patient does not, in fact, have binocular diplopia or a disorder of ocular motility.
- *Slit lamp examination.* This is essential for seeing whether there is a corneal cause of monocular diplopia. Dilated examination will enable the position of the natural lens or intraocular lens to be assessed.

### Investigations

Most causes of monocular diplopia will be identified through systematic examination of the ocular system. However, monocular diplopia may sometimes be of a sensory and not an optical origin. Such cases may be secondary to brain trauma or stroke, and do not improve with a pinhole. In such cases neuro-imaging (CT, MRI) may be necessary to confirm the diagnosis.

> Monocular diplopia may be a functional symptom. However, be sure to exclude all possible causes of monocular diplopia before coming to this conclusion. In any case following trauma, neuro-imaging is advisable to exclude a sensory cause.

## B. BINOCULAR DIPLOPIA

Binocular diplopia is caused by a disturbance of the ocular motility system. Basically the two eyes either do not move together in synchrony, or the point of regard of each eye is too far apart for them to be fused into a single image.

There is some important terminology which needs to be understood:

- Convergent squint – eyes deviate inwards. Also called an esotropia (Fig. 5.1A).
- Divergent squint – eyes deviate outwards. Also called an exotropia (Fig. 5.1B).
- Vertical squint – eyes deviate vertically. Also called hypertropia (if upwards in affected eye) or hypotropia (if downwards in the affected eye).

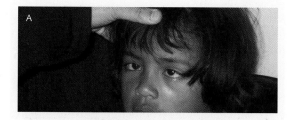

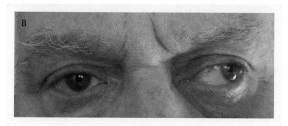

**Fig. 5.1** (A) Left esotropia (convergent squint). (B) Left exotropia (divergent squint).

- The term 'tropia' refers to a manifest squint. This means that during a cover test, the uncovered eye will be seen to take up fixation, moving in the direction away from the deviation (i.e. inwards for exo-, outwards for eso-, downwards for hyper- and upwards for hypo-).
- The term 'phoria' refers to a latent squint and will not be seen during a cover test in the fellow eye, but rather in the cover/uncover or alternate cover test. Once again the same terminology of exo-, eso-, hyper- and hypo- applies.
- Manifest squints may be concomitant, where the deviation is fixed regardless of direction of gaze, or incomitant, where the deviation varies according to the direction of gaze.

It is important to remember that a lot of patients will have a strabismus (a squint) but will not necessarily have double vision. In this circumstance:

- One of the images may be suppressed. This is usually a feature of childhood strabismus where the angle of deviation is constant regardless of direction of gaze (i.e. a concomitant squint).
- The patient has a 'latent' squint – i.e. a 'phoria'. They have a tendency to squint, particularly when tired, but they are able to fuse the images as single.
- The deviation has arisen in a non-fixating blind eye (the patient is therefore effectively monocular).

This chapter concentrates on patients presenting with acquired binocular diplopia. Strabismus is covered in more detail in Chapter 12, Strabismus and paediatrics.

## Differential diagnosis (Fig. 5.2)

### History

Try to establish:

### Nature of the double vision

Is it purely horizontal? If it is worse in the distance, this suggests a sixth nerve palsy. If there is both a vertical and 'torsional' (i.e. off centre, rotating diplopia) component, this could be a fourth nerve palsy or combined third and fourth nerve palsy. Double vision changing during the course of the day, in terms of direction or severity is suggestive of myasthenia. Double vision changing direction or severity over the course of weeks/months may be suggestive of thyroid eye

**Fig. 5.2** Common causes of binocular diplopia

| Type of diplopia | Cause |
| --- | --- |
| Horizontal | Decompensated pre-existing eso- or exo-phoria<br>VI nerve palsy<br>Internuclear ophthalmoplegia<br>Mechanical restriction – medial orbital wall fracture |
| Vertical | Decompensated pre-existing hypo- or hyper-phoria<br>IV nerve palsy<br>III nerve palsy |
| Variable | Thyroid eye disease<br>Myasthenia gravis<br>Orbital myositis, orbital cellulitis, orbital apex lesions |

disease or myasthenia (or both – as autoimmune diseases it is not uncommon for the two disorders to coexist).

## Headache

This is vital in terms of a pupil-involved third nerve palsy as it is a strong indicator of a compressive lesion (particularly posterior communicating artery aneurysm). Headache may also be a feature of a diabetic microvascular third nerve palsy. Temporal arteritis may present with sixth nerve palsy

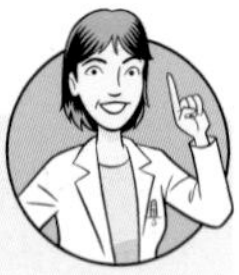

A suspected 'compressive' third nerve lesion is a neurosurgical/neuroradiological emergency and will need to be referred directly. As a matter of urgency it may be necessary to do so before imaging has been performed. Be suspicious of a third nerve palsy with a dilated pupil and headache.

## History of trauma

Blunt trauma to the orbit may cause an orbital fracture. Head injury, perhaps falling off a horse or a road traffic accident, may cause fourth nerve palsy (often bilateral).

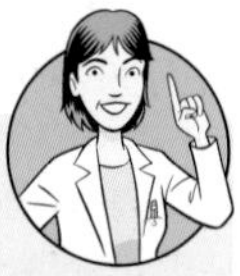

Do not forget the possibility of a sixth nerve palsy being a false localizing sign of raised intracranial pressure. Any history of severe head trauma with loss of consciousness should alert to the possibility of this.

## Previous ophthalmic history

You need to establish if there is a history of childhood squint, or of patching (amblyopia treatment). Myopic subjects have a tendency to exophoria and hypermetropes for esophoria.

## Previous medical history

By far the commonest cause of an acquired third, fourth or sixth nerve palsy in patients over the age of 60 is microvascular. It is therefore essential to find out whether the patient is diabetic or hypertensive. The patient may also volunteer that they have Graves' disease, multiple sclerosis or even myasthenia.

## Examination

### Inspection

Observe the patient for a head posture – these are adopted to compensate for a squint. A face turn may be seen in a sixth nerve palsy, a head tilt may be seen in a unilateral fourth nerve palsy, while a chin-down tilt is seen in bilateral fourth nerve palsy.

Does the patient have a ptosis? If this is variable with fatigue, or bilateral, then it may be suggestive of myasthenia. If the eye under the ptosis is looking down and out, then it is almost certainly a third nerve palsy.

Does the patient have herpes zoster ophthalmicus? A sixth nerve palsy may be a presenting feature.

Observe the patient's orbits and adnexal tissues. Are there features of thyroid eye disease – proptosis, lid retraction, periorbital oedema, injection over the insertions of the horizontal recti? Are the lids red and inflamed, suggestive of orbital cellulitis, or even a cavernous sinus thrombosis?

The direction of the squint, particularly gross convergent or divergent squints, may be obvious on direct inspection. A pen torch may be useful to see the deviation of the corneal reflexes.

## Cover test

Performed at 1/3 metre and 6 metres.

Cover one eye, and observe movement of the fellow eye (look for tropia). Repeat for the other eye. Look for movement of the covered eye when the cover is removed to see if it takes up fixation.

In the alternating cover test, the cover is moved rapidly between the two eyes to see if there is any latent movement (look for phoria).

## Ocular motility

*Versions*, i.e. both eyes moving together, are tested in the six positions of gaze. Remember that the superior and inferior rectus work best on abduction (up and out or down and out) whereas the superior and inferior obliques work best in adduction (down and in or up and in).

*Ductions* are a method of testing the movement of a single eye in isolation (i.e. with one eye covered). They are useful when looking to see whether an eye is truly 'restricted' in gaze. When an eye is mechanically restricted (e.g. following an orbital fracture) it will not be capable of duction in the direction of restriction.

*Saccades*. This is particularly useful for eliciting an internuclear ophthalmoplegia. In this condition, the subject has a limitation in adduction in one eye and abducting nystagmus in the fellow eye. This may be subtle on horizontal versions but can become obvious when you ask the patient to move their eyes quickly from side to side.

## Cranial nerve examination and neurological examination

It is important to identify any coexistant cranial nerve pathology, suggesting a brainstem or orbital apex pathology, or even temporal arteritis. Neurological examination is useful to identify any features suggestive of stroke or space occupying lesion.

## Dilated fundoscopy

It is essential to check whether the discs are swollen, to help to rule out raised intracranial pressure.

## Investigations

### Bloods

- Erythrocyte sedimentation rate (ESR) and creative protein (CRP) in patients over 60 years of age to rule out giant cell arteritis.
- Anti-acetylcholine receptor antibodies are useful in establishing a diagnosis of myasthenia gravis.
- Thyroid function and thyroid antibodies to diagnose thyroid eye disease.
- Blood glucose and lipids when a microvascular cause is suspected.

### Imaging

Computed tomography (CT) of the orbits is useful in diagnosing thyroid eye disease, orbital fractures, orbital myositis, as well as in the management of orbital cellulitis (if an abscess is suspected). B-scan ultrasound may also be useful in diagnosing orbital myositis.

Magnetic resonance imaging (MRI) of the brain is useful in establishing a diagnosis of multiple sclerosis (MS) in a patient with internuclear ophthalmoplegia. MS is by far the commonest cause in the younger age group. In the older age group (over 50), a brainstem stroke/vascular event is far more common. Magnetic resonance angiography (MRA) would be the investigation of choice in a suspected compressive third nerve lesion.

In general, a presumed microvascular palsy does not require imaging. Patients should be followed carefully for 3 months to ensure that there is evidence of improvement. If there is no improvement by this stage then imaging +/– lumbar puncture should be performed. A unilateral palsy in a young patient (<40) is highly unlikely to be microvascular and therefore should be investigated appropriately (imaging +/– lumbar puncture). It is not uncommon for an isolated palsy to be post-viral in origin (particularly in children) but it is essential to perform neuro-imaging prior to making this diagnosis.

### Orthoptic assessment

Orthoptists are specialists in the diagnosis and management of disorders of ocular motility who work alongside ophthalmologists. In general, all patients with double vision will be assessed by an orthoptist. In particular the Hess chart is useful for diagnosing incomitant squint and for monitoring progression or improvement over time.

# Eyelid problems and the bulging eye

## Objectives

You should:

- Be able to differentiate between the causes of ptosis.
- Know the common lid 'lumps and bumps'.
- Be able to identify orbital cellulitis and manage it appropriately.
- Know the features of thyroid eye disease and the related risk factors for visual loss.
- Know the differential diagnosis of proptosis.

## A. EYELID MALPOSITION

The commonest eyelid malpositions are:
- Ptosis – droopy upper lid.
- Entropion – turned in lid margin (Fig. 6.1).
- Ectropion – turned out lid margin (Fig. 6.2).

### Ptosis

#### Differential diagnosis (See fig. 6.3.)

#### History

Ask about symptoms of:
- Headache – important for third nerve palsies.
- Diplopia – third nerve palsy, myasthenia.
- Fatiguability – myasthenia.
- History of contact lens use – commonly can cause aponeurotic dehiscence.

#### Examination

##### Observation
Look for anisocoria (difference in pupil size – important for Horner's and third nerve palsy) and heterochromia (congenital Horner's). Does the patient have an obvious squint, prosthetic eye or features of thyroid eye disease?

##### Ptosis assessment
Using a ruler, you can measure the palpebral aperture (the distance between the upper and lower lids – normally approximately 10–12 mm), the height of the skin crease (low in congenital, high in aponeurotic dehiscence, normally approx 4–5 mm) and levator function (normally approximately >12 mm, reduced in congenital ptosis and in myogenic causes such as myasthenia and myotonic dystrophy). Levator function needs to be checked in isolation, so you need to counteract the action of frontalis; therefore, fix the brow in place and then measure the upper lid margin excursion from down gaze to full up gaze. Look to see if there is fatiguability by measuring the palpebral aperture before and after 1 minute of up gaze; the palpebral aperture will reduce in myasthenia as the levator becomes fatigued.

##### Ocular motility
Check ocular motility to confirm third nerve palsy. Motility will also be disordered in myasthenia.

#### Investigations

MRI should be performed if an intracranial cause is suspected. ACh receptor antibodies are useful to confirm a diagnosis of myasthenia; the 'tensilon' test is very rarely performed these days in the ophthalmology setting.

### Ectropion and entropion

Both of these conditions are extremely common among the elderly where loss of tissue elasticity results in the lid either slipping over the tarsal plate, causing the lashes to point in the direction of the globe (entropion), or to slip downwards, withdrawing the lid margin away from the globe (ectropion).

Lid margin malposition may also be a consequence of trauma, scarring (cicatricial), inflammatory conditions or tumours (e.g. basal cell carcinoma).

Patients may present with epiphora +/– a red eye.

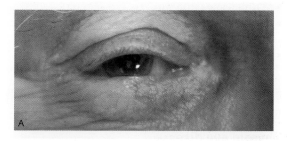

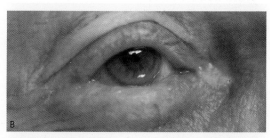

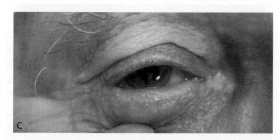

**Fig. 6.1** Right lower lid entropion: (A) lid skin rubbing on cornea; (B) slightly everted lid such that medial eyelashes are pointing upwards; (C) fully everted eyelid into normal position.

## B. EYELID LUMPS AND BUMPS

Common eye lid bumps are:

- Chalazion – or meibomian cyst.
- Hordeolum – stye.
- Inclusion cyst.
- Sebaceous cyst.
- Papilloma.

One must always beware of potentially malignant lesions. The commonest are:

- Basal cell carcinoma.
- Squamous cell carcinoma.
- Melanoma.

Rarer lesions:

- Meibomian gland carcinoma.
- Merkel cell carcinoma.

These should always be suspected in elderly patients with recurrent or atypical lid lumps (may masquerade as a chalazion).

Most lumps and bumps can be excised as a minor operative procedure. Usually this is done on cosmetic grounds at the patient's request. If there is any suspicion of malignancy, the excised material should be sent for histology. In older patients presenting with a suspicious lid lesion a biopsy should be performed first, to ensure that a complete excision can be planned.

## C. EYELID SWELLING

There are many causes of a swollen eyelid:

- Allergy.
- Inflamed cyst – e.g. chalazion.
- Conjunctivitis.
- Bruising/black eye.

The most important condition to be aware of is orbital cellulitis. Red, inflamed lids may be 'pre-septal' only – i.e. involving the most anterior lid tissues. It is important to recognize features suggestive of post-septal (orbital involvement), as this is sight threatening and potentially life threatening (if the sepsis enters the meningeal cavity).

### History

The episode may be preceded by trauma such as a bite. The condition is rapidly progressive. Children may be profoundly unwell – parents may describe the child as being febrile and listless. Ask about double vision or reduced vision.

### Examination

Crucial signs of orbital cellulitis that should not be missed are:

- Proptosis.
- Reduced ocular motility – in some cases the globe may be 'frozen'.

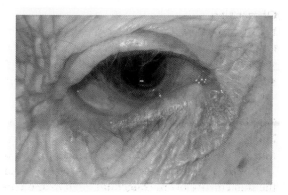

**Fig. 6.2** Right lower lid ectropion.

25

**Fig. 6.3** Common causes of ptosis

| Cause | Features |
|-------|----------|
| Congenital ptosis | Presence since birth, if untreated affected eye may be amblyopic, frontalis overaction (raise eyebrow to lift lid), low skin crease, reduced levator function |
| Aponeurotic dehiscence | Usually older patients, also contact lens wearers<br>High skin crease |
| III nerve palsy | Full ptosis, affected eye deviated down and out +/- pupil dilation |
| Horner's syndrome | Partial ptosis, pupil mioisis, hemifacial anhydrosis<br>If congenital, iris colour may be different in one eye compared to the other (heterochromia) |
| Myasthenia | Ptosis increases with fatigue; variable or bilateral<br>Ptosis improves with application of ice pack to closed lids |
| Pseudo-ptosis | Lid retraction in fellow eye (i.e. in thyroid eye disease)<br>Empty socket syndrome in patients with prosthetic eye |

- Reduced colour vision.
- Reduced vision.
- Swollen optic nerve.

Any children with pre-septal cellulitis should be observed for development of these signs.

## Investigations

Orbital cellulitis is an emergency and requires i.v. antibiotics as soon as suspected. It is therefore likely that treatment will commence before investigations can be performed. Computed tomography (CT) of the orbits is useful for identifying whether there is a periosteal or sinus abscess requiring drainage (usually performed by the ENT surgeons). Blood cultures should also be performed if the patient is febrile.

## D. PROPTOSIS

By far the commonest cause of proptosis, whether bilateral or unilateral, is thyroid eye disease. Other causes include:

- Orbital myositis.
- Orbital cellulitis.

- Orbital apex tumours (e.g. lymphoma).
- Orbital inflammatory disorders (e.g. Wegener's, sarcoidosis).
- Vascular anomalies (orbital varices, carotico-cavernous sinus fistula).

The eye may look proptosed if it is very big, as in high myopia.

## Thyroid eye disease

Features include:

- Adnexal soft tissue swelling – periorbital oedema.
- Lid retraction.
- Proptosis.
- Restriction of eye movement.
- Injection over the horizontal recti insertions, chemosis.
- Raised intraocular pressure, particularly on up gaze.
- Corneal exposure with punctate fluorescein staining.

Patients are at risk of visual loss from:

- Corneal scarring secondary to exposure.
- Glaucoma secondary to raised intraocular pressure.
- Optic neuropathy secondary to compression from engorged orbital contents.

## Examination

1. Exophthalmometry.
2. Ocular motility +/- orthoptic assessment.
3. Visual acuity.
4. Colour vision.
5. Visual fields.
6. Pupils – check for RAPD.
7. Intraocular pressure (both straight ahead and in up gaze).
8. Fundoscopy – look for swollen discs and choroidal folds.

If acute compressive thyroid ophthalmopathy is suspected on clinical grounds, high dose oral steroids (or even pulsed intravenous) should be commenced as soon as possible. This will usually be before imaging, to avoid delay. Once stabilized, the patient can be referred on to an orbital specialist for consideration of surgical decompression.

Orbital CT should be sufficient to recognize all major orbital pathology. It is unusual to require further imaging with MRI.

# Adnexal (eyelids, lacrimal system and orbit)

## EYELID

Disorders of the eyelid are common and affect both adults and children. They frequently present to the general practitioner and may be associated with a conjunctivitis.

The anatomy of the eyelid is shown in Fig. 7.1. Disorders of eyelids can be divided into:

- Eyelash disorders.
- Allergic disorders.
- Infections.
- Benign tumours.
- Malignant tumours.
- Eyelid malpositions.

## Disorders of the eyelashes

### Trichiasis

Trichiasis is a common condition, which is acquired secondary to chronic inflammation and scarring of the lid margin. This is commonly due to chronic blepharitis but other causes include herpes zoster and trachoma.

*Signs*

The classical signs are:

- Posterior misdirection of lashes in the presence of normal lid position.
- Secondary corneal trauma which may stain with fluorescein.
- Chronicity may lead to corneal pannus (Fig. 7.2).

*Treatment*

- Epilation with forceps provides temporary relief and can be performed in the accident department with the aid of a slit lamp.
- Electrolysis is useful for small areas.
- Cryotherapy for larger areas.
- Surgery, which involves excision of the anterior lamella and healing with secondary intention.

Complications of cryotherapy include:

- Skin necrosis.
- Depigmentation.
- Meibomian gland damage.
- Notching of lid margin.

### Distichiasis

This term describes abnormal lashes which originate posterior to the normal lash roots, at or behind the meibomian gland orifices. It can be congenital or acquired. In congenital distichiasis, a partial or

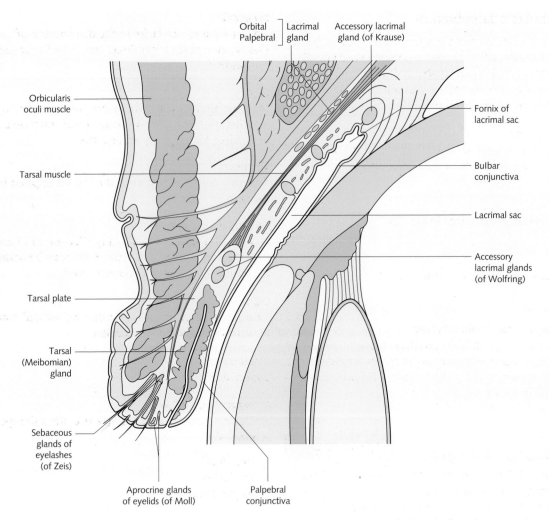

Orbital
Palpebral ] Lacrimal gland
Accessory lacrimal gland (of Krause)

Orbicularis oculi muscle

Tarsal muscle

Tarsal plate

Tarsal (Meibomian) gland

Sebaceous glands of eyelashes (of Zeis)

Aprocrine glands of eyelids (of Moll)

Palpebral conjunctiva

Fornix of lacrimal sac

Bulbar conjunctiva

Lacrimal sac

Accessory lacrimal glands (of Wolfring)

**Fig. 7.1** The anatomy of the eyelid. Note how the conjunctiva starts (palpebral) on the posterior aspect of eyelid and reflects (fornix) on to the sclera towards the corneal limbus (bulbar).

complete second row of lashes emerges at or behind the meibomian gland orifices. Acquired distichiasis

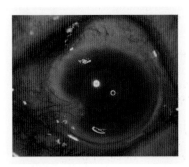

**Fig. 7.2** Left pterygium (nasal conjunctival overgrowth) and superior corneal pannus in a pseudophakic eye.

is the result of metaplasia and dedifferentiation of the meibomian glands, which then become hair follicles. It is usually secondary to a cicatrizing conjunctivitis which may follow a chemical injury, an attack of ocular cicatricial pemphigoid or Stevens–Johnson syndrome.

### Treatment

Treatment is similar for both the congenital and the acquired forms, and is indicated if the lashes rub on the cornea leading to irritation and keratopathy. The options are:

- Lash cut-down and electrolysis for small areas.
- Lamellar division and cryotherapy for larger areas.

## Pthiriasis palpebrarum

This is an infection of the lashes caused by the crab louse *Pthirus pubis,* which can live in pubic hair and from there be transferred to the eyelashes by human contact. It may affect children in poor living conditions and causes irritation, and thereafter presentation to casualty.

*Treatment*
Treatment involves lash trimming or destruction of the lice with topical anticholinesterases.

## Allergic disorders

These are summarized in Fig. 7.3.

## Infections

These may be acute or chronic.

## Acute

### Herpes zoster ophthalmicus
Common, unilateral condition caused by the varicella zoster virus (shingles). It affects the elderly and it is important to consider systemic immunocompromise in the young.

Herpes zoster ophthalmicus (shingles) is uncommon in the young, and should alert the clinician to underlying immunosuppression (e.g. HIV/AIDS or bone marrow suppression). Gentle questioning regarding the patient's bone marrow or immune system can minimize the patient's guilt and improve the rapport between the patient and clinician.

*Symptoms*
Acute pain and headache in the distribution of the first division of the trigeminal nerve. A vesicular rash follows this.

*Signs*
Maculopapular rash, which progresses to crusty vesicles, oedema and swelling. There may be an associated keratopathy and uveitis.

*Treatment*
Systemic aciclovir and topical aciclovir applied to the rash.

### Primary herpes simplex
Uncommon, unilateral, typically affecting children, patients with atopic dermatitis who may be using steroids and the immunocompromised.

*Signs*
Crops of vesicles which are creamy-yellow and may rupture leading to a conjunctivitis.

*Treatment*
Topical aciclovir.

### Other acute conditions
Acute rare conditions which may also affect the eyelids include:

- Impetigo.
- Erysipelas.
- Necrotizing fasciitis.

## Chronic infections

This is most commonly due to chronic blepharitis secondary to *Staphylococcus aureus* and can affect both the anterior and posterior lid margins.

**Fig. 7.3** Summary of allergic disorders of the eyelid

|  | Symptoms | Signs | Treatment |
|---|---|---|---|
| Acute allergic oedema | Sudden onset, itching | Pitting eyelid oedema | Systemic antihistamines |
| Contact dermatitis | Itching, tearing | Eyelid swelling, erythema, crusty skin | Removal of cause, mild topical hydrocortisone |
| Atopic dermatitis (eczema) | Itching | Eyelid crusting, erythema, discharge from secondary infection | Emollients, topical hydrocortisone cream, antibiotics |

### Chronic blepharitis

Chronic blepharitis is a very common condition and tends to be controlled in susceptible individuals rather than cured. It is commonly seen in patients with acne rosacea and atopic eczema.

*Symptoms*
Irritated crusty eyes, excess 'sleep' in the mornings, lacrimation.

*Signs*
Lid margin crusting and scaling, debris around the lash roots, loss of lashes and greasy plugs in the meibomian glands, lid margin erythema, greasy tear film.

Associated ocular signs: these include secondary conjunctivitis and marginal keratitis.

*Treatment*
- Lid hygiene (warm cotton buds dipped in bicarbonate solution or baby shampoo).
- Topical tear film supplements.
- Topical fusidic acid.
- Systemic tetracyclines.

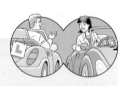

Blepharitis treatment needs to be long term, otherwise there will be recurrence of disease.
Once under control, just lid hygiene may be sufficient.
A good analogy for blepharitis lid hygiene is brushing teeth daily in order to avoid the dentist!

## Benign tumours

## Chalazion

A chalazion (Fig. 7.4) is the most common type of benign eyelid lump. It occurs when a meibomian gland becomes obstructed leading to a granuloma within the tarsal plate.

*Symptoms and signs*
Painless swelling in the posterior lamella, which may discharge either anteriorly or posteriorly.

*Treatment*
Hot compresses encourage discharge and most are self-limiting. It is important to treat any associated blepharitis or cellulitus. Incision and curettage may be required in recalcitrant cases.

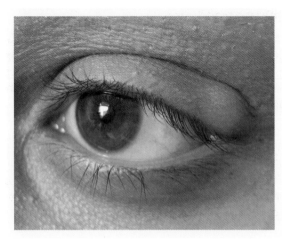

Fig. 7.4 Chalazion – temporal side of upper eyelid.

## Molluscum contagiosum

Molluscum contagiosum is an umbilicated, pearly looking lid margin cyst caused by the pox virus.

*Symptoms and signs*  Irritated red eyes caused by viral discharge from the cysts with a secondary follicular conjunctivitis.

*Treatment*
Excision of the lesion with cautery to the base.

## Other cysts

These are the result of obstruction of the other glandular structures within the eyelid (see Fig. 7.1). They are usually asymptomatic and are excised for cosmetic reasons. They include:

- Cyst of Moll (obstruction of a sweat gland).
- Cyst of Zeiss (obstruction of accessory sebaceous gland).

## Squamous papilloma

A common frond-like structure with a narrow base which is usually asymptomatic and can be excised for cosmetic purposes.

## Xanthelasma

Lipid-containing, yellow, flat lesions, often bilateral, which may occur, but not exclusively, in patients with hypercholesterolaemia. They are asymptomatic and excised for cosmetic reasons.

## Keratoacanthoma

Uncommon, rapidly growing tumour which usually spontaneously involutes and regresses after 2–3 months. There may be a keratin-filled crater. Persistent lesions should be excised, as there may be early squamous cell carcinoma in its base.

## Malignant tumours

### Basal cell carcinoma

This is the most common malignant eyelid tumour and accounts for 90% of all eyelid malignancies. 10% of all basal cell carcinomas occur on the eyelids.

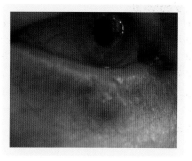

**Fig. 7.5** Right lower lid malignant skin carcinoma.

Main risk factors and predisposing conditions for basal cell carcinoma (BCC) and squamous cell carcinoma (SCC) include fair skin and chronic ultraviolet light exposure. Other BCC risk factors include xeroderma pigmentosum; those for SCC include immunocompromised patients, including those with AIDS, and following renal transplant.

*Symptoms and signs*
Painless lesion which may be nodular, sclerosing or ulcerative ('rodent ulcer'). It is associated with lash loss and a pearly margin. It is slow growing, locally invasive and non-metastasizing.

*Treatment*
Excision biopsy with margin control with either cryotherapy or radiotherapy.

### Squamous cell carcinoma

This is much less common than BCC; however, it is potentially more aggressive with regional lymph node metastasis or perineural spread. It accounts for 5–10% of eyelid malignancies. Clinically, it may be indistinguishable from BCC (Fig. 7.5).

*Treatment*
Excision with margin control.

## Other tumours

### Sebaceous cell carcinoma

This is a very rare, slow-growing tumour which affects the elderly. It arises from the meibomian glands, glands of Zeiss or accessory sebaceous glands.

The clinical diagnosis may be difficult since the lesion often superficially resembles a chalazion. It is important to evert the lid and look for ulcerative changes on the tarsus.

## Eyelid malpositions

### Entropion

This is an in-turning of the lower and, more rarely, the upper lid (Fig. 7.6).

### Ectropion

This is an out-turning of the lower lid (Fig. 7.7).

### Ptosis

There are many causes of ptosis (Fig. 7.8) and each case requires careful history and examination (Fig. 7.9).

*History and symptoms*
Important points are age of onset, duration and associated symptoms such as fatiguability, diplopia and variability.

**Fig. 7.6** Summary of entropion eyelid malpositions

| Cause | Pathogenesis | Treatment |
|---|---|---|
| Involutional | Age-related regeneration of the elastic tissues within the eyelid leads to horizontal laxity | Temporary treatment in casualty – lubricants and eyelid taping to reduce irritation from lashes<br>Permanent treatment is with surgical correction |
| Cicatricial | Severe scarring of the palpebral conjunctiva pulls the lid inwards towards the globe (chemical injuries, trauma and inflammation) | Bandage contact lens prevents eyelash rubbing against the cornea<br>Permanent treatment is with anterior lamellar rotation +/– composite grafts |
| Congenital | Improper development of the inferior retractor aponeurosis | Often self-limiting. In symptomatic cases, surgical correction |

**Fig. 7.7** Summary of ectropion eyelid malpositions

| Classification | Pathogenesis | Treatment |
|---|---|---|
| Involutional | Ageing changes in the elastic tissues within the eyelid leading to lower lid laxity | Surgical correction of the lid laxity |
| Cicatricial | Scarring and contracture of the skin pulling the eyelid away from the globe | Eliminate any chemical cause, for example preserved eye drops. Surgical correction |
| Paralytic | Ipsilateral facial nerve palsy | Lubrication, surgical correction including a temporary tarsorraphy to reduce corneal exposure |
| Mechanical | Tumours on or at the lid margin leading to eversion | Removal of the cause |

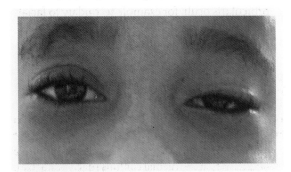

**Fig. 7.8** Left ptosis. Left upper eyelid is covering pupil and may cause amblyopia in children under 8 years of age.

It is important to rule out a pseudoptosis which may be caused by enophthalmos, contralateral lid retraction, ipsilateral hypotropia, brow ptosis or dermatochalasis.

*Signs*

Important measurements are vertical fissure height and levator function. It is important to measure fatiguability and ocular motility, look for jaw winking and check the Bell's phenomenon.

**Fig. 7.9** Summary of categories of ptosis

| Classification | Mechanism | Cause |
|---|---|---|
| Mechanical | The lid is pulled down due to the gravitational effect of a mass or scarring | Large lid lesions pulling down lid<br>Scarring<br>Dermatochalasis (pseudo-ptosis)<br>Oedema |
| Aponeurotic | A defect in the levator aponeurosis | Involutional (senile)<br>Postoperative (perhaps due to stretching from the eyelid speculum) |
| Myogenic | Myopathy of the levator muscle or neuromuscular junction disease | Myasthenia gravis<br>Myotonic dystrophy<br>Congenital ptosis<br>Blepharophimosis syndrome |
| Neurogenic | Innervational defect | III nerve palsy<br>Horner syndrome<br>Marcus Gunn jaw winking |

*Treatment*

Treatment is related to the cause. Medical conditions such as myasthenia, which causes myogenic ptosis, require a neurological referral. There are various surgical options, depending on the age of the patient and the clinical diagnosis.

## LACRIMAL SYSTEM

Tears are trilayered and are predominantly formed by the lacrimal gland. Tears cling and stick to the surface of the eye from conjunctival mucus-secreting glands and do not evaporate from the surface of the eye due to a coating of oil, which is secreted by the meibomian glands. The anatomy of the lacrimal system is shown in Fig. 7.10. It is important to exclude and treat any cause of reflex lacrimation such as trichiasis or blepharitis or dry eyes.

## Symptoms and disorders of the lacrimal system

The main symptom related to the lacrimal system is excess tearing, known as 'watery eye'. This can be caused by two conditions:

- Hyperlacrimation.
- Epiphora.

## Hyperlacrimation

Hyperlacrimation is where there is reflex lacrimal hypersecretion secondary to ocular surface abnormality. Treatment in these cases is to treat the underlying cause.

## Epiphora

Epiphora is the compromise of lacrimal drainage due to:

- Congenital obstruction.
- Eyelid malposition displacing the lacrimal punctum out of the tear lake.
- Lacrimal obstruction along the drainage system which may be partial or complete.
- Lacrimal pump failure due to weakness of the orbicularis oculi, for example secondary to facial nerve palsy.

## Other lacrimal disorders

### Congenital nasolacrimal duct obstruction

This commonly presents to the general practitioner in infancy with symptoms of a recurrent watery, sticky eye with mucus discharge which may be associated with a fluctuant mass at the medial canthus (dacryocstocele). It is common and due to an imperforate end of the nasolacrimal duct. Most are self-limiting and parents should perform firm massage over the medial canthus

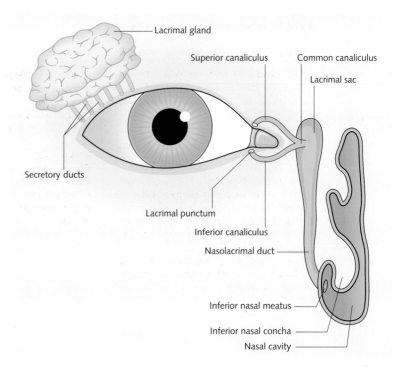

**Fig. 7.10** Lacrimal system. Tears from the lacrimal gland traverse the cornea, enter the puncta, travel along the canaliculi to the lacrimal sac, thence to the nasolacrimal duct, and then pass into the inferior nasal meatus.

Labels: Lacrimal gland · Superior canaliculus · Common canaliculus · Lacrimal sac · Secretory ducts · Lacrimal punctum · Inferior canaliculus · Nasolacrimal duct · Inferior nasal meatus · Inferior nasal concha · Nasal cavity

to encourage development. If epiphora persists after the age of 2, a 'probing' under general anaesthetic can be performed by passing a probe via the punctum through the nasolacrimal duct to perforate the membrane.

## Adult nasolacrimal duct obstruction

*Symptoms*
Sticky, watery eye where the conjunctiva is white. Symptoms worsen in wind or the cold weather.

*Signs*
Include punctual stenosis, blocked system on syringing via the canaliculus with saline. A dacryocystogram may be used to identify the location of the blockage.

*Treatment*
Dacryocystorhinostomy (DCR) connects the mucosal surface of the lacrimal sac to the nasal mucosa by removing the intervening bone.

## ORBITAL DISEASE

The orbit is composed of the bony and soft tissue structures that surround the globe. It has several important functions including protection of the globe, attachments to stabilize ocular movement and connective tissue structures which transmit nerves and blood vessels.

The expression of diseases in terms of clinical signs is often similar despite the large variety of diseases which can affect the orbit. A detailed history and examination is vital (Fig. 7.11).

## Differential diagnosis of orbital disease

### Dysthyroid eye disease
Dysthyroid or thyroid eye disease (TED) is the most common cause of both bilateral and unilateral axial proptosis in adults, and is permanent in 70% of cases (Fig. 7.12). Although associated with thyrotoxicosis, it is uninfluenced by the treatment of hyperthyroidism because patients can be clinically and biochemically euthryoid. TED is an organ-specific autoimmune IgG mediated disease leading to infiltration of muscles and fat surrounding eye. There are two stages:

1. Acute inflammatory (risk of sight loss) – lasts approximately 12–18 months, causing proptosis, and may cause compressive optic neuropathy.
2. Chronic fibrotic – leading to a restrictive myopathy and diplopia.

**Fig. 7.11** History and examination of the orbit

| History | Examination |
|---------|-------------|
| • Onset and duration of proptosis (old photographs may be helpful) – protrusion of the eye caused by a space occupying lesion<br>• Enophthalmos, e.g. due to orbital floor fractures<br>• Pain (due to inflammatory or rapidly progressing disorders)<br>• Diplopia (restriction or inflammation of extraocular muscles or direct involvement of the nerve supply resulting in a palsy)<br>• Visual loss (may be due to exposure keratopathy, optic nerve compression or inflammation or distortion of the macula by a posterior lesion)<br>• Swelling (acute, e.g. infective orbital cellulitis)<br>• Change with Valsalva manoeuvre (suggests a vascular lesion) | Proptosis (can be measured with a ruler or subjectively looking from above the patient)<br>Optic nerve function<br>Pupil reactions including RAPD<br>Fields<br>Visual acuity<br>Colour vision<br>Optic nerve appearance (pallor/swelling)<br>Intraocular pressure<br>Palpation for orbital tenderness and masses |

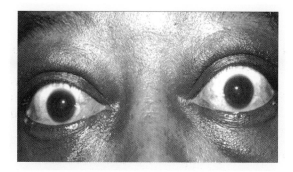

Fig. 7.12    Thyroid eye disease.

Aqueous humour outflow obstruction from the eye may occur leading to increased intraocular pressure, and thus secondary glaucoma. Risk factors include smoking and female gender. Graves' disease affects 2% of females in the UK. Therefore male smokers with TED have the worst prognosis. Fig. 7.13 gives the symptoms and signs of TED. An alternative method of remembering symptoms and examination pointers is to use the acronym of the American Thyroid Association, NO SPECS (Fig. 7.14).

### Investigation
- CT orbit.
- Proptosis (⅔ of globe should lie within the orbital rim).

Raised intraocular pressure (compared to primary gaze) or diplopia (usually up gaze +/– lateral gaze) is due to early inferior rectus muscle tethering and hence difficulty in elevating the eye.

- EOM (extraocular muscle) infiltration and enlargement (inferior rectus (IR) and medial rectus (MR) most commonly involved).
- Thyroid function tests (TSH, T3 and T4).

### Treatment
- Manage thyroid dysfunction.
- Ocular lubricants alone (in mild cases for corneal exposure).
- Glaucoma topical medications (for secondary or post-trabecular glaucoma).
- Acute optic nerve compression (5% of patients).
- Systemic corticosteroids.
- Orbital radiotherapy.
- Surgical orbital decompression.

Chronic phase:

- Diplopia: squint surgery, prisms, botulinum toxin.
- Cosmetic: orbital decompression; lid surgery, e.g. blepharoplasty, lid lowering, etc.

Female thyroid eye disease patients with (mild) proptosis are commonly told nothing more can be done for their cosmetic appearance. Remember that orbital, then squint, then finally eyelid surgery should be performed *in that order*. There are risks and benefits to any surgical procedure and therefore referral to an orbital/thyroid eye disease specialist is advised. Otherwise the result may be Garfield the cat's eyes, i.e. sleepy looking, proptosed eyes following lid lowering surgery without orbital decompression surgery.

## Infective disorders

Orbital cellulitis is an important, potentially visually threatening disorder (Fig. 7.15). The most serious complications are blindness and secondary central nervous system infection leading to a brain abscess.

**Fig. 7.13** Features of thyroid eye disease

Symptoms:
- Nil
- Grittiness (e.g. superior limbic keratoconjunctivitis)
- Redness
- Eyelid swelling
- Diplopia
- Cosmetic appearance, 'bulgy'/'staring' eyes (Kocher sign)
- Visual loss

Signs:
- Lid retraction (Dalrymple sign) – primary due to fibrotic contracture of the levator, secondary due to overaction of the levator/superior rectus complex if there is hyperphoria produced by fibrosis of the inferior rectus
- Lid lag on down gaze (von Graefe sign)

**Fig. 7.14** American Thyroid Association classification for thyroid eye disease

Examination:
NO SPECS – six stages
- (N) No signs or symptoms
- (O) Only ocular irritation (dryness, FB (foreign body sensation))
- (S) Soft tissue involvement (conjunctival chemosis/oedema)
- (P) Proptosis
- (E) EOM (extraocular muscle) fibrosis
- (C) Corneal exposure and ulceration if severe
- (S) Sight loss
  - –Corneal ulceration
  - –Optic neuropathy (compressive)
  - –↑ Intraocular pressure

### Symptoms and signs

Swelling of the eyelid tissues. Preseptal cellulitis is a superficial skin infection, which is anterior to the orbital septum. Signs of orbital cellulitis, which is sight threatening, are pain and conjunctival injection, restriction of eye movements with diplopia, reduced vision and relative afferent papillary defect, feeling systemically unwell with an associated pyrexia.

### Examination

Full ocular and orbital examination must be carried out.

### Treatment

Admit and give intravenous broad spectrum antibiotics until pyrexia resolves and vision returns to normal.

Other conditions which may involve the orbit and should always be considered in the differential diagnosis:
- Inflammatory disease: sarcoid, idiopathic orbital inflammation, Wegener's disease.
- Vascular anomalies: carotid–cavernous fistula, varix, capillary haemangioma.
- Orbital tumours (Fig. 7.16).

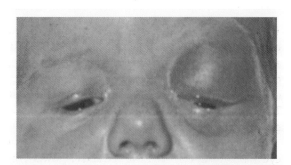

**Fig. 7.15** Orbital cellulitis. Left-sided swollen, tender, erythematous eyelids.

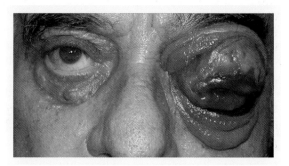

**Fig. 7.16** Left non-axial proptosis and eyelid chemosis. Metastatic orbital disease was later diagnosed.

# Anterior segment (cornea and cataract)

## Objectives (cornea)

You should be able to:

- Describe the structure and function of the cornea.
- Differentiate between bacterial and viral keratitis.
- Describe the clinical signs, ocular and systemic associations of keratoconus.
- Understand the implications of corneal trauma.

## Objectives (cataract)

You should be able to:

- Differentiate between a lens and cataract.
- Counsel a patient prior to cataract surgery.
- Describe the causes of a subluxed/dislocated lens.
- Describe the complications of cataract surgery.

## CORNEA

### Introduction

The cornea is avascular. It has clarity owing to the regular alignment of collagen fibrils, such that parallel light rays can pass through unobstructed. Any compromise from corneal disease leads to corneal opacity, reduced vision and the need for corneal graft. Therefore adequate medical treatment will avoid progression of disease process.

The cornea is the major refractive interface in the eye accounting for $^2/_3$ of the refractive power (the lens providing the other, variable, $^1/_3$ power).

The cornea (Fig. 8.1), particularly involving the stromal layer, is the part of the eye that is operated on during laser refractive surgery (such as photorefractive keratectomy (PRK) and laser in situ keratomileusis (LASIK)).

### Infection

Corneal infection can be a major cause of sight threatening disease (Fig. 8.2). Patients may have bacterial, protozoan or viral disease.

If a painful, red eye with focal corneal opacity is seen, then always consider the possibility of a bacterial keratitis in a contact lens wearer. Advise no contact lens wear in the affected eye for at least 1 month and that they should ideally wear spectacles until the treatment is completed. Some patients have no spectacles at all and are advised to obtain a pair based on measurements for the good eye rather than the two individual eyes.

### Bacterial

These infections are rare in the absence of a corneal epithelial defect. They are therefore seen in the context of contact lens wear and/or ocular surface compromise such as entropion, dry eye, corneal anaesthesia (congenital, diabetes mellitus or acoustic neuroma) or immunocompromise.

Clinical scenarios and ulcer types can help guide initial empiric treatment (Figs 8.3, 8.4). With this information (thus history is important in eliciting

**Fig. 8.1** Description of the five anatomical layers of the cornea

| Corneal layer | Description |
| --- | --- |
| Epithelium | A multicellular layer providing the main external defence to disease (e.g. bacteria) |
| Bowen's membrane | The basement membrane to epithelium |
| Stroma | Approximately 90% of the corneal mass. It is essentially acellular, except for a few keratocytes. A relatively dehydrated state must be maintained to preserve clarity |
| Descemet's membrane | An acellular structure. It provides support for the endothelium |
| Endothelium | A monolayer of non-renewing cells. These very important cells are responsible for maintaining the dehydrated state. They pump fluid actively out of the stroma. Any compromise of the endothelium leads to stromal oedema and clouding, e.g. in Fuch's endothelial dystrophy |

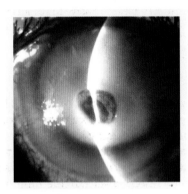

**Fig. 8.2** Microbial keratitis in a contact lens wearer. There is central thinning of the cornea and impending perforation.

any risk factors from the patient), suitable management can be started.

### Management

A corneal scrape is taken and treatment is started. This is usually a quinolone (good broad spectrum cover) such as guttae ofloxacin.

Intensive treatment (hourly drops) continues over 48 hours and clinical response is assessed. Steroids may then be required to reduce stromal scarring.

In extreme cases of corneal thinning and perforation corneal glue or even a tectonic (custom fit) graft may be required. Rapid identification of the organism can prevent endophthalmitis and loss of vision.

### Protozoan

Corneal acanthamoeba infection is associated with soft contact lens wear and poor lens hygiene, particularly the use of tap water.

Infection is characterized by a red eye with intense pain which is out of proportion to the other clinical signs. Classic signs include a ring ulcer with stromal immune ring (Wessely ring), perineural infiltrate and anterior segment inflammation. Diagnosis is obtained with deep corneal scrapes +/− biopsy. Treatment includes Brolene, polyhexamethylene biguanide (PHMB) and ketoconazole. Chronic infection from stromal acanthamoeba cysts can lead to scarring and may require corneal transplantation.

### Viral keratitis

Many viruses may affect the cornea including herpes simplex and zoster. Herpes simplex virus

**Fig. 8.3** Summary of a few candidate organisms in clinical scenarios

| Uncompromised host | Contact lens wearer | Immunocompromised |
| --- | --- | --- |
| Streptococcus | Pseudomonas | Pseudomonas |
| Pseudomonas | Staphylococcus | Staphylococcus |
| Moraxella | Streptococcus | Enterobacter |

**Fig. 8.4** Summary of ulcer patterns

| Ring ulcer | Localized | Purulent |
| --- | --- | --- |
| *Pseudomonas* | *Staphylococcus* | *Streptococcus* |
| *Streptococcus* | | |

(HSV) can affect the epithelium, stroma or endothelium.

### Epithelial disease

This is characterized by the classic dendritic (Fig. 8.5) or geographic (more advanced) forms. The central defect stains with fluorescein and the edges stain with Rose Bengal (stains dead cells). Treatment is with topical antiviral and a cycloplegic.

A neurotrophic ulcer is another form of epithelial disease, this looks like a non-healing corneal abrasion and requires additional treatment such as lubricants, patching, botulinum ptosis or a conjunctival flap.

Reduced corneal sensation (particularly in unilateral disease) is very suggestive of previous HSV infection. Test prior to placement of topical anaesthetic!

### Stromal disease

The classic form is referred to as a disciform keratitis. This may or may not be associated with epithelial or endothelial disease. There is a central ring opacity with corneal oedema and fine keratic precipitates (KPs) (Fig. 8.6). This immune process may progress to scarring with vascularization. Careful treatment with topical steroid and cycloplegic is required.

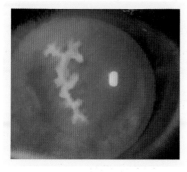

**Fig. 8.5** Herpes simplex keratitis. A dendritic (branching pattern) shaped corneal ulcer is visible glowing green with fluorescein staining (a yellow drop) and blue light.

### Endotheliitis

Focal endothelial inflammation with stromal oedema (temporary decompensation of endothelium).

Any of the above forms may be associated with an iridocyclitis or trabeculitis, and topical steroid and, if required, ocular antihypertensive should be added. With evidence of intraocular inflammation, systemic antivirals are also added.

*Long-term complications* include:

- Corneal scarring (treat with contact lens, long-term, low-strength topical steroid).
- Corneal thinning/perforation (treat with a botulinum ptosis or conjunctival flap).

Either of the above may be treated with a corneal graft. The herpetic disease may recur in the graft.

### Herpes zoster

The multiple epithelial pseudodendrites and anterior stromal infiltrates are responsive to topical steroids. The main treatment is with systemic antivirals (see section on uveitis, Ch. 11).

## Inflammation

The cornea may suffer from non-microbial keratitis which may be due to either local or systemic disease. These conditions classically lead to inflammation, corneal infiltrate and corneal thinning/melting. The mainstay of treatment, in all scenarios, is topical steroid drops (except with extreme thinning) and topical antibiotic, though occasionally systemic steroids are required.

## Ocular disease

There are numerous ocular conditions that may lead to a non-microbial keratitis. Two of these include marginal keratitis and vernal keratoconjunctivitis.

### Marginal keratitis

This relatively common condition is associated with blepharitis, specifically anterior (staphylococcal) blepharitis. Staphylococcal hypersensitivity leads to peripheral (but away from limbus) infiltrate and thinning.

Treatment is topical steroid and lid hygiene (to treat blepharitis).

### Vernal keratoconjunctivitis

This is a superiorly located ulcer found in patients with marked allergic eye disease. It is due to giant papillae under upper lid.

Fig. 8.6 Keratic precipitates on corneal endothelium.

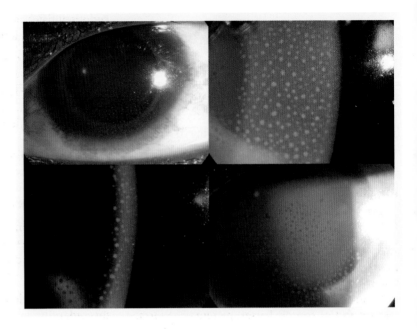

Treatment is with topical steroid and anti-allergic eye drops (e.g. Opatanol (olopatadine)).

## Systemic disease

Rheumatoid arthritis, systemic lupus erythematosus, polyarteritis nodosa, Wegener's granulomatosis and rarely relapsing polychondritis can lead to peripheral necrotizing keratitis (Fig. 8.7).

The management of these diseases is conducted by both the patient's physician and ophthalmologist. Very often local treatment such as steroids, antibiotics and lubricants are not sufficient. Systemic steroid and second line immunosuppressant therapy may be required. The aim is to treat the acute stage and then prevent recurrences on as little medication as possible.

## Some important dystrophies

### Fuch's endothelial dystrophy

This reasonably common dystrophy presents in the 5th to 8th decade with blurred vision, which is initially worse in the morning and improves after a few hours. The loss of endothelial cells causes gradual corneal decompensation. Treatments include hypertonic saline drops (5%) to aid corneal drying and corneal graft.

### Keratoconus

This ectatic dystrophy is characterized by a gradual deterioration in vision (due to worsening astigmatism) in adolescence. It rarely presents in its acute form, corneal hydrops, which is due to a split in Descemet's membrane.

Characteristic clinical signs include:

- Conical cornea (apex usually inferiorly placed).
- Corneal thinning and scarring.
- Vogt's striae (fine lines on posterior corneal surface).
- Fleischer's ring (iron line on corneal epithelium, at the base of the cone).

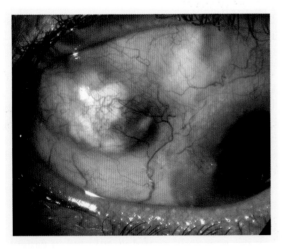

Fig. 8.7 Previous scleritis. Blue choroid showing through overlying thin white sclera.

**Fig. 8.8** Ocular and systemic associations of keratoconus

| Ocular | Systemic |
| --- | --- |
| Blue sclera | Atopy |
| Leber's amaurosis | Down syndrome |
| Ectopia lentis | Marfan's |
| Retinitis pigmentosa | Osteogenesis imperfecta |
| Aniridia | Turner's syndrome |

- Munson's sign (bulging of lower lid on down gaze).
- 'Scissor reflex' on retinoscopy.
- Corneal topography (steep and thin apex).

Ocular and systemic associations of keratoconus are listed in Fig. 8.8.

Treatment of keratoconus is initially refractive (glasses and/or contact lenses: patients need to use rigid lenses to treat astigmatism). If patients become intolerant of contact lenses a corneal graft is offered. Treatment of acute corneal hydrops (which is very painful) is with topical steroid and topical cycloplegic. Corneal graft surgery is very successful (>95% 5 year survival) in this patient group.

Indications for corneal transplantation or penetrating keratoplasty are listed in Fig. 8.9.

## Trauma

## Epithelial abrasion and recurrent erosion

### Epithelial abrasion

Epithelial abrasions are very common and usually easily treated as the epithelium usually heals very quickly.

A green epithelial defect is visible under blue light following instillation of fluorescein stain.

Small abrasions are treated with a short (5–7 days) course of topical antibiotic drops, larger abrasions with ointment (usually chloramphenicol or Fucithalmic (fusidic acid)). Cycloplegics (e.g.

cyclopentolate) and/or patching (for 24 hours; not in children) may be added.

### Recurrent erosion syndrome (RES)

A few patients with previous traumatic abrasions (classically those following fingernail injury or paper cuts) get spontaneous recurrent abrasions (RES).

Patients describe pain on waking and opening eyes; if mild it settles over a few hours. It can be tremendously debilitating. Bilateral RES may indicate a corneal dystrophy.

Treatment is aimed at the acute phase and prevention of recurrences:

- Acute treatment as for abrasion.
- Long-term treatment includes bland eye cream (e.g. lacrilube ointment) at night time, with or without lid taping/patching.

If it is still problematic consider the following, in this order:

- Debridement.
- Bandage contact lens.
- Anterior stromal puncture.
- Phototherapeutic keratoplasty (PTK).

## Perforation

Corneal perforation is a very serious condition and may lead to long-term sight loss. It can be due to acute injury (laceration) or to intrinsic corneal disease, thinning and perforation (e.g. corneal melt secondary to rheumatoid arthritis). This distinction is important as the treatment of the two is quite different.

### Corneal laceration

Lacerations may be partial or full-thickness lacerations.

### Partial-thickness laceration

Be sure of the diagnosis first! Ensure that the wound is Seidel negative (i.e. no wound leak).

Treat as for a corneal abrasion unless there is wound gape, in which case a corneal suture should be placed.

**Fig. 8.9** Indications for corneal transplantation or penetrating keratoplasty

| Corneal structure | Infection | Inflammation | Trauma |
| --- | --- | --- | --- |
| Keratoconus | Herpetic disease | Corneal melt | Trauma |
| Bullous keratopathy | Microbial keratitis | | Alkali burn |
| Corneal dystrophies | | | |

### Full-thickness laceration

*This is an emergency.* The globe should be closed within 24 hours if possible (Fig. 8.10).

*Key signs* are:

- Sudden reduced vision, often following a hammering/drilling injury.
- Low intraocular pressure.
- Shallow anterior chamber.
- Cataract (lens often damaged as well).

Once diagnosed the following treatment should commence:

- Shield or cartella (i.e. NO PAD).
- Patient should be starved ready for a general anaesthetic (avoid local anaesthetic if possible).
- Systemic broad spectrum antibiotics (e.g. oral ciprofloxacin has good vitreous/ocular penetration).
- Check tetanus status and administer as necessary.
- CT scan.
- Corneal repair with 10/0 nylon sutures (see Fig. 8.10).

Long-term management may include contact lens for astigmatism or cataract extraction.

## Alkali burn

Corneal alkali burns are potentially very serious; this is because of the rapid absorption and intraocular penetration of the alkali, leading to both superficial and intraocular complications.

> Early and copious (at least 30 min) irrigation is the crucial first step in treatment. Recheck pH 5 min after irrigation to allow re-equilibration. If still high, re-irrigate.

The key external features are limbal ischaemia and limbal stem cell damage; this will largely account for the longer-term prognosis.

### Treatment

- After irrigation the fornices should be swept with cotton swab or glass rod
- Topical antibiotic and cycloplegic.
- Analgesia (oral).
- Topical steroid if intraocular inflammation.
- Sodium citrate (reduce risk of corneal melt).
- If melting occurs use collagenase inhibitor (acetylcysteine 10–20%).
- Always check intraocular pressure and treat as appropriate.
- Bandage contact lens.
- If persistant epithelial defect consider stem cell failure:
  - Limbal stem cell graft.
- If perforation:
  - Cyanoacrylate glue.
  - Lamellar corneal graft.
  - Penetrating corneal graft (Fig. 8.11).

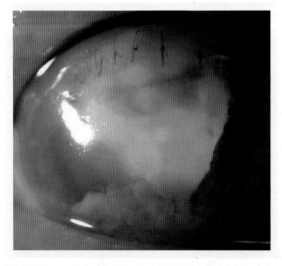

**Fig. 8.10** Corneal sutures (10/0 nylon) visible following primary repair of penetrating eye injury. The lens capsule is breached and soft lens matter is visible inferiorly.

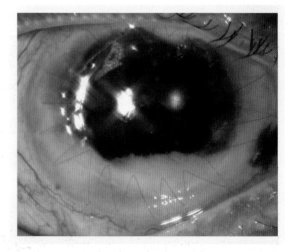

**Fig. 8.11** Penetrating keratoplasty (corneal graft), continuous corneal suture and hypopyon.

## UV keratitis

Also known as 'arc eye'. Most commonly seen in welders who do not wear a protective mask and also seen in UV sun-bed users.

Patients present in great pain and clinically there are multiple small epithelial defects (punctate epitheliopathy).

Treatment is with a short course of topical antibiotic ointment and cycloplegic.

## CATARACT

A cataract is an opacity of the crystalline lens in the eye (Fig. 8.12). The most common operation performed worldwide is cataract surgery. It is also one of the commonest causes of blindness worldwide. The word 'cataract' comes from a Greek word meaning waterfall (i.e. opaque white water). The commonest symptoms are blurring of vision and glare.

### Symptoms

*Blurred vision.* Initially the patient will be able to alleviate their blurred vision by attending their optician more frequently, e.g. every few months, and updating their prescription. This is because of a myopic shift due to increasing cataract. The patient may be able to read unaided, due to being more short sighted, but eventually glasses will not help either for reading or for distance.

*Glare.* The patient notices streaking or dazzling rays of light, particularly when looking at oncoming car headlights at night. It is worse when in dark surroundings when pupils dilate. The patient may have only a slight reduction in visual acuity (e.g. 6/9), but relatively much poorer contrast sensitivity. Updating the spectacles will not have any effect on this symptom from the posterior subcapsular cataract.

### Risk factors

Age (ultraviolet light), diabetes, uveitis, trauma.

UV light is more of a problem in causing cataract in Asia or Africa at younger age than in the cloudy UK.

The treatment of cataract is surgical, to remove the cloudy crystalline lens. Modern cataract surgery is very safe with relatively few complications.

*Other lenticular problems* include:

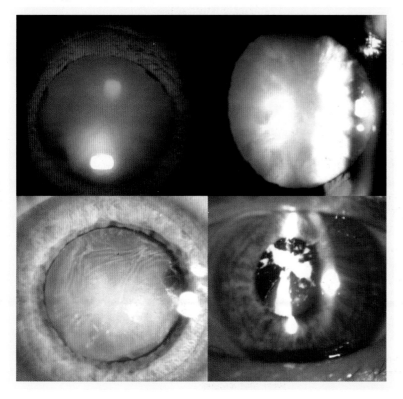

**Fig. 8.12** Different types of cataract. Clockwise from top left: immature, mature, hypermature and Morgagnian.

- Lens subluxation (post-traumatic or spontaneous).
- Phacomorphic glaucoma.
- Phacogenic uveitis.

## Anatomy of the lens

The crystalline lens is situated in the eye between the anterior and posterior segments of the eye. It is suspended in place by zonules, which are fibres that run from the ciliary body to the equator of the lens.

The shape, and thus power, of the lens is varied by ciliary muscle contraction or relaxation. Relaxation of the muscle leads to tightening of the zonules with reduction in the lens curvature and focusing power (for distant vision). During the near reflex, the ciliary muscle contracts, allowing relaxation of the zonules to allow increased lens curvature, and thus increase in focusing power.

The lens gets larger or fatter as we get older with the anterior lens epithelial cells laying down new fibres.

> If the patient has had bilateral cataract surgery at a young age then consider systemic or congenital causes for cataract. Patients usually offer answers if requested by the ophthalmologist.
>
> *Upward decentred lens* occurs in Marfan's syndrome, so politely ask to look inside the mouth and confirm the presence of high arched palate; check the length of the patient's arms, which may reach the knees while standing.
>
> *Downward decentred lens* occurs in homocysteinuria and so is important to ask about previous retinal vein occlusions at a young age (below 40 years). Trauma can cause broken zonules and thus a tilted and decentred lens. It is worth asking about sporting injuries and then gently probe towards a previous history of assault or kicks to the face.

## Common types of cataract

- Nuclear sclerosis (clouding of the central lens, associated with gradual reduction in vision and myopic shift 'index myopia'). This is the commonest form of cataract.
- Posterior subcapsular (opacity, often focal of the posterior lens, which can be quite debilitating and perceived to deteriorate

quickly, even over weeks). This rapid deterioration reflects the site of opacity near the visual axis. They also complain of glare (poor vision in bright light).

> Snellen acuity may overestimate visual function in patients with posterior subcapsular cataract.

- Cortical (radial spoke-like opacity in the anterior lens). These rarely affect vision unless they involve the centre directly.

## Traumatic cataract

Cataract may form following:

- Blunt trauma.
- Penetrating trauma.
- Ionizing radiation.

*Blunt trauma* may lead to a classical anterior subcapsular cataract (Vossius ring cataract) which happens spontaneously or soon after the trauma. A nuclear sclerotic cataract may develop over a longer period. A cataract will follow *penetrating trauma* if the capsule has been breached; this is due to lens hydration (see Fig. 8.10).

*Radiation* to the head may lead to cataract formation over time.

## Postoperative

It is well described that patients will often experience worsening or development of cataract following ocular surgery, such as vitrectomy or trabeculectomy. It is hypothesized that this may be due to postoperative intraocular inflammation. It may also develop following direct trauma to the lens, such as from vitrectomy instruments.

## Systemic disease

### Diabetes

Diabetic patients develop cataracts younger in life than non-diabetic patients and they classically are like senile cataract phenotypically.

*Senile (nuclear sclerosis, posterior subcapsular and cortical cataract).*

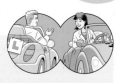

### Snowstorm cataracts

These are rare, characterized by white snowflake opacities in the subcortical area.

### Hypocalcaemia

Small white flecks, seen in severe deficiency.

### Galactosaemia

Galactose-1-phosphate uridyl transferase (GPUT) deficiency; auto recessive.

### Wilson's disease

Cortical, anterior 'sunflower cataract'.

### Myotonic dystrophy

These patients with autosomal dominant disease have a characteristic facies and frontal balding. They demonstrate difficulty relaxing after muscle contraction. Other ocular features include ptosis, external ophthalmoplegia and pigmentary retinopathy. Cataracts are specular and polychromatic in nature; onset is in the 3rd to 4th decade.

## Toxic cataract

Certain medications can lead to cataract formation. They include:

- Systemic steroids (they classically cause posterior subcapsular cataract).
- Anticholinesterases.
- Antipsychotics.
- Amiodarone (cataract and corneal deposits).

## Congenital

Congenital cataracts are discussed in Chapter 12. They can be:

- Inherited (usually autosomal recessive).
- Intrauterine infections (toxoplasmosis, rubella, cytomegalovirus (CMV), herpes).

## Associated with ocular disease

There are certain ocular conditions that are associated with increased frequency and earlier onset of cataract.

## Intraocular inflammation

Patients with chronic uveitis can develop cataract. Fuch's heterochromic iridocyclitis is one condition that can lead to cataract. Topical or systemic steroids, used for uveitis, can themselves induce cataracts.

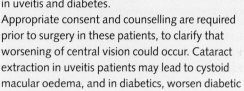

Additional risks can occur following cataract surgery in uveitis and diabetes. Appropriate consent and counselling are required prior to surgery in these patients, to clarify that worsening of central vision could occur. Cataract extraction in uveitis patients may lead to cystoid macular oedema, and in diabetics, worsen diabetic macular oedema.

## Other ocular conditions

Other ocular conditions that lead to cataract include:

- High myopia.
- Angle closure glaucoma (classically leads to anterior capsule opacities, 'glaucomflecken').
- Pseudo-exfoliation syndrome.
- Retinitis pigmentosa (posterior subcapsular cataract).
- Stickler's syndrome.

## Symptoms

### Loss of vision

Patients often complain of gradual loss of vision over 6–12 months. This loss of vision may be absolute (uncorrectable with lenses) or refractive (myopic shift). Occasionally patients will describe a rapid loss of vision with cataract that occurs in the following scenarios:

- Posterior subcapsular cataract.
- Post-traumatic.
- Incidental identification upon covering the better eye (e.g. following ocular exam).

### Glare/reduced contrast sensitivity

Patients may complain of poor vision in bright light, usually associated with posterior subcapsular cataract. Snellen acuity may underestimate real visual handicap.

### Monocular diplopia

This rare symptom of double vision from one eye, while the other is closed, is occasionally reported.

## Signs

Patients are noted to have lens opacity. There may be other signs associated with the cataract such as:

- Inflammation.
- Pseudo-exfoliation syndrome.
- Anterior segment dysgenesis.

## Management of cataract

The definitive management of cataract is surgical removal with an intraocular lens implant. Cataract extraction is the commonest surgical procedure performed worldwide.

### Conservative measures

Occasionally patients decline surgery, or it may not be indicated. The measures employed to maximize vision are glasses, improved light and/or magnifying glasses.

### Surgical removal

Cataract surgery has undergone tremendous advances in the past 10–15 years. The emergence of phacoemulsification has revolutionized the management of cataract. Historically patients were required to have marked vision loss from their cataract before they could have surgery as there were many complications from large incision cataract surgery. The concept of 'mature' cataract is now defunct. The best time to operate is when the patient is having problems with their level of vision, which is disabling and interfering with their daily activities (e.g. reading, driving, television, crossing the road) despite correct and up-to-date spectacles.

Prior to surgery it is essential to counsel patients appropriately. Cataract surgery is a victim of its own success and patients have high expectations from surgery, perhaps more than any other operation. The aim of the microscope-assisted surgery is to remove the cloudy natural lens from the eye and replace it with a plastic (e.g. acrylic) intraocular lens (IOL). The IOL has a lifetime guarantee of being clear and remains in position for the rest of the patient's life.

### Consent

There is a 2% risk of reduced vision from all complications. Patients must be warned of these risks and, as with all surgery, particularly elective surgery, the risk versus benefit ratio for each patient must be discussed. Other potential complications that should be mentioned are:

- Endophthalmitis (0.1% risk).
- Suprachoroidal haemorrhage (0.1% risk).
- Retinal detachment (1:150 risk).

Up to 30% of patients will develop posterior capsule opacification, that will require laser (YAG) therapy at a later date.

### Anaesthetic

The large majority of cataract surgery is performed under local anaesthetic (topical, subtenons, peribulbar or retrobulbar). Occasionally a general anaesthetic is indicated for uncooperative patients.

### Intraocular lens selection

Following removal of the cataract patients have an inert artificial intraocular lens inserted (Fig. 8.13). These are usually selected to make the patients emmetropic following surgery. Lens design has improved greatly from its origins using PMMA (plastic) lenses. Acrylic and silicone lenses are available. Lenses are commonly monofocal but there are increasing selections of multifocal lenses to enable both near and distance vision without glasses.

The power of the lens for insertion is calculated using a biometry formula based on the:

Never force or persuade a patient to have cataract surgery, as there is a small risk of 1/1000 endophthalmitis and of 1/1000 choroidal haemorrhage (devastating infection or bleed, respectively). Risk versus benefit needs to be assessed – all cataract patients could have their surgery done tomorrow if there was no risk at all!

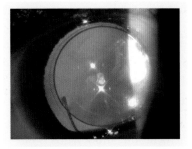

**Fig. 8.13** Pseudophakia. Intraocular lens within capsular bag, which is visible within a well dilated pupil.

- Curvature of the cornea.
- Axial length.
- Refractive index of the lens type.

### Cataract procedure
- Phacoemulsification technique involves a small incision (usually about 3 mm) in the cornea.
- The lens capsule is opened (capsulorrhexis). The cataract is within the capsular bag.
- The cataract is separated and mobilized within the capsular bag with hydrodissection.
- Using the phacoemulsification probe (high frequency ultrasound) the cataract is emulsified and aspirated through the probe.
- An artificial lens is folded and placed into the empty lens capsular bag and unfolded (see Fig. 8.13).
- Usually sutures are not required.

### Postoperative follow-up
Unless there has been an intraoperative complication patients are not seen at day 1 postoperatively. Patients take anti-inflammatory (steroid) and antibiotic drops. They can be given separately or in combination (e.g. Maxitrol™ or Tobradex™). Patients are seen at 3 weeks and they should then have a postoperative refraction when they finish their course of drops.

### Complications
- *Endophthalmitis:*
  Early (onset of a very painful red eye in the first few days postoperatively with a hypopyon).
  Late (chronic inflammation with or without hypopyon).

This devastating complication affects about 0.1% of intraocular surgeries. The management is outlined in Chapter 11.

- *Raised intraocular pressure.*

Most problems with pressure rise relate to retained viscoelastic in the immediate postoperative period. Other causes of raised pressure include inflammation and steroid response glaucoma.

- *Inflammation.*

Some patients experience prolonged or recurrent bouts of inflammation. They can usually be controlled with topical medications; some require oral or peribulbar steroids.

- *Retinal detachment.*

About 1:150 patients experience a retinal detachment postoperatively. This rate increases dramatically if there is a posterior capsular rupture with vitreous loss. High myopia and pre-existing lattice degeneration also increase the risk.

- *Cystoid macular oedema.*

A number of patients experience vision loss, classically stating that their vision was good in the immediate postoperative period and then declined. There is thickening of the macula with classic 'petaloid' pattern of hyperfluorescence on the fluorescein angiogram and cystoid spaces on OCT imaging (Fig. 8.14). Patients are treated with topical steroidal and non-steroidal anti-inflammatory drops. The condition eventually resolves in the majority of cases.

- *Posterior capsular opacification (PCO).*

This is a common complication of cataract surgery but seen less often with the application of newer lens design and materials. The rate with the older PMMA lenses was about 30%. Patients describe a gradual reduction in vision. There is obvious thickening of the posterior lens capsule on slit lamp exam. Treatment is with YAG laser capsulotomy, which punches a hole in the posterior capsule (Fig. 8.15).

The vast majority of patients are very happy with the results of cataract surgery; however, we must always strive to improve outcomes and limit morbidity.

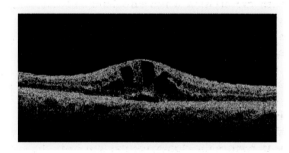

**Fig. 8.14** Optical coherence tomogram (OCT) image showing cystoid macular oedema following cataract surgery in a uveitis patient.

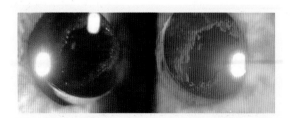

**Fig. 8.15** YAG capsulotomy. An opening is made through the posterior lens capsule.

Additionally we have a responsibility to ensure appropriate patient selection and should only operate when it is necessary.

## OTHER DISEASES OF THE LENS

Apart from cataract formation the lens can play a role in other intraocular pathological conditions.

## Subluxation/dislocation

The lens can be dislocated due to intrinsic ocular disease or following trauma.

*Intrinsic conditions* associated with lens subluxation/dislocation include:

- Marfan's syndrome (an autosomal dominant inherited disorder of connective tissue). The lenses classically lie superotemporally when subluxed. Systemic problems include aortic incompetence, aortic aneurysm, muscular underdevelopment and skeletal malformation.
- Homocysteinuria (an autosomal recessive systemic disease due to a deficiency in cystathione synthetase). There is a general predilection to thromboembolic events. It is associated with downward lens subluxation, central retinal vein occlusions and reaction to general anaesthetic.
- Pseudoexfoliation (associated with zonular laxity and subluxation with minor trauma or surgery).

## Other conditions associated with ectopia lentis

- Stickler's syndrome.
- Ehler's–Danlos syndrome.
- Aniridia.

Subluxed lenses can usually be managed conservatively depending on the extent of the subluxation.

If vision is reduced because of cataract a lens extraction (using an anterior of posterior approach) is performed. If lenses dislocate completely into the vitreal cavity they do not usually cause problems and patients will wear a contact lens. Occasionally the lens will dislocate anteriorly causing pupil block and iris bombe, or into the anterior chamber leading to corneal touch and endothelial damage.

### Phacomorphic glaucoma

When a lens becomes cataractous or swollen it increases in size. This may lead to a pupil block similar to that seen in angle closure glaucoma (Fig. 8.16). Once the intraocular pressure has been managed medically, the cataract should be removed.

### Phacolytic glaucoma

In rare circumstances when a cataract becomes hypermature (see Fig. 8.12; i.e. liquefaction of the cortex) lens proteins may leak into the anterior chamber and block the trabecular meshwork, leading to secondary open angle glaucoma. The treatment is removal of the lens with anterior chamber washout.

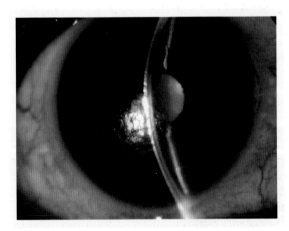

**Fig. 8.16** Phacomorphic glaucoma. Lens thickened, iris bowed forward and narrow angle visible.

# Glaucoma

## INTRODUCTION

*Glaucoma* is a group of diseases defined by a characteristic pattern of progressive optic neuropathy. There is associated irreversible damage to the visual field with the progressive reduction in light sensitivity of peripheral and, later, central vision (Fig. 9.1). Glaucoma is the second commonest cause of blindness world-wide and the commonest cause of irreversible blindness. The only proven treatments are aimed at reduction of intraocular pressure.

## PATHOPHYSIOLOGY

Progressive loss of retinal ganglion cells with a pathognomonic excavation of the optic nerve head leads to a 'cupped' disc (Fig. 9.2). Damage is usually related to the level of intraocular pressure (IOP). The balance between inflow of fluid produced by the ciliary body and outflow through the trabecular meshwork determines the IOP. In most glaucomas the rate of fluid outflow is reduced, e.g. by trabecular meshwork changes or abnormal contact with the iris (Fig. 9.3). The level of IOP required to cause damage varies between individuals. It is influenced by other risk factors such as corneal thickness and vascular factors, and may even be in the normal range (normal pressure glaucoma). The mechanism of ganglion cell damage by high IOP is most likely a combination of mechanical distortion of axons at their exit from the eyeball, causing impaired flow of axonal transport, and localized disturbance of vascular supply. The precise contribution of non-IOP factors (such as vascular) remains disputed.

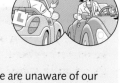

Patients are often unaware of even functionally significant visual loss due to cortical 'filling in' of scotoma (just as we are unaware of our physiological blind spots). It is crucial to explain that we aim to save vision for the future, but cannot repair what is lost, to help patients understand the objectives and limitations of treatment while the disease is still in this asymptomatic stage.

Visual field testing can usually detect damage only when 30–50% of ganglion cells have already been lost. More sensitive techniques (e.g. blue on yellow rather than white on white perimetry) are less specific. Either optic disc or visual field may show detectable change first. Techniques such as three-dimensional laser tomography of the optic nerve or nerve fibre layer thickness measurement by polarized light can also detect early changes. All these technologies can also be used to detect *change*.

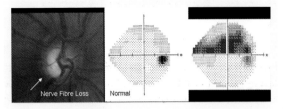

**Fig. 9.1** Right inferotemporal optic disc cupping (or neuroretinal rim loss) is depicted by white arrow. Note that the artery has to climb out of the base of the optic cup towards the retina, while the vein dips into the optic cup. This optic disc corresponds to a paracentral superonasal arcuate field loss as depicted on the automated Humphrey visual field test. A normal visual field test with blind spot is shown for comparison.

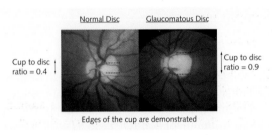

**Fig. 9.2** Normal versus glaucomatous cupped optic disc. Arterioles and venules, respectively, appear and disappear at the centre of the optic disc or optic cup. Look at how the veins and arteries, respectively, climb into and out of the optic cup in the glaucomatous disc. The normal disc is like a saucer, whereas the cupped disc is analogous to a tea cup.

**Fig. 9.3** Cross-sectional diagram indicating the drainage 'angle'.

## GLAUCOMA EXAMINATION

Glaucoma examination may detect:
1. Raised *intraocular pressure* (IOP) – for that individual
2. Optic disc *cupping*.
3. Visual *field* defects.
4. Open or closed *angle* on gonioscopy.

### Aqueous pathway

The aqueous humour is produced by the ciliary body, passes in front of the lens and behind the iris, then through the pupil and over the iris to the periphery towards the angle where it then passes through the trabecular meshwork, the canal of Schlemm, then outwards to the episcleral vessels. The adult eyeball is a rigid box, since the cornea and sclera cannot stretch. If raised IOP occurs, then the pressure is transmitted posteriorly towards the optic disc. The optic disc surface looks like a flat saucer/plate (i.e. plan view), but can be squashed and deformed to become more of a tea-cup shape in three dimensions, hence the term optic disc 'cupping' or 'cupped'.

## PRIMARY GLAUCOMAS

### Primary open angle glaucoma (POAG)

POAG is the commonest form of glaucoma in most races. In most patients idiopathic age-related changes to the trabecular meshwork increase resistance to fluid outflow and the IOP rises. However in up to a third the IOP is within statistically normal limits for that population. Non-pressure-related mechanisms are likely to be more important in these cases.

Slowly progressive damage remains asymptomatic until the late stages. However, objective measures of visual function and performance are affected before patients can notice loss of vision and even asymptomatic patients are more likely to suffer falls and car crashes.

Patients of African origin have a higher prevalence, more severe disease and an earlier onset; increased scarring also makes surgical treatment less successful in this group.

## Primary angle closure glaucoma (PACG) or acute angle closure glaucoma (AACG)

Primary angle closure is defined by abnormal contact between peripheral iris and trabecular meshwork without other additional cause (e.g. vitreous cavity blood pushing the lens forwards).

This is a condition where the pressure in the eye rises acutely to very high levels (typically 65 mmHg). A Goldmann tonometer is used to measure IOP.

### Diagnosing POAG

Primary open angle glaucoma is a *diagnosis of exclusion* that can be made only when other causes, perhaps needing different treatment, have been ruled out (e.g. angle closure, previous trauma). A normal *open angle* (i.e. where iris and cornea meet) on gonioscopy is a requirement for a diagnosis of POAG.

Ocular hypertension is raised IOP without optic nerve damage – approximately 1 in 20 people over the age of 40 have IOP higher than a population-defined normal. Patients may be treated or monitored for signs of change, depending on other risk factors (Fig. 9.4).

### Symptoms

- Headache.
- Severe pain in the eye or over the brow.
- Photophobia, loss of vision.
- Nausea and vomiting.
- There may be a history of seeing 'haloes' around lights which signify sub-acute attacks of angle closure glaucoma.

*Do not always assume nausea and vomiting is from abdominal aetiology.*

### Signs

Screening the first degree relatives of affected individuals increases detection of early disease and can prevent blindness. It is essential to explain the need for all siblings, and children if old enough, to be assessed regularly. This may be a delicate request for patients from cultures that do not openly discuss illness.

Strict visual standards for eligibility to drive are defined by the Driving and Vehicle Licensing Authority (DVLA). Glaucoma patients frequently fail assessments of peripheral vision even while still asymptomatic. It is vital to discuss sensitively the loss of what to many is an important source of freedom while clearly transmitting the legal and moral consequences of continuing to drive when unfit.

**Fig. 9.4** Risk factors for primary open angle glaucoma

| | |
|---|---|
| Greater age | Exponential increase after age 40, to 10–20% over 80 years old |
| Raised IOP | Also increases *rate* of damage |
| Affected first-degree relative | 10–30% increased risk |
| Race | Risk in those of African origin is 5 × that of Caucasians |
| Myopia | Higher risk with greater myopia |
| Thin corneas | Higher risk |
| Larger optic discs | Higher risk |

Visual acuity is severely reduced (typically worse than 6/60 or even counting fingers). Redness and hazy cornea due to oedema is noticeable, particularly when compared to the other side. The pupil is oval, semi-dilated and reacts poorly to light.

Consider *acute angle closure* in any patient with a red eye who is systemically unwell. Rapid marked rises in intraocular pressure cause headache, nausea and even vomiting with a 'vagal-pain' type picture. Another common confusion is with the visual symptoms and nausea of migraine.

## Risk factors

- Elderly (get cataract which may be thicker/ swollen not just cloudy/opaque).
- Hypermetrope (may account for young Mongolian/Singaporian age group).

Remember 'H' for Halifax guy with BIG 'H'ypermetropic eyes, with shorter (axial) eyeball length.

*Topical steroids* can dangerously increase intraocular pressure in susceptible individuals and usage MUST be monitored with regular IOP checks. Unmonitored 'repeat' prescriptions of steroids in primary care are regular causes of litigation.

## What to do

The symptoms and signs of acute glaucoma are so obvious that the diagnosis is easy. Beware of the patient who may not have ALL of the signs and symptoms mentioned, so have a high index of suspicion. Ring the on-call ophthalmologist and discuss whether any treatment is required before the patient is transferred.

## Background/principle

There is not much space between the iris and lens capsule so that aqueous fluid is sequestered/trapped behind the iris and pushes the iris forwards (Fig. 9.5B). The space between the iris and cornea (i.e. the angle – think back to GSCE mathematics days re acute angle) becomes smaller and ultimately closes. A vicious cycle is set up and the pressure in the eye shoots up towards 60–65 mmHg. The retina, iris and cornea become very ischaemic. Hence the drop in vision, poorly reactive pupil and corneal oedema.

The cycle of events is broken by decreasing the eye pressure, improving the view through the cornea to the iris and performing laser iridotomy (Fig. 9.5C) so that the aqueous can gush forwards through the lasered mini-pupil and allow the iris to flop back posteriorly and reopen the angle.

There is about a 4-hour window from the time of extremely elevated IOP until the retina becomes so ischaemic that it dies. Blood is finding it extremely difficult to enter the eye posteriorly to the retina and anteriorly to the iris. This leads to retinal ganglion cell loss and nerve fibre layer loss at the optic disc, which leads to irreversible glaucomatous (optic disc cupping) damage.

## Treatment

1. Carbonic anhydrase inhibitor – i.v. Diamox (acetazolamide).
2. Topical medications (also see POAG section).
   Steroids (e.g. dexamethasone (Maxidex), pred. forte 1%) every 15 min.
   Cholinergic (miotic) – pilocarpine 2% (if blue/ green iris) or 4% (if brown iris).
   B-blockers (e.g. timolol, Betagan).
   $\alpha2$ adrenergic agonists (e.g. Alphagan (brimonidine tartrate), Iopidine (apraclonidine))
   **NOT** Carbonic anhydrase inhibitors (e.g. Trusopt (dorzolamide)) – since already bolus given (as i.v. Diamox (acetazolamide))
   Prostaglandin analogues (e.g. Xalatan (latanoprost), Travatan (travoprost), Lumigan (bimatoprost)).
3. Bilateral peripheral laser iridotomy– to protect the second eye from becoming like the first eye.

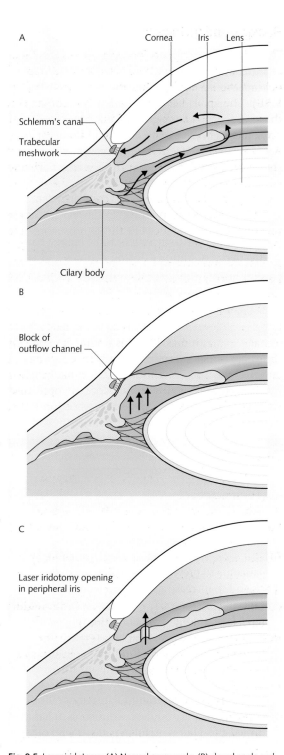

**Fig. 9.5** Laser iridotomy. (A) Normal open angle, (B) closed angle and (C) re-opened angle following laser iridotomy.

## SECONDARY GLAUCOMAS

Secondary glaucomas are all high-pressure conditions due to impaired drainage of aqueous from the eye. They can be classified either by cause (Fig. 9.6) or by site of obstruction:

- *Pre-trabecular*:
  Neo-vascular membranes due to retinal ischaemia obstructing the trabecular meshwork
  Uveitis – viscous aqueous and abnormal adhesions between iris and lens.
- *Trabecular*:
  Steroid-induced changes
  Particulate obstruction (pigment, blood, lens particles)
  Inflammatory trabeculitis, e.g. from herpes simplex.
- *Post-trabecular* – raised episcleral venous pressure, e.g. Sturge–Weber syndrome, carotico-cavernous fistulae.

**Fig. 9.6** Causes of secondary glaucoma

| | |
|---|---|
| Inflammatory – uveitic | Abnormal adhesions may form between iris and trabecular meshwork or lens |
| Post-surgical | After retinal detachment or other intraocular surgery |
| Lens-related | Pseudo-exfoliation (deposition of abnormal extra-cellular matrix) Lens-related angle closure 'phacomorphic' or anterior lens subluxation Leakage of lens proteins into anterior chamber 'phacolytic' |
| Pigment dispersion | From abnormal iris pigment shedding into the anterior chamber |
| Traumatic | Red blood cells in the anterior chamber ('hyphaema') Direct and inflammatory damage to trabecular meshwork |
| Steroid-induced | Topical or periocular steroids, e.g. eczema can increase IOP |
| Vascular | Neovascular – abnormal vessel growth due to ocular ischaemia (e.g. in diabetes) can occlude the trabecular meshwork |
| High episcleral venous pressure | Sturge–Weber syndrome, carotico-cavernous fistula |

Principles of management are the same as for primary glaucomas, with the additional treatment of underlying causes where possible (e.g. carotico-cavernous fistulae or uveitis).

## CONGENITAL GLAUCOMA

Congenital glaucomas are rare but contribute significantly to the total burden of years of blindness, especially in cultures where consanguineous marriages are common. Definitive treatment is mostly surgical (e.g. goniotomy).

## TREATMENT

The only proven treatments are all aimed at reduction of intraocular pressure. Good evidence from large randomized trials supports lowering IOP as the main treatment. Claims for the 'neuro-protective' abilities of some compounds remain unproven.

The principles of treatment are:
- Define the lowest IOP needed to halt or slow progression of visual field loss sufficiently to prevent functionally significant blindness within a patient's lifetime. Pressures in the low teens may be required.
- Treat underlying causes and any angle closure if present.
- Treat in a step-wise fashion with more effective, simpler dosing schedule drugs first.
- Consider surgery, occasionally laser, if maximally tolerated treatment is insufficient.

### Medical

A number of different classes of drugs are widely used (Fig. 9.7).

Drugs applied to the tear film pass down the nasolacrimal duct to the nasal cavity. From here they can be inhaled as an aerosol directly on to the bronchial mucosa. Systemic absorption via nasal vessels (i.e. venous plexus) also bypasses first-pass metabolism by the liver and leads to significant blood levels. Puntal occlusion – pressure on the inner canthus after drop instillation – can reduce the rate of side-effects. A twice daily drop of timolol can have the systemic effects of an oral 10 mg dose.

Concordance and compliance with treatment is the biggest barrier to effective medical treatment of glaucoma – made even more challenging by the initially asymptomatic nature of the disease. Simple treatment regimes minimizing side-effects are vital to achieve good IOP control and to minimize the burden from treatment itself.

Concordance with treatment is the biggest barrier to effectiveness. Simpler dosing regimes and combined drug preparations help. Allergy to drugs or the preservatives used in them also limits usage.

Eye drops can kill patients! Always check if topical beta-blockers are causing reversible airways obstruction or bradycardia. Many a bradycardic or wheezy glaucoma patient has received a pacemaker or started bronchodilator therapy before their beta-blockers were stopped! Local side-effects give swollen lids, injected red eyes and excoriated itchy skin.

### Laser

Several glaucoma laser treatments are used:
- *Laser peripheral iridotomy* is used in angle closure glaucoma to prevent forward bowing of the iris and so increase access of aqueous to the trabecular meshwork.
- *Argon laser iridoplasty* – a ring of peripheral iris is thinned to improve aqueous access to the trabecular meshwork in some angle closure patients where laser iridotomy is insufficient.
- *Laser trabeculoplasty* directly treats the trabecular meshwork and aims to stimulate remodelling of tissues and reduce outflow obstruction. It has a limited effect but is useful in patients who cannot tolerate or use drops due to, for example, arthritis.
- *Trans-scleral diode laser ciliary body ablation* reduces aqueous production through destruction of the ciliary body tissues. It is hard to predict the response and so is used mainly in patients who cannot undergo surgery.

**Fig. 9.7** Medical treatment of glaucoma

| Class of drug and examples | Mechanism of action | Contraindications and side-effects |
|---|---|---|
| Beta-blockers<br>– Timolol<br>– Levobunolol<br>– Betaxolol<br>– Carteolol | Reduce production of aqueous by the ciliary body | Reversible airways obstruction (asthma or COPD)<br>Can cause heart block and bradycardia<br>Reduced exercise tolerance |
| Alpha-2 adrenergic sympathomimetic agonists<br>– Brimonidine<br>– Apraclonidine | Reduce production of aqueous by the ciliary body and small increase in outflow | Contraindicated in severe cardiovascular disease<br>Apraclonidine crosses the blood–brain barrier – causes drowsiness and lethargy in elderly<br>Allergy and skin/conjunctival hypersensitivity |
| Parasympatho-mimetic agents<br>– Pilocarpine | Increases outflow: ciliary muscle contraction opens trabecular meshwork | Pupillary constriction, induced myopia, iris–lens adhesions, brow ache and risk of retinal detachment |
| Carbonic anhydrase inhibitors<br>– Systemic; acetazolamide<br>– Topical dorzolamide or brinzolamide | Reduce production of aqueous by the ciliary body | Allergy and skin/conjunctival hypersensitivity: these are sulphonamide derivatives with risk of Stevens–Johnson syndrome. Systemic – nausea, lassitude, depression, paraesthesiae, renal stones, electrolyte imbalance |
| Prostaglandin analogues<br>– Bimatoprost<br>– Latanoprost<br>– Travoprost | Increase uveoscleral outflow of aqueous | Excess lash growth<br>Periocular and iris pigmentation change |
| ALL DROPS | Preservatives | Risks of preservative allergy and lower subsequent surgical success |

## Surgical

## Trabeculectomy

A flap of sclera is lifted beneath the conjunctiva and a hole made into the anterior chamber.

Releasable sutures close the scleral flap and allow postoperative adjustment to the rate of flow. Antimetabolites such as mitomycin C are used to modify the healing/scarring process (Fig. 9.8). Drainage is into the 'bleb' – a cyst-like structure protected by the upper lid (Fig. 9.8B). Newer 'non-penetrating' surgical alternatives have fewer side-effects (such as postoperative hypotony) but lower rates of success.

### Glaucoma drainage devices – 'tubes'

In some conditions, or after failed trabeculectomy surgery, insertion of a drainage tube may be more successful than a trabeculectomy. A plastic tube drains fluid behind the equator of the globe. Surgical complications in recent trials have been similar to high-risk trabeculectomy.

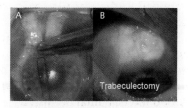

**Fig. 9.8** Trabeculectomy surgery. (A) (Left) Sponges soaked in antimetabolites placed subconjunctivally during trabeculectomy surgery. (B) (Right) Trabeculectomy. Conjunctival bleb and superior placed peripheral iridectomy are visible; eye looks downwards and upper lid is elevated.

## Objectives

You should be able to:

- Describe the structure and function of the retina.
- Describe the complications of vascular retinal disease.
- Differentiate between diabetic maculopathy and retinopathy.
- Understand the importance of diabetic retinopathy screening.
- Classify hypertensive retinopathy.
- Identify wet age-related macular degeneration patients clinically and refer appropriately.
- Understand important symptoms and signs for posterior vitreous detachment and retinal detachment.

The retina is the part of the eye responsible for converting light energy into a nerve impulse (i.e. phototransduction) which is conducted along the optic nerve, chiasm, tracts to the lateral geniculate nucleus, and then onwards to the visual cortex in the occipital lobe of the brain.

The retina is a 10-layered structure (Fig. 10.1) that essentially follows the rules of all sensory nerve pathways (i.e. three orders). The sensory neuron is the photoreceptor cell (cone and rod cells: nuclei in the outer nuclear layer), the secondary neuron is the bipolar cell (nuclei located in the inner nuclear layer), and the tertiary neuron is the ganglion cell axon – grouped together they make up the optic nerve. In addition to the above pathways there are many other integrated cell types that process visual information at the retinal level; they include horizontal cells, amacrine cells and Muller cells.

The retinal vasculature comprises a central retinal artery and vein at the optic disc (Fig. 10.2).

## RETINAL VASCULAR DISEASE

Many conditions that affect the retina primarily affect the retinal vessels, leading to retinal vessel leakage initially (usually due to pericyte loss in diabetes). Eventually the retinal vessels (capillaries) close off, leading to local ischaemia. This results in a rise in vascular endothelial growth factor (VEGF) stimulating abnormal blood vessel growth (neovascularization).

Neovascularization can lead to many complications including:

- Haemorrhage:
  - Vitreous.
  - Pre-retinal.
- Tractional detachment.
- Rhegmatogenous retinal detachment.

## Diabetes

Diabetes is a potentially devastating systemic disease with many organ complications. It is helpful to remember the acronym KNIVES (Figs 10.3, 10.4).

The onset of ocular complications in diabetic patients is variable and is dependant on systemic control (Figs 10.5, 10.6).

Diabetic classification is based on the Early Treatment of Diabetic Retinopathy Study (ETDRS).

Retinal effects of diabetes are divided into *maculopathy* and *retinopathy*.

### Maculopathy (within the major arcades)

These patients may be asymptomatic or present with a gradual (over months) deterioration of vision.

This form is characterized by (Fig. 10.7):

- Microaneurysms
- Leakage (retinal thickening/oedema, hard exudates) with or without macular ischaemia (seen on fluorescein angiogram).

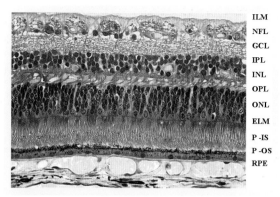

| | ILM |
| | NFL |
| | GCL |
| | IPL |
| | INL |
| | OPL |
| | ONL |
| | ELM |
| | P -IS |
| | P -OS |
| | RPE |

**Fig. 10.1** Ten retinal layers: internal limiting membrane; nerve fibre layer; ganglion cell layer; inner plexiform layer; inner nuclear layer; outer plexiform layer; outer nuclear layer; external limiting membrane; photoreceptors (inner and outer segments); and retinal pigment epithelium.

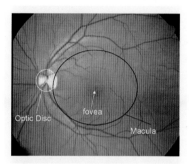

**Fig. 10.2** Normal fundus. The fovea is two disc diameters away from the optic disc (white circle) and also at the centre of the macula area (black circle).

**Fig. 10.3** Organs involved from diabetic complications

### Diabetes and KNIVES

| **K**idney | |
| --- | --- |
| **N**erves | Large |
| | Small |
| **I**nfection | |
| **V**ascular | Macro |
| | Micro |
| **E**yes | (See main text) |
| **S**kin | Secondary in injections |
| | Infections |

**Fig. 10.4** Ocular complications of diabetes mellitus

- Neuro-ophthalmic:
  - Cranial nerve palsy (lll, IV, VI)
  - Papillitis
- Orbital:
  - Mucormycosis
- Corneal
  - Neurotrophic
  - Bacterial keratitis
- Glaucoma:
  - $\uparrow$ Risk of POAG
  - Neovascular
  - $\uparrow$ Risk of steroid response glaucoma
- Cataract:
  - Early senile cataract
    Nuclear sclerosis
    Cortical opacity
    Post-subcapsular
  - Snowstorm cataract
- Retina:
  - Maculopathy
    Not clinically significant
    Clinically significant
  - Retinopathy
    Mild NPDR
    Moderate NPDR
    Severe NPDR
    Very severe NPDR
    Low-risk PDR
    High-risk PDR
  - Other
    Vitreous haemorrhage
    Tractional RD
    Rhegmatogenous RD

**Fig. 10.5** Risk factors for diabetic maculopathy

Risk factors for diabetic maculopathy include:
- Type II > Type I
- Hypertension
- Renal disease
- Hypercholesterolaemia

**Fig. 10.6** Risk factors for diabetic retinopathy

Risk factors for proliferative diabetic retinopathy include:
- Type I > Type II DM
- Poor glucose control
- Ocular surgery (beware post cataract extraction)
- Hypertension
- Renal dysfunction
- Pregnancy
- Anaemia

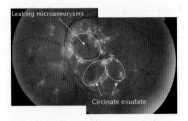

**Fig. 10.7** Diabetic maculopathy, due to leaky blood vessels or microaneurysms in macular region. There is also moderate to severe non-proliferative diabetic retinopathy present.

**Fig. 10.8** Clinically significant macular oedema (three criteria)

- Any thickening within 500 μm (i.e. ⅓ of disc diameter) of the fovea
- Any hard exudate within 500 μm of fovea associated with thickening
- Retinal thickening >1 disc diameter within 1 DD of fovea (DD: usually about 1500 μm)

If the changes are such as to affect vision or imminently threaten vision they are referred to as *clinically significant macular oedema (CSMO)* (Fig. 10.8). If those changes are present, yet do not threaten vision, they are referred to as *not clinically significant*.

The prognosis is poor if:

- The leakage is diffuse.
- There is significant ischaemia on fundus fluorescein angiography.
- There is associated cystoid macular oedema.
- There is coexistent renal failure.

## Retinopathy

Diabetic retinopathy patients are usually asymptomatic until very advanced stages (hence the need for a screening programme). With advanced disease (neovascularization) they may present with a sudden painless loss of vision due to haemorrhage.

Asymmetric diabetic retinal retinopathy (e.g. right mild non-proliferative diabetic retinopathy and left proliferative diabetic retinopathy may be due to ocular ischaemia from ipsilateral/left carotid artery stenosis) may warrant carotid artery duplex ultrasound referral.

*Diagnosing vitreous haemorrhage in a diabetic.*
If a patient is seen with a sudden increase in floaters and loss of vision, it is worth asking and confirming whether the patient is diabetic. There should be no RAPD present. It is most likely that a *vitreous haemorrhage* from proliferative diabetic retinopathy has occurred rather than retinal detachment.

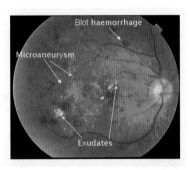

**Fig. 10.9** Background diabetic retinopathy or mild non-proliferative diabetic retinopathy. Macular region changes imply the presence of diabetic maculopathy, but it is not clinically significant diabetic macular oedema.

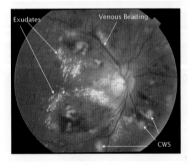

**Fig. 10.10** Pre-proliferative or severe non-proliferative diabetic retinopathy. Signs include cotton wool spots and venous beading.

The characteristic changes include (Figs 10.9, 10.10):

- *Non-proliferative diabetic retinopathy (NPDR)* (Figs. 10.11, 10.12):
  - *Microaneurysms* (an indicator of micro vascular vessel wall changes/weakness: located deep in the inner nuclear layer)

- *Haemorrhages* (flame: in superficial retinal nerve fibre layer; dot and blot: in deeper retinal outer and inner plexiform layers)
- *Thickening/oedema* (intraretinal fluid: a sign of leakage)
- *Hard exudates* (intraretinal lipoprotein deposits: a sign of leakage) They are sharp, well demarcated yellow blobs, which are deeper to superficial retinal blood vessels
- *Cotton wool spots* (reflect leakage of axoplasmic fluid: a sign of ischaemia). They are superficial white fluffy retinal blobs, and are not usually crossed by retinal blood vessels

- *Venous beading* (a sign of ischaemia). They are sausage-like venules of changing calibre along their length
- *Intraretinal microvascular abnormalities* (IRMA; a sign of intra retinal shunts, another feature of ischaemia).
- *Proliferative diabetic retinopathy (PDR)* (Figs 10.13, 10.14): all of the above (i.e. NPDR), *plus*:
  - Neovascularization of the disc (NVD)
  - Neovascularization elsewhere (NVE)
  - Pre-retinal or vitreous haemorrhage
  - Vitreoretinal traction (adhesion between vitreous and retina leading to retinal elevation).

**Fig. 10.11** Non-proliferative diabetic retinopathy classification

- *Mild.* At least one microaneurysm, and criteria not met for moderate.
- *Moderate.* Intraretinal haemorrhages/microaneurysms, and/or cotton wool spots, venous beading, intraretinal microvascular abnormalities (IRMAs), and criteria not met for severe.
- *Severe.* At least one of: intraretinal haemorrhages in 4 quadrants, venous beading ≥ in 2 quadrants, intraretinal microvascular abnormalities ≥ 1 quadrant and criteria not met for very severe.
- *Very severe.* At least two of criteria for severe.

**Fig. 10.12** Relationship between new and old diabetic retinopathy (DR) classification, screening terminology and ophthalmic clinic referral time and clinic follow-up intervals

| New classification | 5 year risk of HR-PDR | Screening terminology | Initial clinic referral time | Appropriate F/U interval | Old classification |
|---|---|---|---|---|---|
| Clinical significant macular oedema (CSMO) | | Maculopathy (M) | 13 weeks | 4 months after laser treatment | Diabetic macular oedema |
| No diabetic retinopathy | | Level 0 | | 12 months | No DR |
| Mild non-proliferative | 15% | Level 1: background | | 12 months | Background DR |
| Moderate non-proliferative | 33% | Level 1: background | | 6-9 months | Background DR |
| Severe non-proliferative | 60% | Level 2:pre-proliferative | 13 weeks | 3 months | Pre-proliferative DR |
| Non-high-risk proliferative | 75% | Level 3: proliferative | < 2 weeks | 2 months or treatment | Proliferative DR |
| High-risk proliferative (HR-PDR) | | Level 3: proliferative | < 2weeks | Treatment | Proliferative DR |

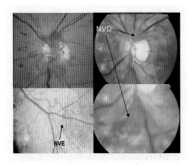

**Fig. 10.13** Proliferative diabetic retinopathy (PDR). Signs include new vessels at disc (NVD) and elsewhere (NVE).

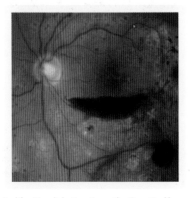

**Fig. 10.14** Proliferative diabetic retinopathy. Preretinal haemorrhage secondary to new vessels elsewhere (NVE) inferotemporally.

Medical students should be able to classify diabetic retinopathy fundus photos into: (a) diabetic retinopathy – background, pre-proliferative, proliferative and treated proliferative; and (b) diabetic maculopathy – present or not present. Following MBBS or equivalent qualification the NPDR classification (see Figs 10.11, 10.12) is used by ophthalmologists.

### Non-proliferative diabetic retinopathy terminology

The '4-2-1' rule arises from the severe category criteria (see Fig. 10.11).

## Screening

Prevalence rates of diabetes is now estimated to be between 5 and 10% in Western societies, so there is a need to screen large populations of at-risk individuals.

The role of screening is to pick up pre-clinical (pre-sight threatening) disease and implement appropriate therapy. Screening can be performed by ophthalmologists, endocrinologists, general physicians, GPs, optometrists, ophthalmic nurses or photographic technicians (using a reading centre). Whichever method is employed, patients with suspicious features should be referred to an ophthalmologist for assessment (see Fig. 10.12).

MACULOPATHY = centre of macula problem, i.e. red (microaneurysm) dots and yellow (hard exudate) blobs close to the fovea. It is not easy to appreciate three-dimensional retinal thickening with the direct ophthalmoscope (a two-dimensional viewing device). Refer if maculopathy is present.

## Treatment

The mainstay of treatment of both maculopathy and retinopathy is laser photocoagulation (i.e. thermal laser).

Laser treatment alone is insufficient to treat or halt the progression of diabetic eye disease. Tight blood glucose and blood pressure control are essential.

The aim of treatment with macular laser is to stimulate the retinal pigment epithelium to pump more fluid out of the retina.

The aim of laser in proliferative diabetic retinopathy (PDR) (Figs 10.15, 10.16) is to ablate and destroy the ischaemic retina, which produces VEGF stimulus to induce NVE and, when severe, the iris (rubreosis) (Fig. 10.17).

Treatment may not work (35% failure rate in maculopathy) and the patients must be consented and counselled regarding this. All treatment is accompanied by counselling regarding patients' general health.

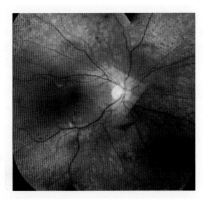

**Fig. 10.15** Pan-retinal photocoagulation laser scars (mildly pigmented). New vessels at disc have regressed and vitreous haemorrhage has resolved.

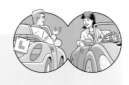

*Principle of diabetic retinal laser.* Diabetic macular laser is for stabilization rather than improvement of vision. Diabetic pan retinal photocoagulation laser is again aiming for stabilization of central vision at the expense of peripheral vision. Explain to the patient that they will notice more tunnel vision following such laser treatment.

### Maculopathy

If a patient has CSMO then focal or grid laser is applied (lightly). The response is assessed 4 months later, and further laser applied if there is still thickening. Usually laser is applied three times, but this may be exceeded if clinically appropriate.

### Retinopathy

If a patient develops high-risk PDR, pan-retinal photocoagulation (PRP) is applied. Some ophthalmologists treat any new vessels, low or high risk. Coexistent maculopathy should be treated first, since PRP itself may exacerbate maculopathy.

The treatment consists of 1000–1500 burns during each of three sessions, to minimize cystoid macular oedema. The response to treatment is assessed at 6–8 weeks. Persistent vitreous haemorrhage, where duration is over 3 months, may require a vitrectomy (removal of vitreous and blood) with internal laser. A tractional retinal detachment (Fig. 10.18) involving the macula would require a vitrectomy and relieving of traction.

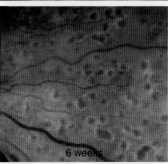

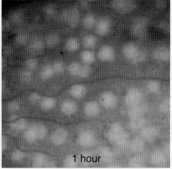

1 hour

6 weeks

**Fig. 10.16** Laser scars initially look yellow (small circles in upper figure) and then become more pigmented with time. Racial pigmentation accounts for the final appearance of each retinal scar (i.e. mild or severe pigmentation).

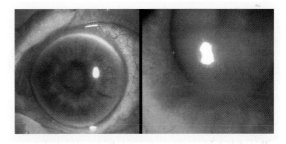

**Fig. 10.17** Rubreosis in a diabetic patient. Rubreosis or new vessels on the iris. This can occur secondary to proliferative diabetic retinopathy or previous central retinal vein occlusion. A poor prognosis following cataract surgery is expected because of underlying proliferative diabetic retinopathy.

## Other complications of PDR

Neovascular (rubreotic) glaucoma may develop in this setting. This involves new vessels growing on the iris and into the angle (rubreosis) with fibrosis leading eventually to secondary narrow angle glaucoma (see Chapter 9). Adequate treatment of the PDR is required to prevent this happening. An end-stage eye may become phthisical (Fig. 10.19).

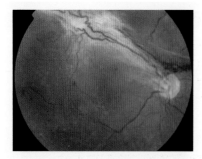

**Fig. 10.18** Tractional retinal detachment secondary to proliferative diabetic retinopathy. Fibrotic scars are visible superonasally and inferotemporally.

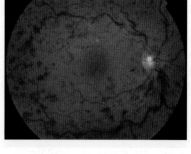

**Fig. 10.20** Central retinal vein occlusion (CRVO). Note the four quadrant (flame) haemorrhages and tortuous vessels. Right swollen optic disc and two cotton wool spots (superior to fovea) are visible.

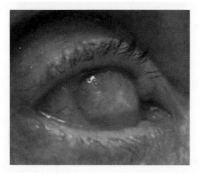

**Fig. 10.19** Phthisis. A scarred and shunken eyeball, due to end-stage diabetic retinopathy.

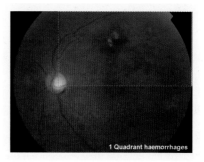

1 Quadrant haemorrhages

**Fig. 10.21** Branch retinal vein occlusion (BRVO). Note only one quadrant is affected, commonly the superotemporal quadrant.

## Non-laser treatments of diabetic eye disease

In recent years there has been a significant amount of research into newer treatments for both maculopathy and retinopathy.

### Maculopathy
- Intravitreal steroid (triamcinolone: to limit leakage).
- Statins (to reduce exudates density).
- Protein kinase C inhibitors (ruboxistaurin).
- Intravitreal anti-VEGF (Avastin (bevacizumab)).

### Retinopathy
- Protein kinase C inhibitors.
- Intravitreal anti-VEGF (Avastin (bevacizumab)).

## Retinal vein occlusion

Retinal vein occlusions (central (CRVO) and branch (BRVO)) are relatively common events leading to painless reduction in vision (mild–severe). The causes of both types overlap; however, the prognosis, clinical course and treatment are different (Figs 10. 20–10.22).

**Fig. 10.22** Causes of retinal vein occlusion

| Central vein occlusion | Branch vein occlusion |
|---|---|
| POAG | Hypertension |
| Hypertension | Arteriosclerosis |
| Arteriosclerosis | Diabetes |
| Diabetes | Inflammatory eye disease with vasculitis (e.g. Behçet's) |
| Hypercoagulable states: <br> • SLE/anticardiolipin syndrome <br> • Polycythemia <br> • Lymphoma <br> • Myeloma | Hypercoagulable states <br> • SLE/anticardiolipin syndrome |
| Inflammatory eye disease: <br> • Sarcoidosis <br> • Syphilis | Oral contraception |
| Oral contraception | |

*Aetiology of vein occlusions.* Always look for other signs of coexistent retinal/choroidal disease, and also vitritis, as vein occlusions may occur with inflammatory eye disease such as Behçet's disease.

Vein occlusions usually occur in the elderly (>55 years) population and can usually be attributed to raised intraocular pressure (commonly CRVO) and/or arteriosclerosis (commonly BRVO). However, vascular occlusions may be an indicator of underlying systemic disease such as diabetes, hypercholesterolaemia or autoimmune disease, thus all patients must be investigated appropriately (Fig. 10.23).

## Central retinal vein occlusion (CRVO)

The critical signs of CRVO are diffuse haemorrhages in all four quadrants and dilated tortuous veins (see Fig. 10.20). Other signs include:

- Cotton wool spots (a sign of ischaemia).
- Disc swelling.
- Macular oedema.
- Neovascularization (a later feature of ischaemic CRVO) of disc, retina and/or iris.

There are two types of central retinal vein occlusion, *ischaemic* and *non-ischaemic*.

### Ischaemic

This type characteristically has a greater reduction in vision (<6/60) with an afferent pupil defect (RAPD). There is much retinal damage. On fluorescein angiogram there are large areas of non-perfusion. 75% develop neovascularization if untreated and 50% develop neovascular glaucoma within 3 months. They invariably develop macular oedema. Follow-up should be frequent (every 2–4 weeks) for the first 6 months.

*Principle of PRP laser.* The aim of pan-retinal photocoagulation laser treatment in a patient with ischaemic central retinal vein occlusion is not to improve vision, but to prevent rubreotic glaucoma (i.e. a blind and painful eye).

**Fig. 10.23** Investigation of retinal vein occlusion

| Systemic investigation |
| --- |
| – Blood pressure |
| – Blood glucose |
| – Lipids (include cholesterol) |
| – Full blood count (FBC) |
| – Chest X-ray (CXR) |
| – Erythrocyte sedimentation rate (ESR) |
| – Cardiovascular work up (ECG, carotid scan, +/– ECHO) |
| – Thyroid function tests |
| – Coagulation screen |
| – Protein C and S |
| – Serum protein electrophoresis (SPEP) |
| – Anticardiolipin antibodies |
| – Autoantibody screen |
| – VDRL |
| – sACE and serum calcium |
| **Ocular investigation** |
| – Complete ocular examination |
| – Fluorescein angiogram |

*Treatment.* If iris vessels develop (rubreosis) then PRP laser treatment should be applied.

Maculopathy due to CRVO does not respond to laser treatment. We currently await the results of clinical trials for newer therapies such as intravitreal steroid (e.g. triamcinolone and Posurdex (slow release dexamethasone) and anti-VEGF agents (e.g. Lucentis (ranibizumab), Avastin (bevacizumab) and Macugen (pegaptanig)).

### Non-ischaemic

These patients have vision better than 6/60 and no relative afferent pupil defect. They usually have milder maculopathy that may resolve spontaneously.

Follow-up is every 4–8 weeks for 18 months, since 10–15% may convert to ischaemic type.

*Treatment.* None required unless converts to ischaemic type (see above).

## Branch retinal vein occlusion (BRVO)

Patients present with painless loss of vision or just vague blurring. The causes are outlined in Fig. 10.22

and are similar to the causes of CRVO, as are the required investigations (see Fig. 10.23). Branch occlusions usually occur at crossing points of retinal arterioles and veins (seen as AV nipping in hypertensive patients) as they share a common adventitial sheath (see Fig. 10.21).

The clinical signs include:

- Sectorial retinal haemorrhage (either flame or blot).
- Cotton wool spots.
- Macular oedema.
- Sheathing (or whitening) of associated retinal arteriole (late feature).
- Retinal/disc neovascularization (in 30% of cases).
- Vitreous haemorrhage.

Visual loss is usually due to macular oedema. Patients are investigated and reviewed with the results of tests at 2–4 weeks. They are then reviewed at 4 months post occlusion. If the macular oedema is unresolved patients are treated with grid laser treatment.

*Treatment.* If patients develop retinal new vessels then sector PRP is applied.

## Hypertensive retinopathy (HR)

This describes a series of classic changes that occur in patients with high blood pressure (a simplified classification is presented in Fig. 10.24). They include:

- Haemorrhages.
- Cotton wool spots (CWS).
- AV (arteriovenous) nipping – a specific feature of HR and not DR.
- Copper/silver wiring (a sign of arteriolar sclerosis).
- Macular oedema/exudates (in a circinate/star pattern).
- Disc swelling (indicator of malignant hypertension).
- Arterial macroaneurysms.
- Choroidal ischaemia (sign of severe hypertension) with patchy infarction (due to pre-eclampsia, DIC or collagen vascular disease).

**Fig. 10.24** Simplified classification of hypertensive retinopathy

| Mild HR | Arteriovenous (AV) nipping |
|---|---|
| Moderate HR | AV nipping and cotton wool spots (CWS) |
| Severe HR | Disc swelling and other features (e.g. AV nipping and CWS) |

If there is disc swelling and high blood pressure (diastolic >110 mmHg) patients must be referred urgently for control of blood pressure (if untreated 90% mortality in 1 year).

## Investigations

- Blood pressure.
- Blood glucose.
- FBC, U&E.
- Fluorescein angiogram.

## Treatment

Treat the blood pressure and observe the retinal changes over a period of weeks. Haemorrhages and cotton wool spots should resolve.

## Retinal arterial occlusion

These may be transient (amaurosis fugax) or permanent (central/branch retinal artery occlusion).

### Transient monocular blindness (TMB) or amaurosis fugax

Patients complain of transient (<24 hours) monocular loss of vision.

The causes of TMB are:

- *Thrombotic.* Cholesterol deposition and atheroma formation within vessel lumen (e.g. carotid artery disease).
- *Embolic.* Platelet, cholesterol, calcific (e.g. carotid artery disease or subacute bacterial endocarditis (SBE) from cardiac valve disease).
- *Haematological.* Sickle cell disease, polycythemia, anaemia, hyperviscosity states.
- *Vasospastic.* Non-embolic idiopathic arterial narrowing.

Emboli typically cause black loss of vision (i.e. 'negative' visual symptom). Grey, white, patchy (i.e. 'positive' visual symptoms) loss of vision or recovery usually indicates non-embolic loss of vision (e.g. vasospasm). A practical way to help distinguish various forms of transient monocular blindness is by their duration (e.g. <1 minute can be bilateral or unilateral 'visual obscurations' which occur in giant cell arteritis (GCA) or papilloedema; Fig. 10.25).

Causes of and treatments for amaurosis fugax are summarized in Fig. 10.26.

**Fig. 10.25** Practical timings for causes of transient monocular blindness

| Transient monocular blindness |
| --- |
| <1 min |
| Postural arterial hypotension |
| Papilloedema, disc drusen |
| Hypoperfusion – hypercoagulability, vasculitis, GCA |
| >1 min |
| Embolic |
| Non-embolic – vasospasm, retinal migraine |

**Fig. 10.26** Causes of and treatments for amaurosis fugax

| Causes | Treatment |
| --- | --- |
| Embolic (heart or great vessels) | Aspirin |
| Carotid stenosis | Carotid endarterectomy |
| Hypercoagulability (e.g. SC) | Anticoagulation |
| Vasculitis (e.g. GCA) | Steroids |
| Postural arterial hypotension | Review BP medications |
| Vasospasm | Nifedipine |

## Signs

There is often no evidence of an embolic event in the retina and the physician relies on the clinical history. Occasionally one can see an embolus (usually at a branching point or arterial bifurcation).

Retinopathy due to poor ocular circulation (e.g. ocular ischaemia) is characterized by multiple mid-peripheral haemorrhages with or without cotton wool spots. Rarely do they develop neovascularization.

## Investigation

It is important to assess the presence of treatable carotid artery stenosis (>70%) or cardiac disease. These patients should be referred for:

- Cardiac work up.
- Carotid Doppler studies.
- ECHO studies.
- Neurological exam (if associated neurological symptoms, e.g. paraesthesiae/paresis).
- FBC, U&E, lipids, blood glucose, ESR, CRP.
- Autoantibody screen.
- Serum protein electrophoresis (SPEP).

## Prognosis

It is important to note that patients with embolic TMB have greater cardiovascular morbidity and associated mortality. Up to 30% of patients with embolic TMB have an acute myocardial infarction. There is a 2%/year risk of a stroke. (If there is a defined embolic event that risk rises to 25% by 3 months.)

## Treatment

Treat the underlying risk factors (e.g. hypertension or diabetes).

Place patients on aspirin (75 mg/day); warfarin may be required if cardiac cause of emboli (e.g. atrial fibrillation). If symptomatic patients have >70% carotid stenosis then carotid endarterectomy is indicated.

# Central retinal artery occlusion (CRAO)

CRAO is an uncommon but devastating event, usually leading to irreversible blindness in the affected eye. It is usually due to thrombus or embolus (Fig. 10.27). This can only be effectively treated if the patient presents within the **first 4 hours** of the onset of the visual loss.

## Symptoms of CRAO

Severe unilateral sudden loss of vision; a past history of recurrent transient visual loss may also be present; there are no systemic symptoms.

## Signs of CRAO

Visual acuity is grossly reduced, relative afferent pupil defect (RAPD) is present The classic retinal appearance is of a pale (swollen) retina with a (foveal) cherry red spot. Occasionally there is central sparing (25%) due to a patent cilioretinal artery. Occasionally it can be bilateral (1–2%); if so, think of systemic causes such as giant cell arteritis (GCA) or vasculitis.

## Investigation

- ESR (urgent to rule out GCA).
- CRP, FBC, U&E.
- Blood pressure.

**Fig. 10.27** Causes of central retinal artery occlusion

| |
| --- |
| Embolus – carotid, cardiac |
| Thrombosis – 65% are arteriosclerotic |
| Giant cell arteritis (GCA) – consider if bilateral |
| Collagen vascular disease – SLE, PAN |
| Hyperviscosity syndromes – polycythemia, myeloma |
| Others |

- Fluorescein angiogram.
- VDRL, SPEP.
- Cardiovascular work-up (see above).
- ERG (to determine prognosis).

**Treatment**

Treatment must be instigated immediately (<4 hours) post central retinal artery occlusion (CRAO). Ideally, transfer immediately to the eye department. The aim of treatment is to dislodge a presumed embolus (by reducing intraocular pressure). This is attempted by:

- Ocular massage (exert firm pressure for 10 seconds, stop for 10 seconds).
- i.v. Acetazolamide (Diamox) 500 mg stat.
- Anterior chamber paracentesis.
- Rebreathing $CO_2$ (from a paper bag) – raises carbon dioxide levels in the blood and may help to improve blood flow.
- ESR needs to be checked anyway to exclude giant cell arteritis (particularly over 65 year age).

These treatments are largely unsatisfactory. If neovascularization develops, then PRP is applied. It is very important to follow-up these patients (including those with branch retinal artery occlusions (BRAO); Fig. 10.28) and manage their co-morbidity. These patients, if untreated, are at high risk of subsequent stroke and myocardial infarction.

## Differential diagnoses

Fig. 10.29 lists common causes for macular oedema. Vascular conditions that may present like diabetic retinopathy include (TIP: Acronym SCORE):

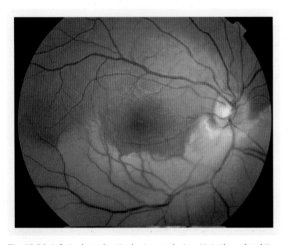

**Fig. 10.28** Inferior branch retinal artery occlusion. Note the pale white retina compared to a normal superior orange-coloured perfused retina.

| **Fig. 10.29** Common causes of cystoid macular oedema |
| --- |
| Postoperative |
| – Cataract |
| – Laser |
| – Cryotherapy |
| Central/branch retinal vein occlusion |
| Diabetic retinopathy |
| Uveitis |
| Rare causes |
| – Retinitis pigmentosa |
| – Retinal telangiectasia |

- **Sickle Cell** retinopathy – usually **SC** disease.
- **Ocular** ischaemic syndrome – reduced carotid blood flow.
- **Radiation** retinopathy – history of orbital/cranial radiation.
- **Eales'** disease.

## AGE-RELATED MACULAR DEGENERATION (ARMD OR AMD)

ARMD is the largest single cause of blind registration in the Western world. The disorder is felt to be a combination of inherited and environmental factors. It is a disorder of the retinal pigment epithelium (RPE) with secondary neural retinal degeneration (Figs 10.30, 10.31).

## Classification

10% of the UK population has ARMD. 90% of patients with ARMD have the *dry* type and 10% have the *wet* type.

*Dry ARMD.* Patients present with a gradual painless reduction in vision often over many years. Characteristically drusen (soft), pigment clumping and macular atrophy (Fig. 10.32, 10.33).

*Wet ARMD.* A sudden loss or distortion of vision (Fig. 10.34) occurs due to the formation of a subretinal neovascular membrane (SRNVM) or due to haemorrhage or subretinal fluid (SRF) or leakage. Although the wet type is less common, it is responsible for >80% of severe visual loss (Figs 10.35, 10.36).

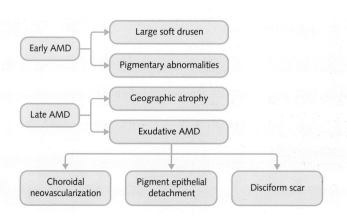

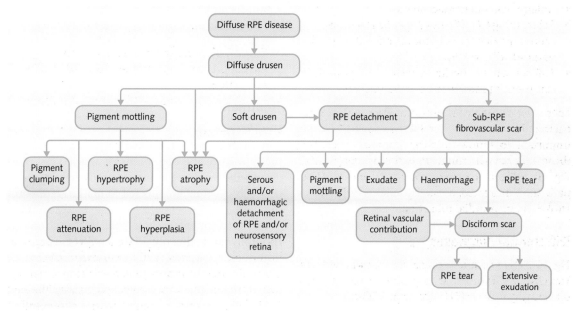

**Fig. 10.31** Pathogenesis of age-related macular degeneration.

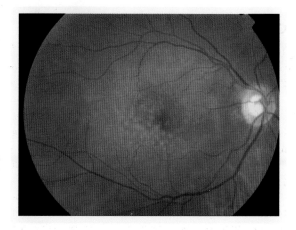

**Fig. 10.32** Macular drusen. They are soft edged with overlying retinal vessels.

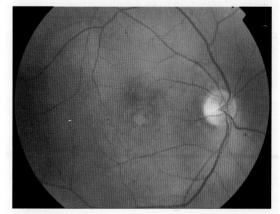

**Fig. 10.33** Geographic atrophy or dry age-related macular degeneration (left eye).

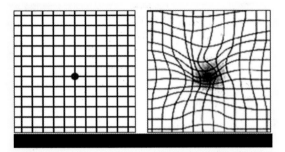

**Fig. 10.34** Amsler grid (left image) becomes distorted (right image) when a patient with macular degeneration looks at the central black spot with the affected eye.

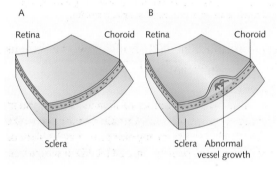

**Fig. 10.35** Choroidal neovascular membrane (right image) in wet age-related macular degeneration causes elevation of the retina and subsequently subretinal haemorrhage and fluid.

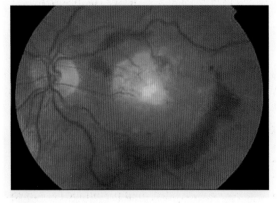

**Fig. 10.36** Wet age-related macular degeneration (left eye). Subfoveal choroidal neovascular membrane with circumferential subretinal haemorrhages at the edge of a dome-shaped subretinal fluid collection.

Patients over 55 years of age experiencing sudden, distorted vision should be referred promptly (<48 hours) for a fluorescein angiogram to assess suitability for wet age-related macular degeneration (ARMD) treatment.

## Investigation

- Full ocular exam. Signs include: drusen (small yellowish deposits), pigment clumps, atrophy, haemorrhage, subretinal fluid, exudates.
- Amsler grid.
- Fluorescein angiogram (to detect and delineate a neovascular membrane and leakage; hyperfluoresces).
- Ocular coherence tomography (OCT).

## Treatment

Until recently the only treatment available for these patients was 'hot' or 'thermal' argon laser to limit the growth of the membrane. It was necessary to destroy the overlying retina as part of the treatment, thus subfoveal treatments led to marked reduction in vision.

Newer treatments include 'cold' laser applications (photodynamic therapy: PDT), anti-VEGF preparations such as Lucentis™ and intra-/periocular steroid. The aim of all these treatments is to limit or reverse neovascular membrane growth and preserve vision.

Pharmacological treatments aimed at preventing visual loss include multivitamins and antioxidants (vitamins A, E and zinc), where there is a 40% risk reduction of having severe visual loss. Other agents include dietary components that are macular pigments (lutein and zeaxanthin) which act as antioxidants and are felt to play a role in maintaining retinal health.

Smokers should not be started on the current commercial preparations with large vitamin A doses due to increased risk of lung cancer. Special formulations exist for smokers (e.g. ICaps).

## POSTERIOR VITREOUS DETACHMENT (PVD)

Floaters and flashing lights are the two most common symptoms.

*Floaters.* These are black or opaque objects that float across the line of vision and are usually less noticeable with time. Patients can describe them as spiders, flies, hairs or nets. They change position with eye movements, and are seen most clearly against a white or bright background. Floaters occur because of a change in vitreous gel consistency.

*Flashing lights (photopsia).* These are lights that flicker in the patient's peripheral field of vision. The cones ('c for central, colour vision') and rods ('peripheral motion or night vision') perform phototransduction (i.e. convert light signals to electrical impulses). Tugging and stretching of the photoreceptor layer by vitreous causes monocular photopsia due to stimulation of rods and cones. It does not matter if the eye is open or closed.

## RETINAL DETACHMENT (RD)

A RD occurs when the (top nine layers of the) retina is separated from the 10th retinal layer, the retinal pigment epithelium (RPE), by subretinal fluid (SRF).

There are three types of RD:

- *Rhegmatogenous.* Retinal tear allows liquid from vitreous cavity to form SRF.
- *Exudative.* Inflammatory and neoplastic lesions (e.g. metastasis, posterior scleritis) lead to serous exudation from leaky blood vessels.
- *Tractional.* Fibrotic or vascular membranes along the posterior vitreous can contract and pull on the retina. Risk factors include: diabetes, central retinal vein occlusion, sickle cell retinopathy, retinopathy of prematurity.

### Rhegmatogenous retinal detachment (RRD)

If the vitreous gel pulls too hard on the retina (in 10-15% of cases) a tear can develop anteriorly near the firm adhesions of the ora serrata. As fluid from vitreous cavity goes through the retinal tear, the retina (top 9 layers usually) lifts off or detaches from retinal layer no 10, the retinal pigment epithelium (RPE).

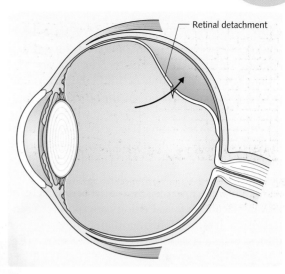

**Fig. 10.37** Rhegmatogenous retinal detachment. The arrow depicts fluid entering the subretinal space through a retinal tear.

This subretinal fluid (SRF) leads to rhegmatogenous retinal detachment (Fig. 10.37).

### Symptoms
Sudden increase in number of floaters and persistent flashing lights (photopsia). Curtain coming across the vision of either eye, from any direction; may be black or grey. 60% of RRD patients have all TRIAD of symptoms.

*Photopsias – intra- or extraocular?* Check whether photopsia occurs in one or both eyes. In common or classic migraine, zig-zag lines or fortification spectra are seen from BOTH eyes (perhaps with aura and headache); monocular photopsia suggests an ocular structural problem.

### Signs
Visual acuity may be normal or grossly reduced; field loss.

### Risk factors
- Acute PVD.
- High myopia.
- Trauma.
- Previous complicated/multiple intraocular surgery.
- YAG laser capsulotomy.
- Past ocular history/family history of retinal detachment.

Brown RPE pigment and red blood cells from torn or avulsed blood vessel can be released into vitreous cavity. This very useful and important clinical sign on slit lamp examination is called *tobacco dust or Schaffer's sign*.

A retinal tear commonly occurs in the superotemporal region (approx 75%) and the other three quadrants (approx 10% each) because gravity causes the superior part of the retina (Fig. 10.37) to fall down in the eye and the vitreous gel is anchored firmly more nasally at the optic disc. Therefore a dark or black curtain or inferonasal field defect can occur which enlarges towards the centre of the field of vision. Macular or foveal vision corresponds to central vision. It is therefore important to note whether the loss of field is small with good central vision (e.g. 6/9 vision) or huge with poor central vision (e.g. CFs vision).

## Rhegmatogenous RD consent issues

- ?VA (visual outcome), multiple operations may be required.
- Red eye (haemorrhage/inflammation postoperatively).

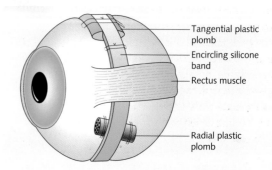

*Retinal detachment consent.* A patient with retinal detachment is often so afraid of losing their vision that they do not understand the different types of surgery that may be planned or actually performed during the consent process. Patients do not realize that RD surgery is very different from cataract surgery. Simple language and principles are helpful during consent, limiting complaints and encouraging realistic expectations from the surgery.

*Retinal detachment referral.* It is worth noting the vision for quicker acceptance of referrals by ophthalmologists; if the macula is unaffected ideally surgery should be performed before it becomes affected. Macula OFF or retinal detachment including the fovea should be operated within 10 days.

- Scleral *buckle* or explant – can cause diplopia.
- 80% success with primary RD repair.
- Cataract – will develop and most likely to need surgery within 5 years.
- GAS – vision change/posture required/no flights for 2 weeks.
- OIL – removal required (usually within 2 years)/raised IOP.

## Summary of rhegmatogenous RD surgery (in order)

1. Correct the structure of eye – by flattening retina, to avoid the eyeball changing shape and becoming phthisical.
2. Regain the peripheral lost field of vision.
3. Stabilize the central vision.
4. If macula OFF, then to try to improve the central vision.

Although subretinal fluid (SRF) is present in all three types of RD, the treatment differs:

- Rhegmatogenous – laser, cryotherapy (to seal up or glue down the original tear) with either scleral buckle (Fig. 10.38) or vitrectomy.
- Exudative – treat the underlying cause (e.g. metastasis, posterior scleritis).
- Tractional – relieve traction by vitrectomy.

Tangential plastic plomb
Encircling silicone band
Rectus muscle
Radial plastic plomb

**Fig. 10.38** Different types of plastic buckles used during retinal detachment surgery.

# Medical ophthalmology and uveitis

It is not easy to remember all of the systemic manifestations of the diseases mentioned in this chapter. We have tried to provide help in the form of clusters of acronyms throughout the tables and text. Patients are most grateful when you confirm their own suspicions, for example their recent respiratory or skin problem is actually related to their known pre-existing condition.

## CONNECTIVE TISSUE DISEASES

### Rheumatoid arthritis

Rheumatoid arthritis (RA) is a chronic systemic inflammatory condition characterized by a persistent, peripheral, symmetrical polyarthritis. It is a common disease affecting females more than males (F>M). Rheumatoid factor (RhF) blood test. General, neuromuscular and ocular features are shown in Fig. 11.1.

### Systemic lupus erythematosus

Systemic lupus erythematosus (SLE) is a **M**ultisystem **a**utoimmune condition characterised by **A**uto-antibodies to double stranded **D**NA (dsDNA) (ACRONYM: MAD).

Antigen–antibody complex deposition may result in the kidneys being affected. Females are affected more than males (F>M). General, renal, ocular and retinopathy features of SLE are shown in Fig. 11.2.

### Scleroderma

Chronic disease dominated by cutaneous manifestations. Females are affected more than males (F>M). SCL70, anti-centromere antibody blood tests. It can be part of CREST syndrome. General, CREST syndrome and ocular features are shown in Fig. 11.3.

**Fig. 11.1** General, neuromuscular and ocular features of rheumatoid arthritis. (TIP: ACRONYMS: RUN, VAN, LAP, MAN.SPEK)

| General features | | Neuromuscular | Ocular |
|---|---|---|---|
| **V**ascular: (RUN)<br>(i) **R**aynaud's phenomenon<br>(ii) **U**lceration of skin<br>(iii) **N**ailfolds splinter haemorrhages | **L**ung nodules and fibrosis | Proximal **M**yopathy | **S**cleritis (MCQ: not iritis) |
| **A**rthritis: predominately peripheral and symmetrical | **A**myloidosis of kidneys | **A**tlantoaxial subluxation (cervical vertebra level 1 and 2) may result in spinal cord compression | **P**eripheral corneal thinning– may perforate if very severe |
| **N**odules: tendons, internal organs and pressure points (TIP) | **P**ericarditis | Sensory **N**europathy | **E**piscleritis |
| | | | **K**eratoconjunctivitis sicca– 'Dry eyes', also associated with Sjögren's syndrome |

**Fig. 11.2** General, renal, ocular and retinopathy features of systemic lupus erythematosus. (TIP: ACRONYMS: BRAN, Renal PRHO, PEN.SPEK.)

| General features | | Kidneys | Ocular features | Retinopathy |
|---|---|---|---|---|
| Facial **B**utterfly rash | **P**ericarditis | **P**roteinuria | **S**cleritis | 'Primary' retinal vasculitis (with cotton wool spots, disc oedema and haemorrhages) |
| **R**aynaud's phenomenon | **L**ungs: pleurisy, **E**ffusions and fibrosis | Chronic **R**enal failure | **P**eripheral corneal thinning | |
| Poly**A**rthralgia symmetrical and migratory | **P**eripheral **N**europathy | **H**ypertension | **E**yelid erythema | |
| **N**ailfold infarcts | Psychosis | Nephritic syndrome (i.e. **O**edema) | **K**eratoconjunctivitis sicca | 'Secondary' to hypertension |

**Fig. 11.3** General, CREST syndrome and ocular features of scleroderma. (TIP: ACRONYM: MI.renalPRHo.CREST.SPEK,LER.)

| General features | CREST syndrome | Ocular features |
|---|---|---|
| **M**icrostoma – 'purse string mouth' | **C**alcinosis | Tight **S**kin over eyelids causing **P**unctal **E**ctropion |
| Nailfold **I**nfarcts | **R**aynaud's phenomenon | **K**eratoconjunctivitis sicca |
| Lungs: fibrosis | O**E**sophageal and small intestine fibrosis, causing dysphagia and malabsorption | **L**agophthalmos |
| Heart: myocarditis and **P**ericarditis | **S**clerodactyly | **E**piphora |
| Kidneys: **R**enal failure and **H**ypertension | **T**elangiectasia | **R**etinopathy usually caused by renal hypertension |
| Musculoskeletal: polyarthralgia and myositis | | |

## Polymyositis and dermatomyositis

Insidious, symmetrical, proximal muscle weakness results from muscle inflammation. This is a rare condition more common in females than males (F>M). Blood tests: CK, ANA, smooth muscle and Jo1 autoantibodies. General and ocular features are listed in Fig. 11.4.

## Sjögren's syndrome

This is a chronic inflammatory autoimmune disorder affecting the lacrimal and salivary glands. Inflammation and infiltration by plasma cells and lymphocytes lead to subsequent fibrosis. General features and management of this disorder are shown in Fig. 11.5.

There are two types: primary and secondary (Figs 11.6, 11.7).

## VASCULITIDES

## Giant cell arteritis

Giant cell arteritis (GCA) is an arteritis affecting any extracranial medium and large muscular arteries. It is a medical emergency since the vertebrobasilar arteries can be affected, leading to a brain stem infarct and thus death.

Patients are usually more than 60 years old. ESR (>60 in 80% patients) and CRP blood tests are both usually elevated. General and ocular features of this disorder are listed in Fig. 11.8.

**Fig. 11.4** General and ocular features of polymyositis and dermatomyositis. (TIP: ACRONYM: CREST.FANISH.ROPED. (N.B. Scleroderma CREST syndrome is different.)

| | General features | | Ocular features |
|---|---|---|---|
| **C**ardiomyopathy | | | |
| **R**aynaud's phenomena | Lung **F**ibrosis | | **R**etinopathy with cotton wool spots |
| **OE**sophageal dysphagia and dysphonia from laryngeal and pharyngeal muscle involvement | **A**rthralgia | | Periorbital **O**edema |
| (**S**houlder and hip) muscular girdle weakness | **N**ailfold **I**nfarcts | | Purple **E**yelids – or a heliotrope rash |
| **T**elangiectasia | **S**kin: purple (**H**eliotrope) rash (in 25% patients) | | **D**iplopia – resulting from ocular myopathy |

**Fig. 11.5** General features and management of Sjögren's syndrome

| General features (ACRONYM: DEMP) | Management |
|---|---|
| | Treat associated conditions |
| **D**ry **E**yes (xerophthalmia) | Tear supplements |
| Dry **M**outh (xerostomia) | Topical mucolytic agent |
| Dys**P**areunia and chest infections | Vaginal lubricants |

**Fig. 11.6** Primary Sjögren's syndrome – the 'sicca' complex with no associated disease

| Associated blood tests | Detection rate |
|---|---|
| Rheumatoid factor (RhF) | Positive 80% |
| Anti-nuclear factor (ANA) | Positive 80% |
| Hypergammaglobulinaemia | 50% |
| Anti-Ro/La autoantibodies (salivary gland, gastric parietal cell, and smooth muscle) positive | |

**Fig. 11.7** Connective tissue and other associations of secondary Sjögren's syndrome

| Connective tissue disease associations | Other associations |
|---|---|
| Rheumatoid arthritis | Graves' disease |
| Systemic lupus erythematosus | Chronic active hepatitis |
| Polymyositis/dermatomyositis | Primary biliary cirrhosis |
| Scleroderma | Myasthenia gravis |
| Polyarteritis nodosa | Coeliac disease |
| Mixed connective tissue disease | Non-Hodgkin's lymphoma risk increased × 40 in Sjögren's syndrome |

Temporal artery biopsy is usually performed within 1 week to confirm diagnosis. Histology shows:

- Artery wall thickened by inflammatory cells (histiocytes, lymphocytes, and giant cells, fibrinoid necrosis); skip lesions.
- Discontinuous internal elastic lamina (IEL) can be detected not just within 1 week, but as long as 28 days later.

## Polyarteritis nodosa

Polyarteritis nodosa is a systemic vasculitis affecting medium-sized and small arteries. Males are affected more than females (M>F). General and ocular features are listed in Fig. 11.9.

## Wegener's granulomatosis

Wegener's granulomatosis is a potentially fatal disease caused by necrotizing vasculitis. Serum antineutrophil cytoplasmic antibodies (c or p - ANCA) blood tests are helpful to diagnose the condition. Fig. 11.10 lists general and ocular features.

## Down's syndrome

This is caused by trisomy or translocation of chromosome 21; incidence is 1/700 live births. General and ocular features of Down's syndrome are shown in Fig. 11.11.

## UVEITIS

Uveitis is a term used to describe inflammation of the uveal tract (Fig. 11.12). Uveitis may occur in isolation, secondary to another intraocular problem or as part of systemic disease (Figs 11.13–11.15).

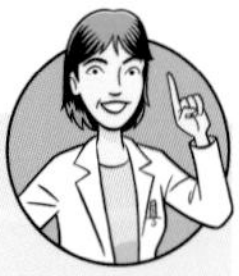

There are three types of uveitis: *anterior*, *intermediate* or *posterior*. It is therefore important to dilate the pupil, view the retina and check whether cells are present in the vitreous cavity and to ascertain if the posterior segment is involved.

**Fig. 11.8** General and ocular features of giant cell arteritis. (TIP: ACRONYM: FM.WATCH.MAP.CAMB.MAN.)

| | General features | Musculoskeletal | Arteritis | Ocular features: |
|---|---|---|---|---|
| **F**ever | **W**eight loss | Muscle weakness and pain | **C**erebral infarction | Ocular palsies-caused by **M**uscle or nerve ischaemia |
| **M**alaise | **A**norexia | **A**rthralgia | **A**ortitis | Central retinal **A**rtery occlusion (CRAO) |
| | Tender superficial **T**emporal arteries (and scalp ulceration) | **P**olymyalgia rheumatica (PMR) syndrome: main feature is proximal limb girdle weakness and pain | **M**yocardial infarction | Anterior ischaemic optic **N**europathy (AION) as a result of occlusion of posterior ciliary arteries |
| | Jaw **C**laudication (pathognomonic for GCA) | | **B**owel infarction | |
| | **H**eadaches | | | **A**nterior segment ischaemia |

**Fig. 11.9** General and ocular features of polyarteritis nodosa. (TIP: ACRONYM: Renal PRHO.MAP.BAN.SIR.)

| Kidney | Heart | General | Ocular features |
|---|---|---|---|
| **R**enal failure | **M**yocardial infarction | **B**owel infarction | Necrotizing **S**cleritis (and keratitis) |
| **H**ypertension (malignant) | **A**ngina | **A**rthritis | **I**schaemic optic neuropathy |
| Nephritic or nephrotic syndrome (**O**edema) | **P**ericarditis | Peripheral **N**europathy | **R**etinopathy: (i) 'primary' vasculitis with occlusion (ii) 'secondary' due to hypertension |

**Fig. 11.10** General and ocular features of Wegener's granulomatosis (TIP: ACRONYM: LUCK.PEN.SCORN.)

| General features | | Ocular features |
|---|---|---|
| **L**ungs | **P**yrexia | **S**cleritis and episcleritis |
| **U**pper respiratory tract – saddle nose and haemoptysis | Middle **E**ar and sinus lesions | **C**orneal infiltration and ulceration |
| **C**erebral vasculitis | Peripheral **N**europathy | **O**rbital involvement: proptosis, painful ophthalmoplegia, chemosis, retinal venous congestion, optic nerve involvement |
| **K**idneys (renal failure major cause of death) | | **R**etinopathy: arterial narrowing, venous tortuosity, cotton wool spots, choroidal thickening, cystoid macular oedema, and choroidoretinitis |
| | | **N**asolacrimal duct obstruction |

**Fig. 11.11** General and ocular features of Down's syndrome. (TIP: ACRONYM: SNIP.A.BEAK-BIRCH.NEST.)

| General features | Ocular features | | |
|---|---|---|---|
| **S**hort stature | **B**lepharoconjunctivitis | **B**rushfield's spots on **I**ris | **N**ystagmus |
| **N**ose – poorly developed bridge | **E**picanthic folds with Mongoloid slant of eyelids | | **E**ctropion |
| **I**nward curved (clinodactyly) short fingers | **A**cute hydrops (may be presenting feature of) **K**eratoconus | **R**efractive errors (mostly myopic) | **S**trabismus |
| Single **P**almar crease (hand) | | **C**ataracts | Hyper**T**elorism |
| Heart lesions (**A**trial or ventricular septal defects) | | **H**ypoplastic optic disc | |

**Fig. 11.12** Anatomy of the uveal tract: iris, ciliary body and choroid.

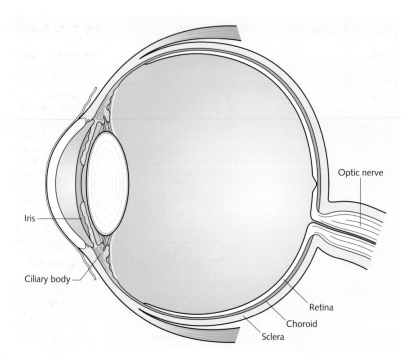

Iris

Ciliary body

Optic nerve

Retina

Choroid

Sclera

## Classification of uveitis

Uveitis may be classified in a number of different ways (see Fig. 11.13):

- Acute or chronic.
- Anatomically (see Fig. 11.14).
- Age of onset.
- Presence of granulomas.
- Immunocompetence.

Using each of these classifications it is possible to put each case of uveitis into a distinct group: those that require investigation immediately and those that do not. Patients are not usually investigated after their first episode of anterior uveitis. They are treated and then discharged after the inflammation has settled.

**Fig. 11.13** Classification of uveitis

**Anatomy**
- Anterior
- Intermediate
- Posterior
- Panuveitis

**Duration**
- Acute
- Chronic

**Age of onset**
- Infantile
- Juvenile
- Adult

**Granulomas**
- Granulomatous
- Non-granulomatous

## Anatomical considerations

The uveal coat comprises the iris, ciliary body, pars plana and choroid (see Fig.11.12).

When all parts of the uveal tract are inflamed it is referred to as panuveitis and may be an indicator of underlying systemic disease.

## Anterior uveitis

This refers to iritis or iridocyclitis, and is the most common form seen in practice. The majority of patients only ever have one episode with no recurrences. Patients typically complain of a painful, red eye with photophobia (Fig. 11.16), because the iris is moving in a sticky environment. Therefore dilatation or cycloplegia relieves the discomfort. The signs of uveitis are outlined in Fig. 11.17.

**Fig. 11.14** Causes of uveitis by location.

**Anterior**
Idiopathic
HLA-B27 +ve
Ankylosing spondylitis
Postoperative
Fuch's iridocyclitis
Reiter's syndrome
Autoimmune
Rheumatoid arthritis (including juvenile
idiopathic arthritis-associated uveitis)
Inflammatory bowel disease
Psoriatic arthritis
SLE
Behçet's disease

**Posterior**
Sarcoid
Behçets disease
POHS
AMPPE
MEWDS
Birdshot chorioretinopathy
Serpiginous chorioretinopathy
Multiple sclerosis
Toxoplasmosis
TB
Syphilis
Leprosy
Acute retinal necrosis
Herpetic
Endophthalmitis
Exogenous
Postoperative
Trauma
Endogenous
Immunocompromised
IV drug abuser

**Fig. 11.15** Causes of uveitis.

**Non granulomatous**
Idiopathic
HLA-B27 +ve
Ankylosing spondylitis
Postoperative
Fuch's
Reiter's syndrome
Autoimmune
Rheumatoid arthritis (including juvenile
idiopathic arthritis-associated uveitis)
Inflammatory bowel disease
Psoriatic arthritis
Behçet's disease
Multiple sclerosis
Behçets disease

**Granulomatous**
Sarcoid
TB
Syphilis
Phacoanaphylactic
Leprosy
POHS
Sympathetic ophthalmitis

**Masquerade syndromes**
Lymphoma
Reticulum cell sarcoma
Malignant melanoma
Retinal tear/detachment
Leukaemia
Retained IOFB

**Fig. 11.16** Symptoms of uveitis

| **Pain** |
| Inflammation |
| Raised IOP |

| **Red eye** |
| +/− Hypopyon |

| **Photophobia** |

| **Blurred vision** |

| **Floaters (intermediate and posterior uveitis)** |

| **Headache** |

| **Associated symptoms** |
| Rash |
| Cough |
| Dyspnoea |
| Arthritis |
| Urethritis |
| Mouth ulcers |
| Genital ulcers |

## Investigation

Do not forget a dilated fundus exam to exclude any posterior segment involvement. Granulomatous, recurrent or bilateral uveitis episodes (Fig. 11.18) warrant referral to ophthalmologists and further investigations (Fig. 11.19).

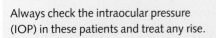
Always check the intraocular pressure (IOP) in these patients and treat any rise.

## Fig. 11.17 Signs of uveitis

**Anterior**

Cells in the anterior chamber (AC)
Flare in the AC
Keratic precipitates (KP) fine or 'mutton fat',
i.e. granulomas
High/low or normal IOP
Posterior synechiae (PS)
Peripheral anterior synechiae (PAS)
Iris bombé
Angle closure glaucoma
Cataract

**Intermediate**

All of above
Snowball opacities in vitreous
Snowbanking (creamy peripheral exudate)

**Posterior**

All of above
'White dots'/choroidal infiltrate
Vasculitis
Periphlebitis
Disc swelling
Ischaemia
Retinal neovascularization

Key point: There is usually little inflammation in an immunocompromised patient, e.g. HIV positive patient with toxoplasmosis.

## Fig. 11.19 Investigation of uveitis

**History**

**Exam**

**Ocular tests**

Fluorescein angiogram (FFA)
Ocular coherence tomography (OCT)
Intravitreal tap
Endophthalmitis (C&S)
Cytology (e.g. for lymphoma detection)
Toxoplasmosis PCR
CMV PCR

**Blood tests**

Basic
FBC, U&E, LFT, ESR, CRP, sACE, $Ca^{2+}$
Immunological
AutoAb screen (Rh Factor, ANA)
HLA testing (B27, B5, A29)
Syphilis
HIV test
Toxoplasmosis antibodies
Lyme titres

**X-rays**

CXR (sarcoid and TB)
Lumbosacral spine (ankylosing spondylitis)
MRI brain and optic nerve (MS)

**Skin test**

Mantoux

**Lumbar puncture**

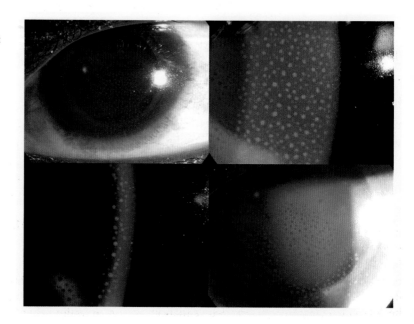

Fig. 11.18 Keratic precipitates. Use the magnification of the slit lamp and the orientation of the slit beam to confirm that the lymphocytic white cell deposits are on the corneal endothelium.

**Fig. 11.20** Treatment of acute iritis

**The principles of treatment**
Cycloplegia (pain relief and to prevent posterior synaechiae)
Anti-inflammatory drops (reduce activity, usually use steroids)
Control any rise in IOP (avoid prostaglandin analogues)
Add systemic/local steroid if indicated (see text)
Treat any underlying cause, e.g. sarcoidosis

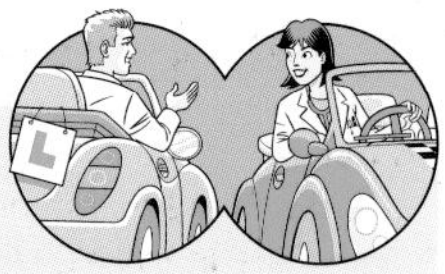

If snowballs and/or snowbanking are detected then an appropriate history should be sought, e.g. episodes of previous optic neuritis or any other neurological symptoms disseminated in time and place. Try to avoid the term multiple sclerosis (MS) and if necessary use the term demyelination instead.

## Treatment

See Fig. 11.20 for basic treatment. Beware secondary glaucoma which may be open or closed angle. Topical steroids may also cause steroid response glaucoma.

## Follow-up

All new patients should be referred and then seen within 1–2 weeks to assess response to treatment. If the inflammation has settled, then the steroid drops can be tapered (reduce frequency by 1 drop a day every week). Patients are then assessed at 6 weeks for resolution of inflammation.

Fig. 11.21 details systemic causes of uveitis and treatment modifications.

Most patients do not require further treatment, but are seen again if symptoms recur.

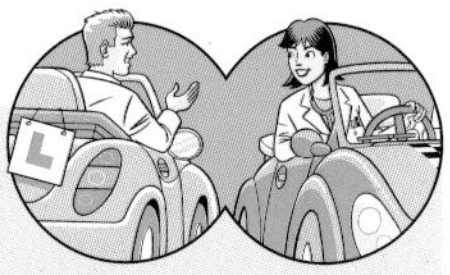

Ask about shingles and previous cold sores affecting lips or even the eye. Anterior uveitis is only one of many causes of a red eye. These patients should not be started solely on topical steroids, since viruses love to replicate in a steroid environment. Bottom line, if uveitis is suspected, give cycloplegic for pain relief and refer to the ophthalmologist.

## Intermediate uveitis

Intermediate uveitis is usually idiopathic. These patients present with floaters due to vitreous opacities and/or visual loss predominately due to cystoid macular. A subgroup of these patients, termed 'pars planitis', have snowballs and/or snowbanking, and the differential diagnoses include demyelination.

Visual loss from cystoid macular oedema (CMO) can be documented by fundus fluorescein angiogram (FFA) and/or an optical coherent tomography (OCT) test (Figs 11.22, 11.23). Macular oedema is treated with systemic or locally administered steroid (i.e. orbital floor injection, posterior subtenons or intra-vitreal). The goal of treatment is to limit visual loss from macular oedema.

## Posterior uveitis/choroiditis

Posterior uveitis may present with any of the symptoms and signs of anterior or intermediate uveitis. Floaters or reduced vision are the primary presenting symptoms.

The causes of posterior uveitis are numerous (see Figs 11.14, 11.15). When managing these patients it is very important to manage both the ocular and systemic condition, often between ophthalmologist and physician.

The investigation of these patients is outlined in Fig. 11.19. The treatment principles are detailed in Fig. 11.24.

## Scleritis

This is a granulomatous vasculitis affecting the sclera and occasionally the cornea (sclerokeratitis). Symptoms include a dull boring ache, such that the patient is "unable to sleep" (Fig. 11.25).

Phenotypes of scleritis are described in Fig. 11.26.

## Causes of scleritis

- Idiopathic.
- Postoperative.
- Systemic vasculitis (e.g. polyarteritis nodosa: PAN; Wegener's granulomatosis; rheumatoid arthritis).
- Infections (herpes zoster, syphilis, TB).

**Fig. 11.21** Identification of systemic cause of uveitis and treatment modification

| Systemic cause of uveitis | Modification of therapy |
| --- | --- |
| Sarcoidosis | Respiratory physician referral and systemic steroids +/− disease modifying agent may be added later |
| Ankylosing spondylitis | Rheumatology physician referral and may require systemic non-steroidal anti-inflammatory drug |
| Reiter's syndrome | Treat the urethritis, e.g. with doxycycline Rheumatology physician referral for arthritis |
| Juvenile idiopathic arthritis (JIA) | Rheumatology referral and systemic steroids +/− disease modifying agent may be added later |

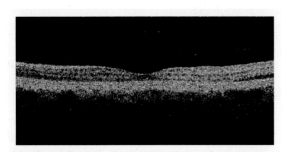

**Fig. 11.22** Optical coherent tomography (OCT) imaging shows a cross-section through the macula. A normal macula with a 'V'-shaped valley or depression is visible.

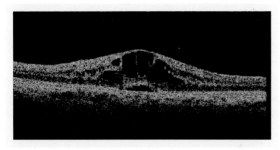

**Fig. 11.23** Cystoid macular oedema. The black regions are fluid-filled cystic spaces. Note the humped or volcano-shaped macula.

**Fig. 11.24** Treatment of posterior uveitis

**The principles of treatment**
Treat any underlying infection
       Toxoplasmosis (clindamycin)
       Syphilis (penicillin)
Anti-inflammatory treatment
       Reduce activity
       Reduce macular oedema
       Limit retinal/choroidal neovascularization
Steroids usually sufficient
Local steroid if unilateral disease
       Intra vitreal
       Sub tenons
       Orbital floor
Systemic steroid if bilateral or associated with systemic disease
       E.g. sarcoidosis
If uncontrolled or complications with steroid add second line agent
       Ciclosporin
       Azathioprine
       Cyclophosphamide
       Mycophenolate
Monitor the following on treatment
       Blood pressure
       Blood sugar
       Full blood count
       Urea and electrolytes
       Liver function

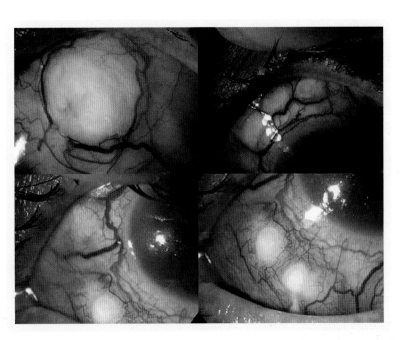

Fig. 11.25 Necrotizing scleritis. Avascular ischaemic ('cream cheese') sclera surrounded by prominent scleral vessels.

## Treatment of scleritis

Systemic steroids are the mainstay of treatment. Second-line agents may need to be added, e.g. ciclosporin, CellCept (mycophenolate mofetil), or cyclophosphamide.

## Specific causes of uveitis

### HLA-B27 +ve

Patients with this particular haplotype are more susceptible to iritis. There is no specific treatment other than for the iritis. They should be investigated for ankylosing spondylitis.

### Ankylosing spondylitis

This is an inherited arthritis affecting the axial skeleton. Patients present in the 2nd or 3rd decade with ocular signs and/or back pain with reduced mobility. Early signs include iritis and sclerosis of the sacroiliac joints. End-stage disease is characterized by kyphosis and a 'bamboo' spine on X-ray. Treatment is with anti-inflammatory drugs and

**Fig. 11.26** Phenotypes of scleritis

| Type of scleritis | Typical appearance |
| --- | --- |
| Anterior diffuse | Painful, sectoral scleral injection with overlying congested conjunctiva |
| Nodular | Single or multiple nodules |
| Necrotizing (with inflammation) | Very painful, active inflammation at the edges, may be bilateral |
| Necrotizing (without inflammation) | Usually in rheumatoid patients Elderly females Scleromalacia perforans (painless loss of scleral tissue with uveal exposure) |
| Posterior scleritis | Thickened sclera (>2 mm) on ultrasound Overlying exudative retinal detachment, swollen optic disc and/or proptosis |

physiotherapy to prolong adequate mobility. A cardiology review should be considered in these patients (increased incidence of heart block and aortic insufficiency).

## Postoperative

The anterior segment is usually inflamed following ocular surgery and therefore treatment with steroid drops is routinely given. Persistent inflammation may occur and prolonged treatment may then be required (Fig. 11.27). If inflammation is excessive, e.g. a hypopyon is present, then endophthalmitis (i.e. infection) should be considered and appropriate management commenced (see below).

## Autoimmune conditions

### Juvenile idiopathic arthritis-associated uveitis
This is a seronegative (Rh factor negative) arthritis affecting children. The eyes are affected in the pauciarticular form commonly. These children develop a chronic uveitis with cataract and glaucoma as common complications. They often require systemic therapy and the ocular prognosis is poor.

### Psoriatic arthritis
Psoriasis alone is not associated with iritis; patients must also have arthritis (affects distal interphalangeal joints). See medical ophthalmolgy section earlier in this chapter.

### Inflammatory bowel disease
Both Crohn's disease and ulcerative colitis may be associated with iritis or episcleritis.

### Behçet's disease
This is a rare condition, typically found in Mediterranean/Japanese males. It is associated with HLA-B51 haplotype. Patients present with a severe uveitis (hypopyon may be present), disc swelling and retinal vasculitis (Fig. 11.28). Associated features include mouth ulcers, genital ulcers, erythema nodosum or arthritis. These patients require aggressive systemic therapy (steroids and disease modifying agents, e.g. cyclophosphamide). The prognosis is poor.

## Sarcoidosis

30% of patients have ocular involvement from their disease; uveitis is often their presenting complaint. Other examples of ocular involvement include:

- Episcleritis.
- Scleritis.
- Optic neuritis/atrophy.

**Fig. 11.27** Giant cells deposited on the intraocular lens (IOL) (B) 2 months after cataract surgery in a patient with previous recurrent anterior uveitis. The red reflex was obscured and intensive topical steroid drops were started. (C) 2 weeks and (A & D) 4 weeks later. All deposits cleared by 8 weeks and the patient remained on maintenance of once daily topical steroid drop.

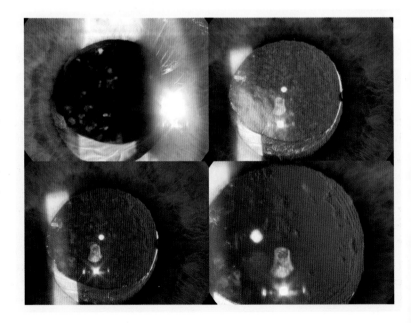

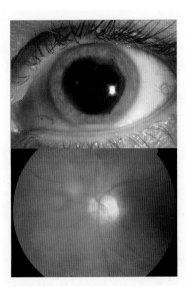

**Fig. 11.28** Behçets disease. (A) Left eye with small hypopyon. Irregular pupil shape due to two small anterior synaechiae (at 8 and 12 o'clock). Note the good, clear view of the pupil and lack of red eye appearance. There is a history of persistent mouth and recurrent groin ulcers. (B) Artery and veins are inflamed in focal areas (nasal to left optic disc). Hazy view of optic disc and retinal vessels is due to mild vitritis.

- Retinal vasculitis (haemorrhages and exudates) incl BRVO.
- Vitritis with 'snowballs'.
- Choroiditis.

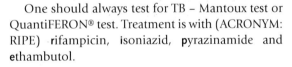

All patients with posterior uveitis should be asked about symptoms of sarcoidosis, e.g. skin rashes (erythema nodosum), arthritis and dyspnoea.

## Investigations

Investigations ('must know') include:

- Serum ACE (may not be raised in exclusively ocular disease).
- Serum $Ca^{2+}$.
- Chest X-ray.
- High-resolution CT chest.
- Biopsy of any skin or chest lesions.

Treatment is local or systemic depending on the extent of involvement. First-line systemic treatment is steroid.

## Infectious causes of uveitis

### Tuberculosis

Tuberculosis is a granulomatous disease and about 2–5% of patients have ocular uveitic manifestations, including:

- Mutton-fat keratic precipitates.
- Panuveitis.
- Choroidal granulomas.
- Multifocal choroiditis.
- Retinal ischaemia/neovascularization.
- Optic disc oedema.

Enquire whether patient is from, or is in contact with, people from endemic TB regions such as the Indian subcontinent. You may gently enquire about any breathing problems then continue with weight loss, night sweats and haemoptysis. Furthermore, think of TB in AIDS patients with eye signs described above (remember they may be Mantoux negative).

One should always test for TB – Mantoux test or QuantiFERON® test. Treatment is with (ACRONYM: RIPE) **r**ifampicin, **i**soniazid, **p**yrazinamide and **e**thambutol.

### Syphilis

The eye can be involved in syphilis (secondary and tertiary disease). Secondary syphilis can lead to:

- Iridocyclitis (granulomatous (gumma)/non-granulomatous).
- Cornea (interstitial keratitis).
- Chorioretinitis:
  - Multifocal or diffuse
  - Massive pigmentary change
  - Neuroretinitis (disc and macular oedema, cotton wool spots and haemorrhages).

Syphilis can be diagnosed with an FTA-Abs test. Treatment is with penicillin or doxycycline.

### Toxoplasmosis

Toxoplasmosis is a parasitic infection that can infect the eye in utero (congenital) and postnatally.

Congenital toxoplasmosis can affect the eye (e.g. choroid and then retina) and the rest of the embryo (e.g. brain and chest). Infected children may be normal or have multiple birth defects depending on the age of inoculation.

Adult toxoplasmosis may be primary (rare) or a reactivation of an old locus of infection.

'**P**'rimary toxoplasmosis is usually acquired from the ingestion of undercooked/raw meat. These patients have an ill defined '**P**'ale chorioretinitis with a mild-to-moderate amount of vitreous activity.

'**S**'econdary/reactivated toxoplasmosis has a classic appearance of a pigmented '**S**'car (Fig. 11.29) with adjacent white fluffy infiltrate. There is often an intense vitritis making the view of the retina difficult. Vision may be reduced from cystoid macular oedema, direct or indirect foveal involvement (e.g. branch retinal artery or vein occlusion).

Patients are treated if they have:

- Lesions within the macula (particularly between disc and fovea).
- Lesions adjacent to the disc.
- Lesions overlying a major vessel (risk of vein occlusion).

*Treatment*   Treatment is with one of two regimens:

- Pyrimethamine, sulfadiazine, folinic acid and oral steroid.
- Clindamycin and oral steroid.

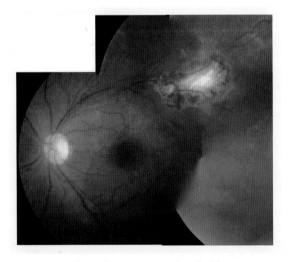

**Fig. 11.29** Toxoplasma chorioretinitis scar, along the left superotemporal arcade.

## Herpes zoster

Herpes zoster can affect any part of the eye. It is a DNA virus that lies dormant on the ganglia of sensory nerves (e.g. trigeminal ganglion in herpes zoster ophthalmicus (HZO) or the dorsal root ganglion in shingles).

Herpes zoster ophthalmicus classically presents with a tingling sensation over the scalp and forehead of affected patients. The rash subsequently develops, not crossing the mid-line. Direct ocular involvement may follow any time after the appearance of the rash. There is increased likelihood of intraocular involvement if there are vescicles on the tip of the nose (Hutchinson's sign) or lid margin.

The diagnosis tends to be made clinically (Fig. 11.30) though antibodies may be tested.

Consequence of herpes zoster infection to eye are shown in Fig. 11.31 (see also Fig. 11.32). Glaucomatous consequence of herpes zoster infection to eye are listed in Fig. 11.33.

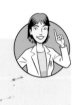

The pressure is nearly always raised in zoster-related uveitis. Corneal oedema obscuring the iris view may also be present.

*Treatment*   If patients have posterior segment disease or an orbital apex syndrome, systemic antiviral treatment should be commenced immediately, as there is a risk of developing encephalitis. Aciclovir 800 mg 5/day i.v. can be given.

### Cytomegalovirus

Cytomegalovirus (CMV) is a ubiquitous virus that is usually non-pathogenic. However, in immunocompromised individuals (e.g. AIDS or post-transplant) CMV retinitis may occur. This is seen clinically as a progressive retinitis (see Fig. 11.32) with cotton wool spots and haemorrhages. Retinal thinning and secondary rhegmetogenous retinal detachment may develop. The diagnosis is made clinically or with vitreous biopsy and PCR.

Treatment is with systemic and intraocular antiviral agents (e.g. ganciclovir, foscarnet, cidofovir). If retinal detachments develop they usually require silicone oil insertion.

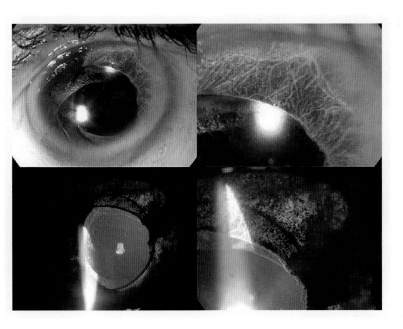

**Fig. 11.30** Herpetic uveitis in a pseudophakia patient. (A & B) Usually there is no obvious iris depigmentation. (C & D) Iris sector atrophy on transillumination is an important sign for this diagnosis.

**Fig. 11.31** Consequence of herpes zoster infection to the eye

| Region of eye affected | Consequence of herpes zoster infection to eye |
| --- | --- |
| Lids | Rash<br>Ptosis (isolated or part of a III nerve palsy or Horner's syndrome) |
| Extraocular muscle | Motor nerve palsy, single or multiple<br>Part of orbital apex syndrome |
| Conjunctiva | Follicular conjunctivitis |
| Scleritis | Necrotizing scleritis<br>Sclerokeratitis |
| Cornea | Epitheliopathy with reduced sensation (small erosions)<br>Stromal disease including interstitial keratitis<br>Endotheliitis |
| Iris | Iritis<br>Ischaemia (iris sector atrophy) |
| Lens | Cataract formation |
| Vitreous | Vitritis |
| Retina | Retinitis (acute retinal necrosis: ARN; progressive outer retinal necrosis: PORN – see Fig. 11.32)<br>Central/branch vein occlusion (CRVO BRVO)<br>Retinal detachment |
| Optic nerve | Optic neuritis<br>Ischaemic optic neuropathy |

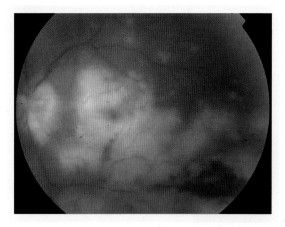

**Fig. 11.32** Left fundus photo showing deep retinal creamy-yellow coalescing lesions with inferotemporal retinal haemorrhages. This is a necrotizing herpetic retinopathy called progressive outer retinal necrosis (PORN). Differential diagnosis includes cytomegalovirus (CMV) retinitis. There is, however, very little vitritis and hence a good view of the optic disc and retinal vessel details. The patient was found to have a low CD4 white cell count and subsequently was newly diagnosed to be HIV positive.

**Fig. 11.33** Glaucomatous consequence of herpes zoster infection to eye

| Type of glaucoma | Mechanism |
| --- | --- |
| Open angle | Due to inflammatory debris Trabeculitis |
| Closed angle | Peripheral anterior synechiae Iris bombé |

Many HIV patients know their CD4 level and generally have a separate set of hospital notes for the HIV clinic. Rather than plunging into their HIV/AIDS status, you may wish to ask whether their CD4 count has been, or is, less than 50. This way you can quickly ascertain relevant information without offending the patient.

## HIV

HIV infection may affect the eye directly, or secondary opportunistic infections may cause problems. Fig 11.34 shows some HIV-related eye signs and Fig. 11.35 lists opportunistic diseases affecting the retina in HIV patients.

**Fig. 11.34** A small selection of HIV-related eye signs

| Part of eye | Some HIV-related eye signs |
| --- | --- |
| Conjunctiva | Conjunctivitis Kaposi sarcoma (may be hidden in fornix) |
| Retina | Mild retinitis with occasional haemorrhages and/or cotton wool spots |

**Fig. 11.35** Opportunistic diseases affecting the retina in HIV patients

| Part of eye | Opportunistic diseases |
| --- | --- |
| Retina | Cytomegalovirus |
| | Herpes zoster/simplex |
| | Toxoplasmosis |
| | Syphilis |

Patients are now aggressively treated with antiretroviral therapies and additional appropriate treatment should be added if a coexistent disease is found.

HIV patients often have atypical response patterns to disease. They may have a low threshold for vitreous biopsy and PCR analysis in any retinitis/choroiditis.

## Candida

Candida infection typically affects the immunocompromised or i.v. drug abusers. If the eye is affected treatment (local and systemic) should be commenced, e.g. intravenous and intravitreal amphotericin. Ocular features following candida infection are detailed in Fig. 11.36.

ITU patients who develop blurry vision in one or both eyes need their vision documented and appropriate referral.
Central line tips can develop candida infection, which then embolizes and spreads to the eye, causing blurry vision.

**Fig. 11.36** Ocular features following candida infection

| Part of eye affected | Ocular features |
|---|---|
| Anterior chamber | Iritis +/– hypopyon |
| Vitreous | Vitritis<br>Vitreal opacities ('string of pearls') |
| Retina | Focal retinitis (small white elevated lesions)<br>Risk of tractional (vitreous organization) or rhegmatogenous (necrosis) detachment |
| Choroid | Deep pale/creamy lesions |

**Fig. 11.37** Causative organisms for exogenous endophthalmitis

| Type of endophthalmitis | Causative organism |
|---|---|
| Acute | Staphylococcus epidermidis, Staphylococcus aureus, streptococci, Pseudomonas, Proteus |
| Chronic | Propionibacterium acnes, Staphylococcus epidermidis, fungi |
| Trauma | Staphylococcus epidermidis, streptococci, fungi, Gram-negative organisms |
| Bleb-related | Streptococci |

## Endophthalmitis

This term describes inflammation of one or more coats of the eye with contiguous cavity inflammation. It is usually reserved for infections of the eye, and can be classified according to cause, onset or causative organism.

> Any postoperative acute red eye (e.g. cataract surgery in past 2 weeks) with increasing pain and/or decreased vision is suggestive of infection and should be referred immediately for ophthalmic review. Always check the vision to have an early point of reference.

Endophthalmitis may occur following:

- Intraocular surgery (risk is about 0.1–0.2%).
- Penetrating trauma (up to 10% risk of endophthalmitis).
- Draining glaucoma bleb (increased risk in mitomycin C blebs).
- Endogenous (very rare, occurs in septic patients).

Causative organisms for exogenous endophthalmitis are listed in Fig. 11. 37 and for endogenous endophthalmitis in Fig. 11.38.

Patients presenting soon after surgery or following trauma with very painful red eyes should be referred urgently. If they develop a hypopyon they should be managed as an endophthalmitis (Fig. 11.39). The prognosis is often poor for these patients, especially if there is any delay in diagnosis.

### Investigation and management of endophthalmitis

- Appropriate history and ocular exam performed (check for hypopyon).
- Patients should be prepared for aqueous and vitreous tap and intravitreal antibiotic injection.
- Vitreous tap performed with local anaesthesia (topical and subtenon injection).
- 0.1 ml of aqueous and 0.1 ml of vitreous aspirated.
- Intravitreal vancomycin (1 mg/0.1 ml) and amikacin (0.4 mg/0.1 ml).
- If fungal infection suspected intravitreal amphoteracin (10 µg) is also given.
- Topical and oral ciprofloxacin (good intraocular penetration) commenced.

**Fig. 11.38** Causative organisms for endogenous endophthalmitis

| Type of endogenous endophthalmitis | Causative organism |
|---|---|
| Fungi | Candida, Aspergillus |
| Gram-positive organisms | Staphylococcus aureus, group B streptococci, Streptococcus pneumoniae and Listeria monocytogenes |
| Gram-negative organisms | Klebsiella spp., Escherichia coli, Pseudomonas aeruginosa, and Neisseria meningitidis |

**Fig. 11.39** Hypopyon in a patient with previous glaucoma drainage tube surgery. (A) Injected conjunctiva and scleral vessels. (B) Right eye, superotemporal conjunctival epithelial defect (stained yellow with flourescein) allowing entry of bacterial organisms into the eye. (C) Misty view of pupil (due to anterior chamber cells). (D) Bloodstained level within hypopyon, which is posterior to corneal endothelium.

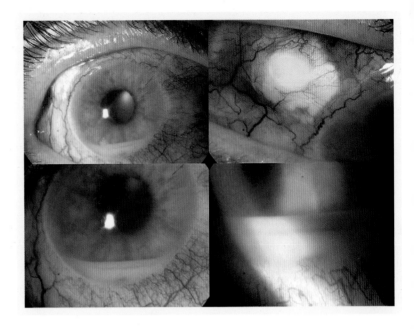

## Masquerade syndrome (i.e. non-inflammatory and non-infectious causes)

There are a number of conditions that may present like uveitis and their diagnosis should be considered when there is no response, or a poor response, to therapy.

Adequate examination should rule out:

- Retinal detachment/tears.
- Retained intraocular foreign body (IOFB).
- Malignant melanoma.

Vitreous biopsy may be required to rule out:

- Ocular lymphoma.
- Reticular cell sarcoma.
- Leukaemia.

Consider masquerade syndrome if disproportionate panuveitis is observed without the usual signs of inflammation: red, painful, photophobic, and posterior synaechiae. Particularly if the episode occurs at an age of late onset.

## Multifocal choroidopathies

This term describes a group of similarly appearing conditions that affect the RPE and/or the choriocapillaris. Classically patients present with blurred

Ask about specific joint problems, for example low back ache, which may be pivotal in identification of spinal prostate metastasis and multiple myeloma. Try to use the term 'neoplasm' rather than the hated 'cancer' word, which is generally much more upsetting to patients.

vision (central lesion), floaters (vitritis) or incidentally ('white dot' lesions noted at opticians). These patients may also describe visual field defects.

There are many causes of uveitis (Figs. 11.14, 11.15). Remember the basic principles of history taking, examination and investigation to manage patients appropriately and safely.

The prognosis is still poor for many patients as the underlying pathogenic mechanisms are poorly understood. More directed therapies are being formulated, so be sympathetic with patients with chronic or recurrent episodes of uveitis.

## Objectives

You should be able to:

- Define the terms 'binocular single vision' and 'amblyopia'.
- Understand the causes of and differences between amblyopia and leukocoria.
- Describe the importance of diagnosing a congenital cataract or cloudy cornea at birth.
- Understand there are many causes of congenital cataract that may require detection and treatment.
- Understand the importance of retinopathy of prematurity screening.
- Describe the wider implications of neonatal conjunctivitis.
- Describe some systemic and ophthalmic features of phakomatosis.

Paralytic squint is covered in Chapter 13.

## VISUAL DEVELOPMENT AND BINOCULAR SINGLE VISION

Binocular single vision (BSV) is the simultaneous use of two eyes to give a single mental impression. Therefore requirements include that the eyes need to be aligned towards the same object and presence of reasonably good vision in each eye. Worth has described three grades of BSV: simultaneous perception (two images from two eyes), fusion (two-dimensional view) and stereopsis (three-dimensional view). BSV offers an increase in the field of vision, elimination of individual blind spots, binocular visual acuity (often better than monocular) and accurate depth perception.

## NON-PARALYTIC STRABISMUS

Children can often present with strabismus or amblyopia ('lazy eye') after a routine health visitor check or after their first school vision test. The nerve connections at the lateral geniculate nucleus (i.e. relay from the retinal ganglion cells and optic tracts to the visual cortex) cease to be plastic around age 8. Therefore visual acuity develops during early childhood, usually until 8 years of age. If the ocular images are not aligned in childhood, then the brain concentrates on the better seeing eye at the expense

of the other eye. The result is suppression of visual development of the misaligned eye or amblyopia.

Non-paralytic strabismus may be primary or secondary.

### Primary

It develops in a child with otherwise normal ocular examination. It is thought to be due to a central developmental anomaly and there may be a family history.

### Secondary to ocular disease

- *Refractive error.* If this is different between the two eyes (anisometropia), one ocular image will be blurred. Generally, correcting hypermetropia typically improves a convergent squint or esotropia and correcting myopia improves a divergent squint or exotropia.
- *Media opacity.* For example corneal opacity, cataract, vitreous haemorrhage (Fig. 12.1).

### History

- Parental recall/observation.
- Pre-school/health visitor screening.
- Note age of onset/constant or intermittent/eye(s) turning in or out.
- Past medical history including viral infections and immunization history.
- Family history of squint/eye surgery in childhood/'lazy eye' (amblyopia).

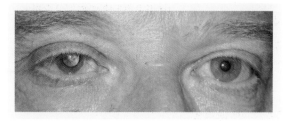

**Fig. 12.1** Right leukocoria due to cataract.

A squint may be classified as

1. *Esotropia*. A manifest convergent squint.
2. *Exotropia*. A manifest divergent squint.
3. *Accommodative*. Near vision entails both accommodation and convergence. If this reflex is abnormal then focusing on a near object may result in excessive convergence and therefore an 'accomodative esotropia'. This condition will be completely corrected by glasses.
4. *Mixed*. Both a manifest (eso- or exotropia) and accommodative component. The accommodative element of this condition will be corrected by glasses.

## Examination

Observation for the following:
- Manifest squint and constancy, alternation.
- Facial features including any suggestion of chromosomal syndromes.
- Epicanthic folds which may contribute to the appearance of a pseudosquint.

Active examination (see also Chapter 14):

- Visual acuity (e.g. forced choice preferential learning, Cardiff cards, Kay's pictures, Sheridan–Gardiner test).
- Corneal reflections with a pen torch.
- Cover test.
- Extraocular movements.
- Cycloplegic refraction (this paralyses accommodation to allow measurement of true degree of hypermetropia).
- Dilated eye examination for media opacity and retinal disease.

## Treatment

This is aimed at maximizing visual acuity and minimizing amblyopia.

- Correction of any significant refractive error with glasses.
- Removal of any obstruction in the visual axis which may be giving rise to stimulus deprivation amblyopia, e.g. cataract, correction of ptosis.
- Amblyopia treatment with graded occlusion of the better eye (e.g. patching or atropine).
- Surgery. This may be undertaken to maximize the potential for binocular single vision and stereopsis in a young child. Alternatively it may be for cosmetic reasons when children reach school age. The extraocular muscles are recessed (moved backwards from their insertion) to reduce their action or resected to increase their action.

# OTHER IMPORTANT PAEDIATRIC OPHTHALMIC CONDITIONS

## Congenital cataract

The incidence of congenital cataract is about 3:10 000 live births and two-thirds are bilateral. Congenital cataract is an important cause of amblyopia due to stimulus deprivation. (see above). It may present with a cloudy pupil or white pupillary reflex (leukocoria) at screening following birth (Fig. 12.2).

It is therefore important to manage the following:

- The visual significance of the cataract and the effect on visual development.
- Treatment of any underlying cause (summarized in Fig. 12.4).

### Management of congenital cataract

**Visual development**

Cataract density must be assessed with direct, indirect and portable slit lamp examination. Associated ocular pathology such as glaucoma, microphthalmos and aniridia must be excluded.

| **Fig. 12.2** Differential diagnosis of leukockoria |
| --- |
| Congenital cataract |
| Retinoblastoma (Fig. 12.3) |
| Persistent primary hyperplastic vitreous |
| Familial exudative vitreoretinopathy |
| Coat's disease |

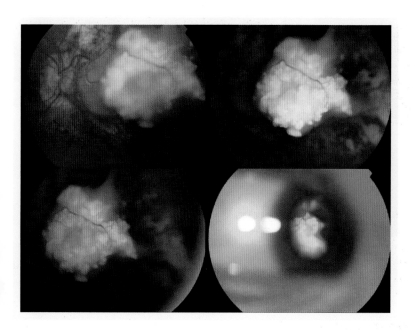

**Fig. 12.3** Retinoblastoma. (A) Nasal to right optic disc; (B & C) protruding into vitreous cavity with overlying retinal blood vessels; and (D) visible through pupil, giving impression of leukocoria (white pupil reflex).

| **Fig. 12.4** Causes of congenital cataract |
|---|

Hereditary:
- Autosomal dominant
- Autosomal recessive
- X-linked

Chromosomal abnormalities:
- Down's syndrome

Metabolic abnormalities:
- Galactosaemia
- Galactokinase deficiency
- Lowe's syndrome
- Hypoparathyroidism

Intrauterine infection (TIP: ACRONYM: ToRCH)
- **TO**xoplasmosis
- **R**ubella
- **C**ytomegalovirus
- **H**erpes simplex
- Varicella zoster

Associated with other developmental disorders

Although measurement of vision in neonates is difficult, important indicators of reduced vision include nystagmus and strabismus. Special investigations such as electrodiagnostic tests may be useful.

## Surgery

Timing is crucial in visually significant cataract to prevent amblyopia. Bilateral dense cataracts require early surgery whereas mild cataracts may be observed if vision develops normally. Unilateral dense cataracts require urgent surgery.

Parents need to be counselled since these neonates require intense antiamblyopia management following surgery and results may be disappointing.

## Treatment of any underlying cause

Any infant with congenital cataracts should have the following investigations, unless there is a clearly established inheritance pattern:
- 'ToRCH' screen – TOxoplasmosis, Rubella, Cytomegalovirus, Herpes simplex (Figs 12.4, 12.5) – varicella zoster antibody titres.
- Urinalysis for reducing substance for galactosaemia.

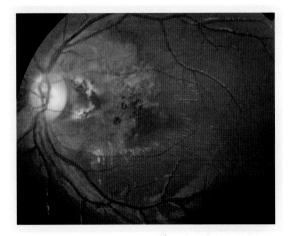

**Fig. 12.5** Intrauterine or neonatal infection can result in retinal scarring.

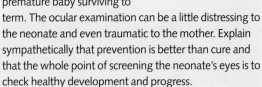

Remember the mother is anxious and worried about her premature baby surviving to term. The ocular examination can be a little distressing to the neonate and even traumatic to the mother. Explain sympathetically that prevention is better than cure and that the whole point of screening the neonate's eyes is to check healthy development and progress.

- Urine chromatography for amino acids.
- Fasting blood glucose.
- Serum calcium and phosphorus.
- Red blood cell GPUT.
- Serum galactokinase.
- Referral to a paediatrician if there is any suggestion of other systemic abnormalities.

## Retinopathy of prematurity (ROP)

This is a proliferative vitreoretinopathy affecting infants born pre-term with low birth weight. The retinal vessels start to develop at 4 months' gestation. The vessels reach the nasal periphery at 8 months gestation but do not reach the temporal periphery until 1 month after birth. In pre-term infants, the incompletely vascularized retina is susceptible to damage, particularly by high oxygen concentrations. Management of ROP is particularly important because screening and treatment of certain stages of the disease may halt progression and preserve vision.

### Screening

There are two main criteria:

- Babies born ≤ 32 weeks' gestation.
- Babies weighing ≤ 1500 g.

Screening for these infants should begin at 6 weeks' post-natal age or 34 weeks' post-conceptual age and subsequently at 2-weekly intervals until the retina is fully vascularized.

## Management

ROP is graded according to location, extent, stage and 'plus' disease.

There are five stages (TIP: ACRONYM: DR.FReD):

Stage 1: **D**emarcation line between vascularized and non-vascularized retina.

Stage 2: Demarcation line develops into a **R**idge.

Stage 3: Ridge with **F**ibrovascular proliferation.

Stage 4: Sub-total **RE**tinal detachment.

Stage 5: Total retinal **D**etachment.

Features of 'plus' disease (TIP: ACRONYM: PVD):

1. Poor **P**upillary dilatation.
2. **V**itreous haze.
3. **D**ilatation of retinal vessels.

Features of threshold disease are shown in Fig. 12.6.

## Treatment

Treatment is usually performed when threshold disease has been reached. Recent studies have shown that some infants with pre-threshold disease may benefit from treatment. Laser treatment to ablate the ischaemic retina is successful

**Fig. 12.6** Features of threshold disease

**Threshold disease**

All of the following should be present:
Stage 3
'Plus' disease involving:
5 contiguous or 8 non-contiguous clock hours
Location: Zone 1 (60° circle around optic disc, posterior retina) or Zone 2 (from zone 1 to nasal ora serrata)

in about 85% of infants with threshold disease. Vitreoretinal surgery is indicated in those with advanced disease.

## Other retinal conditions

Coat's disease and familial exudative vitreoretinopathy (FEVR) (Fig. 12.7) may present with visual loss or in pre-verbal children a squint or leukocoria. They must have a dilated retinal exam. Coat's disease can lead to massive amounts of subretinal fluid and exudates. It is usually a unilateral disease and usually affects boys. FEVR is an uncommon autosomal dominant condition that is inherited and is similar in appearance to retinopathy of prematurity. There is dragging of the vessels, with or without fluid leakage, with or without exudates.

## Primary congenital glaucoma

This is a rare condition affecting 1:10 000 live births; 60% are boys. It is due to maldevelopment of the angle of the anterior chamber which impairs aqueous outflow. Clinical features include corneal haze, buphthalmos (a large eye due to high intraocular pressure leading to stretching), Halb's striae and optic disc cupping.

Fig. 12.8 shows a cloudy, opaque cornea and possible causes are listed in Fig. 12.9.

### Management

Surgery consists of a goniotomy as first choice, followed by medical management and further surgery if necessary. Follow-up is long term to monitor visual development and reduce amblyopia.

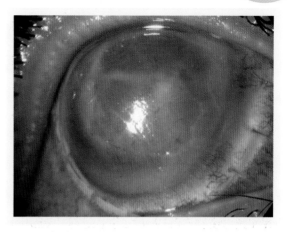

**Fig. 12.8** Cloudy opaque cornea.

**Fig. 12.9** Causes of a cloudy cornea at birth

Congenital glaucoma
Birth trauma
Congenital rubella
Mucopolysaccharidoses
Congenital hereditary endothelial dystrophy (CHED)

## Neonatal conjunctivitis

Conjunctivitis within the first month of life is a notifiable disease in the UK. Chlamydial conjunctivitis is the most common cause of neonatal conjunctival infection. There may be associated systemic features such as pneumonitis and otitis.

It is worth noting when the sticky eye conjunctivitis infection started. Gonococcal conjuncticvitis typically presents at 2–4 days, chlamydial at 5–14 days post partum.

Treatment is with topical tetracycline ointment and oral erythromycin. It is important that oral tetracyclines are not administered to children under 12 years of age as this leads to staining of the adult dentition. Gonococcal conjuncticvitis is less common and potentially extremely serious as it can cause corneal ulceration and perforation.

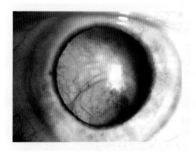

**Fig. 12.7** Familial exudative vitreoretinopathy – a differential diagnosis of leukocoria. Note the white reflex is from behind the clear lens of the eye towards the retina.

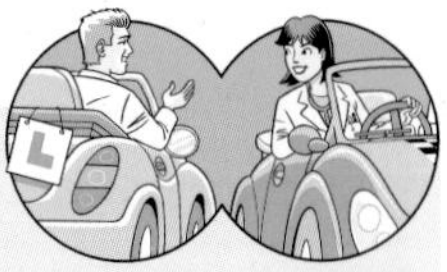

Explain to both parents that the underlying source for neonatal conjunctivitis needs to be identified. Therefore they both need to be examined for evidence of a genital infection, because the infection was transmitted from the mother to the baby during vaginal delivery. (Be careful to check that a caesarian was not performed!)

# Phakomatosis

This is a group of hereditary disorders with skin, other organ, retina and neurological manifestations. They include autosomal dominant ( AD) conditions such as tuberous sclerosis, von Hippel–Lindau syndrome, and neurofibromatosis. The ophthalmic findings in these disorders are summarized in Fig. 12.10.

Recent pathophysiology has demonstrated that Sturge–Weber should not be considered a true phakomatosis, but a syndrome resulting from cortical vein or dural sinus dysplasia.

**Fig. 12.10** Ophthalmic findings in phakomatosis

| Condition | Systemic and ophthalmic features |
| --- | --- |
| Neurofibromatosis 1 | Two or more of the following:<br>≥ 6 café-au-lait spots<br>≤ 2 neurofibromas/1 plexiform neurofibroma<br>Axillary/inguinal freckling<br>Bone dysplasia/defect<br>Optic nerve glioma – in 15% cases<br>Lisch (iris) nodules – in 95% cases |
| Neurofibromatosis type 2 | Bilateral acoustic neuroma or VIII nerve neurofibromatosis, meningioma, cataract and other nervous system tumours such as glioma and schwannoma |
| Von Hippel–Lindau disease | Isolated cases: two or more haemangioblastomas (retinal or CNS) or a single haemangioblastoma in association with a visceral tumour, e.g. renal carcinoma or phaeochromocytoma Familial cases: single haemangioblastoma or visceral complication |
| Tuberous sclerosis | Multiple features including **S**hagreen patches, **A**denoma sebaceum, **C**afé-au-lait spots, cardiac **R**habdomyoma, **A**sh leaf patches, **S**ubungual fibromas, retinal astrocytic **H**amartomas (in 50% patients) (ACRONYM: SA.CRASH) |
| Sturge–Weber | Triad of cutaneous (naevus flammeus), meningeal and choroidal haemangiomas. Glaucoma occurs in 50% patients |

# Neuro-ophthalmology

## Objectives

You should be able to:

- Define the causes of papilloedema.
- Describe the visual field patterns of optic pathway disease.
- Describe common causes of optic atrophy.
- Understand appropriate investigations for optic atrophy and third nerve palsy.
- Distinguish between a pupil-involving and pupil-sparing third nerve palsy.
- Describe the aetiology and principal features of third, fourth and sixth nerve palsies.

Neuro-ophthalmology describes the interaction between the eye and the rest of the nervous system. Broadly, the eyes can be directly affected in neurological disease or act as an indicator of central nervous system problems such as tumours or vascular events such as stroke.

## ANATOMY

Neuro-ophthalmic diagnosis relies on a good knowledge of anatomy. This relates in particular to the optic nerve pathway (Fig. 13.1), pathways governing eye movement (see Fig. 13.2 for horizontal eye movements) and control of the pupil (Fig. 13.3). Fig. 13.4 summarizes important visual field defects that occur along the visual pathway.

### Optic nerve

The optic nerve is made up from approximately 1.5 million ganglion cell axons (first order neurons). The nerve courses posteriorly and medially through the orbit to enter the anterior cranial fossa through the optic canal and then onwards to the optic chiasm. Fibres derived from the nasal retina decussate at the chiasm while temporal fibres remain ipsilateral (see Fig. 13.1).

The chiasm lies above pituitary gland and is thus the portion of the pathway affected by pituitary tumours.

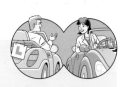

*Visual fields.* The patient's right visual field projects to the left occipital cortex and vice versa. Try not to get confused between the examiner's and the patient's perspective of left or right. When examining and talking to the patient always use the patient's perspective. For example, a right homonymous hemianopia is when half of the visual field is missing on the right or ipsilateral side from the patient's point of view. Draw the visual field defect on paper or in the notes again as though it is from the patient's point of view (see Chapter 14). In this way communication errors between doctors can be avoided.

### Optic tract

Fibres run from optic chiasm to the lateral geniculate body to synapse with the second order neurons, which then form the optic radiations. A group of fibres (about 10%) leave the tract to synapse directly in the pretectal nucleus (part of the autonomic system) which drives pupillary responses via the third cranial nerve.

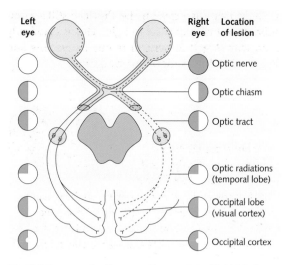

Fig. 13.1 Summary of optic nerve pathway and visual field defects.

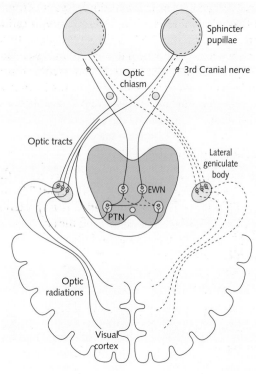

Fig. 13.3 Schematic of light reflex and visual field pathway. Pretectal area (PTN) and Edinger–Westphal nucleus (EWN) are both at the level of the midbrain.

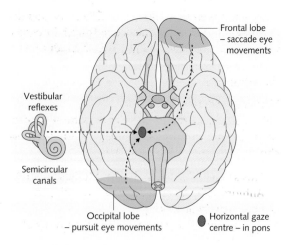

Fig. 13.2 The horizontal gaze centre, which lies in the pons, coordinates signals originating from the vestibular system, frontal and occipital lobes.

**Fig. 13.4** Visual field defects according to location of lesion along visual pathway

| Location of lesion | Type of field defect |
| --- | --- |
| Optic nerve | Complete monocular |
| Optic chiasm | Bitemporal hemianopia |
| Optic tract | Homonymous hemianopia |
| Optic radiations (temporal lobe) | Homonymous superior quadrantianopia ('pie in the sky') |
| Occipital lobe (visual cortex) | Homonymous hemianopia |
| Occipital cortex | Homonymous hemianopia with macular sparing |

## Optic radiations

Following synapse in the lateral geniculate body, the nerve fibres fan out and run through the parietal and temporal lobe. These fibres then recongregate within the occipital lobe cortex (see Fig. 13.1).

## Horizontal eye movement

Horizontal eye movement is mediated via the para median pontine reticular formation (PPRF) in the pons. This nucleus lies in the pons adjacent to the sixth nerve nucleus. The PPRF also coordinates signals originating from the vestibular system, frontal and occipital lobes (see Fig. 13.2). Communicating fibres run from the PPRF to the contralateral third nerve nucleus via the medial longitudinal fasciculus (MLF). Effectively the contralateral medial rectus activity is driven at the same time as the ipsilateral lateral rectus; thus we have 'comitant', i.e. linked, eye movement.

## Vertical eye movement

Vertical eye movement is mediated higher up the brain stem in the rostral interstitial (ri) MLF in the upper midbrain. The communication is via posterior commisure fibres which run behind the aqueduct of Sylvius. These fibres extend to both third nerve nuclei and drive vertical gaze.

## Autonomic control of the pupil

The pupil size is controlled by the autonomic nervous system (there is both parasympathetic and sympathetic innervation).

## Parasympathetic nervous system

The parasympathetic fibres originate in the Edinger–Westphal (EW) nucleus which sits adjacent to the third nerve nucleus. Fibres (10%) from the optic tract synapse in the EW nucleus. Fibres from the EW nucleus run with the third nerve and innervate the ciliary muscle and constrictor pupillae (see Fig. 13.3).

## Sympathetic nervous system

The sympathetic fibres innervate the dilator pupillae, Müller's muscle (in lid), lacrimal glands and orbital vessels.

## PUPILLARY DISORDERS

The pupil reacts (gets smaller) to light and convergent stimulus. Light induces pupillary constriction through the light reflex (mediated through the optic nerve (afferent) and parasympathetic fibres (efferent) (see Fig. 13.3). The near reflex is a triad of convergence, accommodation (near focusing) and miosis. The near reflex is mediated through the parasympathetic system; however, the centre mediating the response is poorly defined, thus some conditions affecting the parasympathetic fibres between the pretectal nucleus and Edinger–Westphal nucleus lead to 'light-near dissociation', i.e. they can still accommodate but cannot react to light. This is classically seen with Argyll Robertson pupils in syphilis and Parinaud's (dorsal midbrain) syndrome.

*Abnormal pupils.* Ask the patient when the abnormal pupil is noted, for example in bright or dim light. The large pupil in bright light and the small pupil in dim light is usually the abnormal pupil. This is helpful prior to formally testing direct, consensual pupil response and relative afferent pupil defects.

## Specific conditions affecting the pupil

Before considering a pathological cause of anisocoria it must be remembered that up to 10% of the population have physiological anisocoria (pupil difference >2 mm that is constant in light or dark conditions).

## Small pupils

### Horner's syndrome

This is characterized by the classic clinical triad of PAM (ptosis, anhidrosis, miosis), or for multiple choice questions try PACME(H)N:

- **P**tosis (slight due to paralysis of Müllers muscle).
- **A**nhidrosis (ipsilateral decreased sweating in post-ganglionic lesion).
- **C**iliospinal reflex (lost; a rarely known vestigial reflex).
- **M**iosis.
- **E**nophthalmos (apparent; not true if lid elevated by 1 mm).
- **H**eterochromia (in congenital cases).

A painful (i.e. headache) Horner's syndrome is an emergency and the patient should be referred fore investigation of a carotid artery dissection.

*Diagnosis and differentiation of Horner's syndrome.* If there is doubt about the diagnosis 10% cocaine drops are instilled in both eyes, the normal pupil will dilate. To differentiate pre- and post-ganglionic lesions 1% hydroxyamphetamine drops are used; this will dilate a pre-ganglionic Horner's pupil but not a post-ganglionic lesion.

*Other investigations.*

- Physical examination specifically looking for supraclavicular lymph nodes, thyroid enlargement or a neck mass.
- Chest X-ray (to identify lung tumour/mass).
- CT or MRI imaging of brain, midbrain or thorax.
- MRA may be indicated if carotid dissection is suspected.

### Argyll Robertson pupil (ARP)

This is a small, irregular pupil that reacts poorly to light. The near reflex is intact.

Argyll Robertson pupil (ARP) – **A**ccomodation **R**eflex is **P**reserved.

Argyll Robertson pupil is due to tertiary syphilis and an appropriate work-up (i.e. FTA-Abs testing) should be performed.

Treatment is dependant on the presence of active disease.

Other ocular manifestations of syphilis should be sought, such as:

- Interstitial keratitis.
- Chorioretinitis.

### Other causes of small pupils

- Use of miotic drops (e.g. pilocarpine in glaucoma patients).
- Due to posterior synechiae in iritis patients.
- Drug use, e.g. opiates.

### Large pupils

A dilated pupil is a common referral to ophthalmic emergency departments and is usually due to inadvertent pharmacological dilation which should be sought on history. It can also be a marker for serious conditions such as an intracerebral aneurysm or haemorrhage causing a third nerve palsy.

### Adie's pupil

Patients present with a dilated pupil and often blurred vision. This may come on after a viral illness which affects the ciliary ganglion. There is a very slow reaction to light and slow reaction to accommodation.

If there is associated loss of deep tendon reflexes it is referred to as Holmes–Adie's syndrome. Classically the iris has vermiform movements when examined on the slit lamp. They exhibit supersensitivity (i.e. they constrict to very low concentrations (<0.1%) of pilocarpine). Chronic Adie's pupils become small and unreactive with time.

### Trauma

Following globe trauma the iris sphincter may be damaged leading to a large pupil that reacts poorly. Clinically there may be iris transillumination defects seen and angle recession on gonioscopy. These patients are at risk of developing glaucoma.

## MOTILITY DISORDERS

Motility disorders refer to any disorder of eye movement. This includes extraocular muscles (isolated nerve palsies, multiple nerve palsies or myogenic causes), brainstem lesions, central brain lesions and nystagmus.

## Third cranial nerve palsy

The third cranial nerve innervates the superior, inferior and medial recti, inferior oblique and levator palpebrae superioris (LPS), which opens the eyelid. The parasympathetic third nerve, from the Edinger–Westphal nucleus, supplies the pupil and ciliary body.

### Clinical appearance

The key discerning feature in assessing patients with third nerve palsy is the presence or absence of pupil involvement (dilated). Should the pupil be involved there is a greater likelihood of a compressive lesion (such as an aneurysm of the posterior communicating artery) and a CT scan or MRI angiogram should be attained immediately. In third nerve palsy without pupil involvement the incidence of a compressive lesion is far less and the usual cause is microvascular disease in patients over 50 years old.

A painful, pupil-involving third nerve palsy is a neurosurgical (not an ophthalmic) emergency until proven otherwise.

The affected eye is exotropic, intorted and hypotropic (i.e. 'down and out'), due to unopposed action of the fourth and sixth cranial nerves. There may be a ptosis (a droopy lid), diplopia (horizontal and vertical) due to limited ocular movements, abnormal head posture (chin elevation + face turn in direction of palsy) and dilated pupil. There may or may not be all of these features, depending on the extent of palsy (i.e. complete or incomplete palsy).

### Causes of a third nerve palsy
*Aetiology*
- Pupil-involving: compression from posterior communicating artery aneurysm, intracranial tumours, closed head trauma.
- Pupil-sparing: microvascular (ischaemia from diabetes and hypertension), giant cell arteritis, multiple sclerosis and cavernous sinus disease.

### Differential diagnosis of third nerve palsy
- Myasthenia gravis (classically a fluctuating diplopia, fatiguability).
- Orbital inflammatory lesions (e.g. orbital lymphoma, orbital myositis, thyroid eye disease).
- Chronic progressive external ophthalmoplegia.
- Midbrain disease (abnormal ocular motility, e.g. with an internuclear ophthalmoplegia looks like a medial rectus weakness).

Convergence is not possible with a third nerve palsy but is possible with brain stem disease.

### Management of third nerve palsy
Most extraocular motor nerve palsies are microvascular in origin and they usually improve spontaneously. The classic natural history is a worsening over 2 weeks with steady improvement over 4–6 months.

Patients can be managed with occlusion or special prisms on their glasses to overcome the diplopia.

For third nerve palsies due to trauma, mass lesion, or that do not fully recover, surgery can be performed (the motility should be stable for at least 6 months).

All patients should have the following tests:

- Blood pressure.
- Blood glucose.
- Erythrocyte sedimentation rate (ESR: in older patients, i.e. >70).
- Brain imaging (if patients have pupil involvement and/or are less than 50 years old (regardless of medical history) they should have cranial imaging (CT brain or magnetic resonance angiogram: MRA)).
- A tensilon test may be indicated if myasthenia gravis is suspected.

## Fourth cranial nerve palsy

Fourth nerve palsy affects the superior oblique muscle (SOM) leading to its paresis. The SOM is responsible for intorsion, abduction and downgaze. SOM is the major intorter, i.e. rotational movement around the z-axis such that the superior globe rotates medially and the inferior globe rotates laterally. The superior rectus has a limited intorting role.

### Causes
The nerve is fine with a long intracranial course and is thus susceptible to damage from head trauma. Other causes of palsy are:

- Congenital. Patients may be asymptomatic for years. They typically have large vertical fusional amplitudes, tested with a synoptophore, unlike traumatic fourth nerve palsies.
- Vascular (diabetes, hypertension).
- Demyelination.
- Tumour (intracranial).
- Giant cell arteritis.
- Aneurysm.

### Clinical features
The features/signs of a fourth nerve palsy can be quite subtle and unless specifically tested for may not be detected.

- Diplopia (on depression, mainly vertical and torsional).
- Abnormal head posture (head tilt and face turn to unaffected eye and chin depression).

- Diagnosis is made with a head tilt test (tilting the head to the ipsilateral side induces an upward movement of the globe. This is due to unopposed superior rectus action: the other intorter of the eye).

### Differential diagnosis

The differential list is the same as for a third nerve palsy (see above). Additionally the following may present like a fourth nerve palsy:

- Orbital trauma with inferior rectus entrapment.
- Skew deviation nystagmus (see nystagmus section below).

### Management

The management of fourth nerve palsy is essentially as for third nerve palsy. A baseline BP and BS and ESR should be attained. Patients >50 years old and children with an acquired fourth nerve palsy require imaging studies.

Treat the cause if possible.

Patients with microvascular fourth nerve palsies typically improve over 3–4 months. A temporary prism may be incorporated into their glasses.

Non-resolving or permanent fourth nerve palsy may be treated with muscle surgery. These patients must have stable motility for 6 months.

## Sixth cranial nerve palsy

This is probably the most commonly recognized nerve palsy and can be quite dramatic for the patient and their family. The sixth nerve innervates the lateral rectus muscle responsible for abduction of the eye.

### Causes

Causes of sixth nerve palsies depend on site of the lesion and are largely the same as those causing third and fourth nerve palsy. The sixth nerve is particularly vulnerable to damage caused by raised intracranial pressure and is therefore often described as a 'false localizing sign' because it provides no information as to the site of the lesion. Other causes include Gradenigo's syndrome, where there is a bacterial infection of the middle ear.

### Clinical features

Sixth nerve palsies are often quite apparent with an obvious ipsilateral convergent squint due to unopposed medial rectus action. This esotropia deviation is worse on distance fixation. Horizontal diplopia and abnormal head posture (face turn towards affected eye) may also be present.

In a sixth nerve palsy, diplopia is more noticeable in the distance compared to near. It is worth checking the range of eye movements and asking the patient when maximal side by side diplopia is present. The angle of the squint or esotropia is greater for distance viewing and is incomitant (i.e. the angle of the squint is greater on ipsilateral gaze).

### Management

Sixth nerve palsies are investigated as for third and sixth nerve palsies. Young patients (<50 years old) require imaging.

Treat the cause where possible. If the palsy is stable for 6 months and the patient cannot be managed conservatively with prisms, then squint surgery may be considered.

## Nystagmus

Nystagmus is repetitive involuntary to and fro oscillation of the eyes. An ophthalmological referral should be made. It may be horizontal, vertical or torsional. The most common type seen is horizontal nystagmus. Note the description of the direction of the nystagmus is based on the fast phase (jerk) component (e.g. downbeat nystagmus has a slow upward drift with a rapid downward movement). Occasionally there is no fast and slow phase, but phases of equal speed; this is pendular nystagmus.

Nystagmus on looking right and most marked in the right eye is caused by an *ipsilateral cerebellar* or *brainstem lesion* or *contralateral (i.e. left sided) vestibular lesion*.

## Types

Nystagmus can be physiological (i.e. may be induced in normal individuals) or pathological (i.e. exist as a specific entity or part of an associated condition).

### Physiological nystagmus

In certain situations or conditions it is normal to have mild nystagmus.

- Caloric testing refers to the instillation of warm and/or cold water into the ear of patients to induce a nystagmus.
- Gaze evoked nystagmus. It is normal to have a mild nystagmus on extreme left or right gaze. When testing eye movements with nystagmus, just move the eye about 30° from the midline.

### Congenital nystagmus

Congenital nystagmus is seen in children up to 1 year old. Initially they have horizontal pendular movement and later acquire the 'jerk' component.

This may be inherited as an X-linked or autosomal recessive feature or as feature of poor vision in the child as seen in:

- Ocular albinism.
- Retinal dystrophies.
- Optic nerve hypoplasia.

Congenital nystagmus is an indicator of poor vision in a child and referral should be made to an ophthalmologist.

*Management.* Children with congenital nystagmus should be monitored for refractive error (usually present), amblyopia and strabismus. Each component should be addressed to attain and preserve the maximal visual potential for the child.

In the presence of nystagmus, check visual acuity with both eyes together, not individually, or blur one eye (e.g. with a frosted lens). Total occlusion induces increased contralateral nystagmus and gives a falsely low measure of acuity.

### Acquired nystagmus

Unlike congenital nystagmus patients, those with recent onset nystagmus may complain of oscillopsia, i.e. 'everything moves around'. This may be seen with:

- Recent visual loss (e.g. trauma).
- Toxicity (e.g. alcohol, phenothiazines or Wernicke's encephalopathy).
- Cerebral disease (stroke, MS or tumour).

*Management.* Patients presenting with recent onset nystagmus need to have:

- Full history.
- Full physical exam (especially neurological system).

- Toxicity screen if history is indicative.
- Neurological imaging.

Once identified, the cause should be treated, as appropriate.

### Associated with neurological disease

The presence of nystagmus, particularly a new onset of nystagmus, should alert you to possible underlying disease. Some key examples of the nystagmus type and their associations are:

- Convergence retraction nystagmus, i.e. the eyes converge and are drawn back into the orbit on upgaze (this is indicative of dorsal midbrain disease, e.g. Parinaud's syndrome).
- Downbeat nystagmus, i.e. the jerk component is down (this is indicative of lesions at the foramen magnum, e.g. Arnold–Chiari malformation).
- Upbeat nystagmus (indicates possible cerebellar lesions).
- See-saw, i.e. an alternating vertical nystagmus (possible chiasmal lesion).

## OPTIC NERVE DISEASE

A number of clinical features should be sought if optic nerve dysfunction is suspected. They include:

- Reduced visual acuity.
- Abnormal visual field (constricted in glaucoma, caecocentral (scotoma between central fixation and the blind spot) field loss).
- Reduced pupillary response (afferent pupil defect).
- Poor colour vision (tested with Ishihara plates or red desaturation test).

## Clinical features

When examining an optic nerve the following features of the disc should be observed and commented on:

- Neuroretinal rim.
- Swelling (may just be apparent as a hyperaemic disc initially).
- Haemorrhages.
- Atrophy.
- Notches.
- Cup/disc ratio (CDR).
- Glaucoma.
- Disc vessels.
- Retinal vessels.
- Peripapillary (area adjacent to the disc) zones.

Based on these features an optic neuropathy may be classified as:

- *Optic neuritis* (inflammation).
- *Retrobulbar neuritis*. This is the most common, with the disc appearing normal in the acute stage of the process; it becomes atrophic with time (i.e. pale neuroretinal rim 2 months later). This is often associated with demyelinating disease.
- *Papillitis* is disc inflammation. Haemorrhages and swelling are observed on the disc itself. This may be a presentation of demyelination but is more commonly seen with viral infections in children or in young type I diabetic patients.
- *Ischaemic optic neuropathy* (ION: due to an infarction of the optic nerve head). This may be arteritic (i.e. associated with giant cell arteritis: GCA), non-arteritic (embolic) or autoimmune (systemic lupus erythematosis: SLE). The nerve is acutely swollen with haemorrhages.
- *Compressive optic neuropathy* (presents as optic atrophy and progressive visual loss). These patients may have other signs of orbital (proptosis) or intracranial (headache, contralateral disc swelling, sixth nerve palsy) disease.
- *Traumatic optic neuropathy* (following head trauma which may be trivial patients can experience visual loss due to nerve compression from bony fragments or swelling and inflammation). The prognosis for vision is poor.
- *Hereditary optic neuropathy* (rare), e.g. dominant optic atrophy or Leber's optic atrophy.
- *Toxic neuropathies* (e.g. ethanol or vitamin $B_{12}$ deficiency).
- *Retinal disease* (patients with extensive retinal disease, e.g. retinitis pigmentosa or a laser ablated retina, will have optic atrophy also).
- *Radiation optic neuropathy* (may be seen in patients that have received facial, orbital or cranial radiotherapy. Onset is usually delayed >1 year).

## Management

If an optic neuropathy is suspected the following investigations should be performed:

- ESR (especially in a patient >70 years old with ION to exclude GCA).
- FBC.
- Visual field test (identify caecocentral field loss or associated bitemporal loss seen with pituitary tumours).

- Vitamin $B_{12}$ and folate levels.
- Autoantibody screen.
- Orbital and brain imaging if a compressive optic neuropathy is suspected.
- Temporal artery biopsy is performed in cases of suspected GCA.

Once an underlying diagnosis is made appropriate treatment can be implemented.

> Once optic nerve dysfunction has occurred it does not recover fully. The visual acuity of optic neuritis patients usually returns but there is a permanent defect in contrast and colour vision.

## OPTIC DISC SWELLING

Optic disc swelling is a common referral to ophthalmologists and there are many causes. They can be broadly divided into:

- Intracranial (papilloedema).
- Ocular.
- Systemic.

> *Optic disc swelling is not the same as papilloedema.* Papilloedema is bilateral swollen discs due to raised intracranial pressure (ICP). This is an important concept medico-legally when counselling patients about possible differential diagnoses.

## Papilloedema

Papilloedema is bilateral disc swelling due to raised intracranial pressure (ICP).

### Symptoms

These patients may be asymptomatic or present with one or more of the following:

- Visual obscurations (transient loss of vision on standing up).
- Headache, nausea, vomiting or double vision (sixth nerve palsy).

- Reduced visual acuity.
- Reduced colour vision.

### Signs

The signs of papilloedema are:

- Bilateral swollen hyperaemic discs.
- Disc haemorrhages.
- Visual field defect (specific if lesion affects optic pathway, enlarged blind spot initially or constricted field if papilloedema is longstanding).
- Absent spontaneous venous pulsations at the disc.
- 'Champagne cork' appearance in chronic papilloedema.
- Optic atrophy.

### Causes

The common causes are:

- An intracranial tumour.
- Benign intracranial hypertension (BIH), an idiopathic condition affecting young overweight females, classically). They usually have a normal CT scan (+/− dilated ventricles).
- Meningitis (patients have a fever +/− neck stiffness).
- Brain abscess (patients are moribund with a high fever).
- Sagittal sinus thrombosis.

The differential diagnosis for papilloedema is lengthy and is covered in the sections below on ocular and systemic causes of optic disc swelling.

### Investigation

The investigations required are:

- Urgent CT scan to assess presence of a mass lesion.
- MRI scan may also be indicated to aid specific diagnosis.
- Lumbar punctures (high opening pressures in the presence of a normal CT scan may indicate BIH).

Other tests to consider to rule out differential causes include:

- Blood sugar.
- Blood pressure.
- Thyroid function test (orbital disease).
- Tests for uveitis (see uveitis chapter).

The management of papilloedema is directed towards the underlying cause and its treatment.

## Ocular causes

Many intrinsic ocular conditions may lead to disc swelling and are covered in more detail in other parts of the book. They include:

- *Central retinal vein occlusion* (retinal haemorrhages are also present in all four retinal fundus quadrants).
- *Uveitis* (particularly with posterior uveitis or scleritis; there may be contiguous optic nerve inflammation and swelling).
- *Ocular hypotony* (if the intraocular pressure is low the nerve may swell).
- *Anterior ischaemic optic neuropathy* (AION).
- *Optic disc infiltration* (can be granulomatous as in sarcoidosis or malignant as with leukaemia or metastases).
- *Leber's optic neuropathy* (affects men owing to mitochondrial inheritance).
- *Optic nerve tumours* (e.g. glioma or meningioma; disc is swollen if there is rapid growth).
- *Orbital thyroid disease* (due to acute inflammation and swelling of the orbit).

## Systemic causes

The most common and serious systemic condition associated with disc swelling is hypertension. Disc swelling indicates grade IV (or severe) hypertensive retinopathy and urgent treatment is required.

Other causes include:

- Anaemia.
- Uraemia.
- Hypoxia.

Thus investigation of disc swelling should include blood pressure measurement and a full blood count.

## Pseudopapilloedema

There are a few conditions that can give the appearance of a prominent swollen disc, known as pseudopapilloedema. None of these conditions actually lead to nerve fibre layer swelling (clinically seen as blurring of the disc margin). Causes of pseudopapilloedema include:

- Hyperopia (small eyes are often associated with small 'crowded discs').
- Disc drusen (small hyaline deposits giving a 'lumpy' appearance to the disc).
- Myelinated nerve fibres (an embryological remnant due to incomplete demyelination of the nerve fibre layer). Present in 1% of UK population.

## CHIASMAL DISEASE

### Symptoms

Disorders near the chiasm can affect the visual system, with patients complaining of:

- Blurred vision.
- Constricted field (bitemporal hemianopia – 'I bump into things doctor').
- Headache.

### Ocular signs of chiasmal disease

- Bitemporal hemianopia.
- See-saw nystagmus.

### Causes

- Pituitary tumour (compresses from below, thus supero-temporal field affected first).
- Meningioma.
- Craniopharyngioma (compresses from above, thus infero-temporal field affected first). Usually seen in younger patients.

#### Types of pituitary tumour

##### Adenomas
A detailed description of pituitary adenomas can be found in the Crash Course book on Medicine.

##### Pituitary apoplexy
This is a rare and potentially life-threatening condition. It is due to haemorrhage into a pituitary adenoma, often occurring in pregnancy. Patients present with severe headache +/– multiple motor nerve palsies.

#### Investigation of pituitary tumours

##### Imaging
- CT scan.
- MRI scan (better at detailing the relationship of the enlarged gland to the surrounding structure).

##### Endocrine tests
- Serum prolactin.
- FSH.

- TSH.
- Growth hormone.

These tests help identify the cell type in the tumour, explain systemic effects of the tumour (e.g. acromegaly) and monitor response to treatment.

### Treatment

#### Pharmacological
Bromocriptine is used to treat prolactinomas.

#### Surgery
Patients may have their tumours removed by a trans-sphenoidal approach.

#### Radiotherapy
*Meningiomas* are slowly growing, histologically benign tumours which may affect any part of the meninges. The presentation of these tumours depends on their location:

- Tuberculum sellae (ipsilateral optic atrophy and contralateral junctional scotoma).
- Sphenoidal ridge meningioma (optic nerve compression and atrophy).
- Olfactory groove meningioma.
- Optic nerve meningioma (may affect any part of the nerve with ipsilateral optic nerve compression).

These lesions are treated by resection when accessible, with or without radiotherapy.

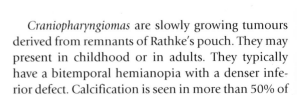

Any newly documented visual field defect and/or optic atrophy should be imaged to exclude a mass lesion.

*Craniopharyngiomas* are slowly growing tumours derived from remnants of Rathke's pouch. They may present in childhood or in adults. They typically have a bitemporal hemianopia with a denser inferior defect. Calcification is seen in more than 50% of these lesions.

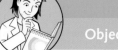

# Ophthalmic examination techniques

## 14

**Objectives**

You should be able to:

- Describe the five methods used to test optic nerve function.
- Understand and perform: visual acuity and direct ophthalmoscopy.
- Perform a test to identify a relative afferent pupil defect and understand its implication.
- Describe two methods to test for colour vision defects.
- Test eye movements and describe the nerve supply of extraocular muscles.

This chapter discusses how to perform a thorough ophthalmic examination. **A**cuity, **F**ields, **R**elative afferent pupil defect (RAPD), **R**ed colour, **O**ptic disc appearance and eye **M**ovements are covered (ACRONYM: AFFROM). It should be noted that all the tests do not need to be done on every patient: the history should direct you to which tests you need to concentrate on.

> There are five main tests of the optic nerve (ACRONYM: AFRRO): **A**cuity, **F**ields, **R**elative afferent pupil defect (RAPD), **R**ed colour and **O**ptic disc appearance.

## VISUAL ACUITY

## Measuring visual acuity

Visual acuity is the single most important part of the examination yet is the one piece of information that non-ophthalmic practitioners leave out. This is largely due to unfamiliarity with the Snellen chart. Distance vision is checked with these charts at 6 m (20 feet in the USA). The letters gradually decrease in size in a very specific way that relates to the angle it subtends at the subject's macula. Remember that we are looking for the best corrected vision and so ask the patient if they wear glasses for distance and to use them. If the vision is 6/9 or worse then you should test the vision again using a pinhole (this should be used with glasses if the patient wears glasses). The Snellen chart is traditionally made to test vision at 6 m, although there are reduced distance charts for 3 m which are commonly used in undergraduate examinations (Figs 14.1, 14.2).

Encourage the subject to try the smaller letters, even if they are not sure. This is important to record the best possible vision. If the patient reads part of a line then a minus sign is used for the number of letters missed on the line or a plus sign added to the line above. An example would be, if a patient reads all of the letters 6/12 line and three numbers on 6/9 line this would be recorded as 6/12 + 3 or 6/9 – 3. Measuring visual acuity is summarized in Fig. 14.3.

> A patient with no perception to light (NPL) and no red reflex on opthalmoscopy is likely to have an artificial or prosthetic eye (like Peter Falk, aka Columbo). So always test visual acuity in both eyes INDIVIDUALLY and do not assume good vision in one eye means good vision in the second eye.

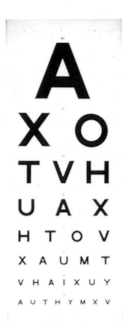

**Fig. 14.1** Snellen chart. The largest letter A, at the top of the chart, is labelled 60. Similarly, the lines below are labelled 36, 24, 18, 12, 9, 6 and 5. Some charts have lines designated 4 and 3 which can be read by people with better than 6/6 vision.

## Recording vision

The recording of vision is confusing but is quite simple when you think about it.

Each record has two numbers. The first is the distance (in metres) that the chart is read at – normally 6 m. If the patient can not see any letters at 6 m, then you would move them closer to 3 m and then 1 m. This number is the top number of the fraction used (e.g. **6**/6).

The second is the distance (in metres) at which a normally sighted person could read the number (if moved away from the chart). This number is the bottom number of the fraction and 6/**6** is the line traditionally for normal vision. Therefore, 6/60 would be the line a normal sighted patient could see at 60 m and a poor sighted patient see at 6 m.

How to record visual acuity is summarized in Fig. 14.4.

> *The vision ruler.* Remember a scale of vision (like a ruler from 0 to 30 centimetres).
>
> 6/5, 6,6, 6/60, 3/60, 1/60, CF, HM, PL, NPL
>
> Test each eye twice: essentially you need to choose one of these options and then repeat with a pinhole. This 'vision ruler' will remind you to write 6/60 rather than 60/6, which can be a reason to be failed in undergraduate OSCE exams. It serves as a reminder to bring the subject at 3 m and then 1 m if 6/60 cannot be read. Finally, it reminds us about the possibility of the prosthetic eye when NPL is encountered.

## Testing near vision

After measuring distance vision you should record near vision using a near vision chart such as the Faculty

**Fig.14.2** A pinhole only allows through a central ray of light (dotted line) to the retina. In this example of a myope, with a longer 'rugby ball' shaped eye compared to the normal, round, 'football' shaped eye, the image is anterior to the retina and needs spectacles to push the image more posteriorly on to the retina. Therefore, if the subject's acuity is improved by using a pinhole, then some of their poor visual performance is due to refractive error (i.e. they are either long- or short-sighted).

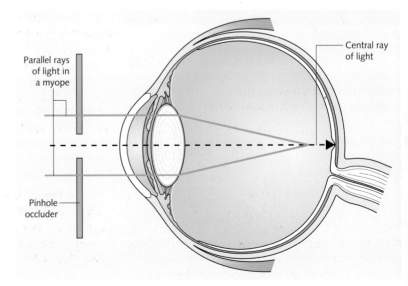

Parallel rays of light in a myope

Pinhole occluder

Central ray of light

**Fig. 14.3** Measuring visual acuity: summary

| | |
|---|---|
| **Patient** | Sit patient on chair 6 m from the Snellen chart (or 3 m if using the reduced Snellen chart) |
| **Doctor** | Introduce yourself and explain the procedure<br>Ask the patient if they are wearing contact lenses<br>Ask the patient if they are glasses for distance – if so ask them to put them on<br>Warn the patient their left eye is to be covered<br>Occlude left eye (do not get them to close this eye) |
| | **First measurement (with distance spectacles, contact lens or unaided)**<br>Ask the patient to read the letters (line by line) on the chart, starting from the top towards the bottom |
| | **Second measurement – pinhole test**<br>Ask the patient to hold the pinhole in front of their right eye<br>Ask the patient to look through the small hole and read the lowest line of letters that they find manageable<br>Record the results |
| | **Repeat the test for the left eye (two measurements) by occluding the right eye** |
| | **If the patient cannot read the top letter of the chart at 6 m (i.e. 6/60)**<br>• Reduce distance to 3 m then 2 m then 1 m (this is recorded as 3/60, 2/60, 1/60)<br>• If unable to read top line at 1 m, test in turn ability to count fingers, to see hand movements, to perceive light. This is recorded as CF, HM and PL respectively. If they cannot perceive light it is recorded as NPL |

**Fig. 14.4** How to record visual acuity: summary

**Visual acuity is recorded as a fraction**
The numerator is the distance from the chart in meters
The denominator is the number written on the chart
i.e. 6 (metres) / 12 (line reached on chart)

**The acuity recorded must reflect how this measure was achieved**
If glasses were worn the number is followed by – C gl
If glasses were not worn (but usually are) the number is followed by – S gl
If contact lenses were worn, the number is followed by – C CL
If acuity is achieved by pinhole, the number is followed by – C PH

*Example:*

| | |
|---|---|
| R. eye 6/12 C gl | L. eye 6/9 C gl |
| 6/6 C PH | 6/6 C PH |

**Fig. 14.5** Testing near vision: summary

| | |
|---|---|
| **Patient** | Put on the glasses you use *for reading*. Hold Test Type book at a comfortable distance and read the smallest print possible |
| **Doctor** | Cover each eye in turn, warning the patient first (do not simply get them to close eye)<br>Record the result using the prefix letter N |

*Example:*
R. eye N5     L. eye N6

*Note:* Newspaper print is usually N8 and small headlines are N12. (*This may be useful for a bedside assessment*)

## DIRECT OPHTHALMOSCOPY

Direct ophthalmoscopy is taught in all medical school curricula but it is a very difficult skill to acquire and is only done well with a considerable amount of practice.

Examination using an ophthalmoscope (Fig. 14.6) with a patient or a model head is described in Figs 14.8 and 14.9. Anterior ocular structures can also be examined. This is often omitted from undergraduate OSCEs, but consider +20 D for cornea and +15 D for iris.

There are five optic discs that you should recognize for MBBS: normal, cupped (glaucoma), pale (optic atrophy), new vessels at disc (diabetes or CRVO) and swollen optic discs (Fig. 14.7).

of Ophthalmologists Test Type N Chart. To perform this test the following points should be noted:

• Test reading at 30 cm using appropriate (reading) glasses.
• Test one eye at a time.
• Smallest writing readable? N5, N8, N12?

For assessing vision in children, picture tests are used, such as the Sheridan–Gardiner test. This type of test can also be done with illiterate patients or with patients who do not know the English alphabet. Testing vision in very small children is difficult and involves a careful history, watching the child perform visual tasks, covering the better eye and using special test types to get an objective measurement. These tests are usually done by orthoptists and paediatric ophthalmologists.

Testing near vision is summarized in Fig. 14.5.

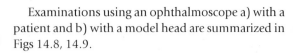

If swollen disc is observed then think of 'Surgical sieve' causes: Vascular, Infective, Inflammatory, Neoplastic, etc. In this manner you should ask the patient systematic and direct questions to elicit any of the following causes: AION, CRVO, papilloedema, TB granuloma, sarcoid granuloma, optic nerve glioma, meningioma, etc.

Examinations using an ophthalmoscope a) with a patient and b) with a model head are summarized in Figs 14.8, 14.9.

It takes 2 months to develop a pale or atrophic disc – i.e. an old CNS lesion. So current neurological signs (e.g. cerebellar signs or recent hemiparesis) with optic atrophy may suggest two CNS lesions separated in time and place, with the diagnosis of multiple sclerosis.

## VISUAL FIELDS

Visual field testing is a crucial part of the ophthalmic exam, particularly if neurological disease is suspected. See Fig. 13.1 for the specific field defect for each lesion. The type of visual field assessment corresponds to the visual acuity. This is why so many different types of field testing are encountered: counting fingers, wiggly fingers, red and white pins. If acuity is just count fingers or hand motions, just test the quadrants grossly with counting fingers or finger movement respectively. Compare the patient's visual field with your own (assuming yours is normal!). Always consider whether the defect fits a pattern. What could the cause be?

### Screening visual field test

Ask the patient, with both eyes open, to look at your eyes. Can they see your face? Any part missing? Place both hands out wide, midway between you and the patient, just within the outer limits of your temporal field. Ask the patient to point to the finger that moves. Move the right index finger, then the left, and then both index fingers together. If only one fingers is seen moving rather than both left and right hand index fingers, then 'sensory inattention' or a right parietal lobe lesion is present. Fig. 14.10 shows the visual field, central fixation and blind spot.

Then move on to testing the eyes individually.

### Testing eyes individually

- Sit opposite the patient, 1 m away, with your eyes level with the patient's.
- Examiner closes right eye, while patient closes or covers left eye.

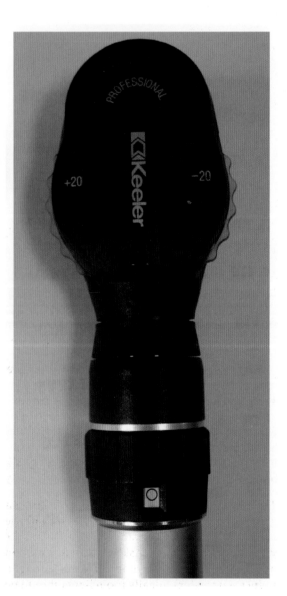

**Fig. 14.6** Direct ophthalmoscope.

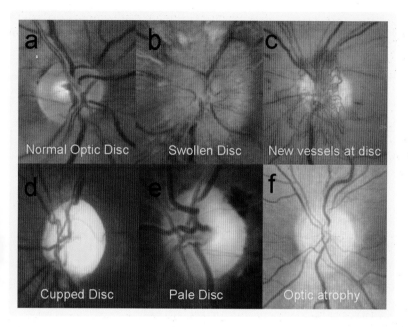

**Fig. 14.7** There are five optic discs to remember and distinguish from each other: (A) normal, (B) swollen, (C) new vessels at disc, (D) cupped, and (E & F) pale optic discs or optic atrophy.

- Look into each other's open eye.
- Consider performing all three steps below, in the set order, regularly to get into a routine ready for examinations.

1. Test with counting fingers in each of the four quadrants of the visual field (Fig. 14.11). One eye at a time at 0.5 m from the patient. Gross hemianopia, quadrantianopia or altitudinal defect will be identified at this stage.
2. Test central 30° with red pin and then in each of the four quadrants of visual field (see Fig. 14.11). One eye at a time at 0.5 m from the patient. Ask whether the red pin looks red, pink, grey or black. This is a very useful way to detect red desaturation, an early sign of optic nerve disease, or subtle field defects and scotomas during field testing. The blind spot can be identified by slowly moving the red pin temporally from fixation centre, and the patient reveals to the examiner when the red pin disappears and then reappears. The pin can be placed along the centre of this blind zone and then moved vertically to map out the size of the blind spot. Blind spots are enlarged in optic neuritis or swollen discs.
3. White pin or finger wiggling movements test peripheral field, again at 0.5 m from the patient. This is a rather insensitive manner of field

testing but excellent when the visual acuity is hand movements or in conditions with tunnel vision such as advanced glaucoma or retinitis pigmentosa.

To make the test easier the following points will help:

- Make sure patient always looks at your eye.
- Try to avoid wiggly fingers or hand movements visual field testing. It is commonly used, generally insensitive and hence bad practice.
- Make sure your hand always lies half-way between you and the patient (Fig. 14.12). There is a tendency to move it towards the patient as you move it inwards.
- To further delineate defects always move the pin from non-seeing area to seeing area (see Fig. 14.12).

## PUPILS

To asses pupils you need to understand the light and near pathways and reflexes. You should use a good pen torch (nice and bright). Introduce yourself to the patient. Ask the patient to fix on a distant target (this is important so as not to induce near reflex). Ideally room lights should be dimmed.

**Fig. 14.8** Examination using an ophthalmoscope with a patient

| Patient | Sit on a chair (pupils, ideally, should be dilated so a darkened room facilitates the examination) |
|---|---|
| Doctor | Switch on the ophthalmoscope<br>Shine the light on your hand and select a large aperture (unless small pupil)<br>Rotate the focusing wheel and set it on zero<br>Keep your index finger on the focusing wheel<br>Ask the patient to remove their glasses (not contact lenses)<br>Try to keep wearing your own spectacles or contact lenses rather than taking them off<br>Ask the patient to look at a distant object straight ahead<br>Warn the patient that you will shine a light into their eye |
| | To examine the **Right** eye, hold the ophthalmoscope in your **Right** hand and use your **Right** eye. (**'Right, Right, Right'**) |
| | Stand at arm's length from the patient (gently rest your other hand on the patient's forehead with your thumb on their eyebrow)<br>Look through the ophthalmoscope and illuminate the pupil<br>The pupil should glow orange-red. This is the **red reflex**<br>Comment whether the red reflex is absent or present<br>While looking at the red reflex move towards your thumb resting on the patient's eyebrow and focus on the retina (by rotating the focusing wheel) |
| | Examine the retina:<br>Locate the **optic disc** → assess the colour and the margins (e.g. normal, pale or swollen), any abnormal other findings (e.g. cupping or new vessels at disc)<br>Follow the major vessels → assess tortuosity and dilation<br>Locate the fovea by asking the patient to look at the light → assess presence of exudates, haemorrhages, drusen or atrophy<br>Examine the peripheral retina by asking the patient to look up, down, left and right → assess pigmentation |
| | Proceed to examine the **Left** eye in similar manner. (**'Left, Left, Left'**). This is the more difficult eye to examine. So practise!! |

*Notes: The retinal view is magnified × 15 by the lenses of the ophthalmoscope and only a small field is viewed with the ophthalmoscope beam. Therefore it is important to get as close as possible to the patient's eye/eyebrow*
*The view of the retina is affected by the patient's refraction*
*When examining a myopic patient the retinal image is enlarged so there is only a small field of view*

Observe the pupils:

- Round or irregular?
- Equal size (unequal pupils called anisocoria)?
- Associated ptosis (Horner's/third nerve palsy), or strabismus (third nerve palsy)?

Bring the light in from outside the visual axis. There are four components to the pupil examination:

- Direct light reflex.
- Indirect (consensual) light reflex.
- Swinging (Marcus Gunn) reflex.
- Near reflex.

## Direct response

Only observe the illuminated eye. You should observe for constriction and comment whether it is brisk or sluggish and if the reaction is big or small. No response may suggest an absolute afferent pupil defect (seen for example in optic nerve transection) or an efferent defect (seen for example in third nerve palsy). This should then be repeated for the fellow eye.

**Fig. 14.9** Using an ophthalmoscope with a model head

A darkened room facilitates the examination

Try to wear your own spectacles or contact lenses rather than taking them off

Switch on the ophthalmoscope (green button and rotate collar)

Shine the light on your hand and select a large aperture (next to target/graticule)

Rotate the focusing wheel and set it on zero

To examine the **Right** eye, hold the ophthalmoscope in your **Right** hand and use your **Right** eye. ('**Right, Right, Right**')

Stand at arm's length from the model head/patient (gently rest your other hand on the patient's forehead with your thumb on their eyebrow)

Look through the ophthalmoscope and illuminate the pupil

The pupil should glow orange-red. This is the **red reflex**

Comment whether the red reflex is absent or present

If model head is back illuminated with table lamp then switch off the direct ophthalmoscope

While looking at the red reflex, move towards your thumb resting on the model head

Examine the retina:

Locate the **optic disc** → assess the colour and the margins (e.g. normal, pale or swollen), any abnormal other findings (e.g. cupping or new vessels at disc)

Follow the major vessels → assess tortuosity and dilation

Locate the macula → assess presence of exudates, haemorrhages

Then proceed to examine the **Left** eye in similar manner ('**Left, Left, Left**')

## Indirect (consensual) light response

Only observe the non-illuminated eye. The light is shone in one eye and the pupil response in the fellow eye is observed. You may need to increase the background illumination to perform this test in patients with dark irides. This test helps to discriminate an efferent from an afferent defect. The consensual response is intact in a eye with an afferent (i.e. optic nerve) problem.

The following points should be noted and will help you understand the pupil responses:

- The efferent output is bilateral (at the Edinger–Westphal nucleus) following unilateral afferent input.
- If there is no absolute afferent pupillary defect (rarely seen, occurs in optic nerve transaction or other severe optic nerve damage), look for a relative afferent pupillary defect (RAPD).

## Swinging (Marcus Gunn) light reflex

This test is used to test for a relative afferent pupil defect, i.e. the transmission of impulses through one optic nerve is slower than the other. This can be due to ('surgical sieve') diseases such as infection (tuberculous granuloma), inflammation (optic neuritis, sarcoid granuloma), neoplasm (optic nerve meningioma or glioma), trauma (fractured bone spicule) involving or compressing the optic nerve.

**Fig. 14.10** Visual fields.

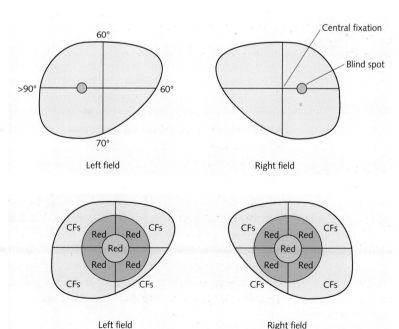

**Fig. 14.11** An example of visual fields documented in notes. Note that the left field is recorded to the left side of the page, as opposed to ophthalmic examinations which have right eye findings on the left side of the page.

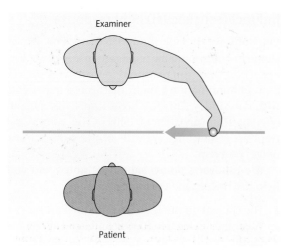

Examiner

Patient

**Fig. 14.12** Movement of a pin into the examiner's and the patient's visual field.

Shine the light to one eye for 3 seconds then swing quickly to other eye. Observe any pupil movement, while counting to 3. NO pupil movement implies NO RAPD. If there is any change in pupil size then there is a RAPD present. If bigger pupil occurs, while counting to 3 seconds, then the side of the RAPD is on the illuminated side. If the pupil becomes smaller, while counting to 3 seconds, then the RAPD is on the opposite side to the illuminated eye. Repeat the steps until you are happy that they are normal or a true RAPD has been detected.

Relative afferent pupil defect (RAPD) – remember that 'B'IG pupil(s) occur, while counting to 3 seconds, when illuminating the 'B'AD optic nerve side (i.e. the side of the RAPD).

### Near reflex

Focus on a distance object then ask to look at a near target (e.g. policeman or budgie on lollipop stick) at approximately 15 cm. Watch for constriction of pupils and convergence (the other two elements of the accommodative response).

Light-near dissociation, where pupils react to accommodation but not to light stimulus, occurs in Argyll Robertson (tertiary syphilis) pupil, Adie's pupil and Parinaud syndrome.

## COLOUR VISION

Colour vision testing is very important in assessing the integrity of optic nerve function. Red is the first colour to be diminished by optic nerve lesions and is often affected before acuity. The most commonly used test is the Ishihara colour plates (Fig. 14.13). This test was originally designed for checking for congenital colour vision deficits such as red/green colour loss, which affects 3–5% of males.

If Ishihara plates are not available get the patient to compare the appearance of a bright red target, such as a hat pin ('if good eye is 100% what percent brightness does the affected eye see?' offer choices 100, 80, 50 or 20%); this gives a good impression of 'red desaturation', an indicator of reduced optic nerve function.

## EYE MOVEMENTS

Before assessing a patient it is important to know the definitions used in relation to eye movement. These are listed in Fig. 14.14.

Introduce yourself to the patient. *Observe* the eyes – are there any clues to underlying cause and/or co-existent problems?

- Ptosis/'down and out' eye – third nerve palsy.
- Proptosis – orbital disease, e.g. thyroid eye disease, orbital myositis, orbital tumour.
- Nystagmus – internuclear ophthalmoplegia.

*Check the corneal light reflex.* Ask the patient to look straight ahead at a pen torch. Are both eyes looking in the same direction? Observe corneal light reflexes (Hirschberg's test). Asymmetry demonstrates subtle deviation. It can also help rule out a pseudostrabismus, where eyes appear to be deviated but the corneal reflex is symmetrical (e.g. broad epicanthal folds and wide interpupillary distance).

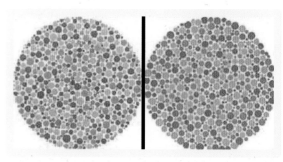

**Fig. 14.13** Ishihara test plates have numbers hidden among coloured dots.

**Fig. 14.14** Definitions used in relation to eye movement

| Term | Meaning |
|------|---------|
| Vergences | Binocular movement of the eyes in opposite directions |
| Convergence | Eyes move medially |
| Divergence | Eyes move laterally (away from each other) |
| Diplopia | Double vision (true double vision is binocular and due to a misalignment of the eyes) |
| Tropia | Manifest deviation |
| Exotropia/esotropia | Deviation away from/to midline |
| Phoria | Latent deviation |
| Exophoria/esophoria | Deviation away from/to midline |

It is beyond the remit of the medical student to formally assess the size of the deviation (squint angle, which is measured in prism dioptres).

## Cover test

The aim of the cover test is to determine if there is a manifest squint. Patients should be tested looking at a target at 6 m (distant) and ⅓ m (near: both with and without glasses). This assesses any difference in squint angle at near and distance.

Cover one eye and watch for movement of other eye (Figs 14.15, 14.16). If the eye was deviated, it will move to take up fixation while the other eye is covered. This may be slow if vision in the deviated eye is poor. Repeat for the other eye. If the deviated eye is covered, the other 'fixing' eye should not move.

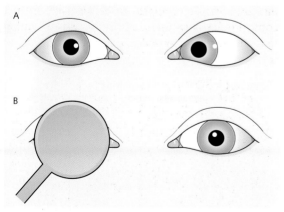

**Fig. 14.15** (A) Left convergent squint or esotropia confirmed by left corneal reflection. (B) Cover test: when covering the right eye, the left eye moves outwards to take up fixation.

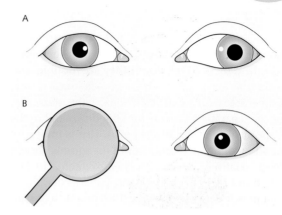

**Fig. 14.16** (A) Left divergent squint or exotropia confirmed by left corneal reflection. (B) Cover test: when covering the right eye, the left eye moves inwards to take up fixation.

## Alternate cover test

This test detects latent deviations – 'phorias' – present when binocular vision is disrupted. These are very common and are illicited by dissociating the eyes (alternate occlusion). They help assess patients, for example, with intermittent diplopia or with diplopia following illness.

Cover one eye for a few seconds then quickly move occluder to cover the other eye. Repeat covering of each eye, watching for the eye moving back to regain fixation when uncovered (Fig. 14.17). Observe for horizontal (most common) and vertical phorias.

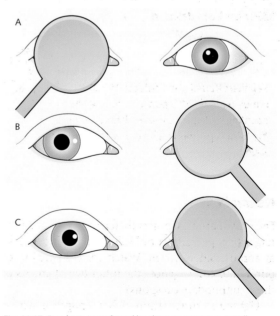

**Fig. 14.17** Exophoria is confirmed by alternate cover test. Initially the eyes are straight and not apparently deviated. (A) The right eye is covered and the left eye remains straight. (B) The occluder is moved to cover the left eye. The uncovered right eye is noted to be deviated outwards, and then (C) moves inwards to take up fixation.

# Extraocular muscle movement

Hold a pen torch at 40 cm. Ask the patient to keep their head still and follow the light with their eyes. Ask the patient to tell you if they see 'double' and where the 'maximum double vision' or image separation is (e.g. with a fourth nerve palsy the maximum image separation is while looking down and to the opposite side of the affected eye). This is indicative of an incomitant squint. Comitant squints should have a relatively full range of eye movement. Use Figs 14.18 and 14.19 to try to identify patterns of extraocular muscle deficits, following third or fourth or sixth nerve palsies.

Then move the pen torch light in an 'H' shape to examine the six cardinal positions of gaze (Figs 14.18, 14.20). The two legs of the H will isolate and test the motion of the superior/inferior rectus pair and inferior/superior oblique pair. The centre part of the H will test the medial and lateral muscles. Test to the extremes of gaze and while moving the light up and down examine for lid lag (thyroid eye disease). The lid does not normally lag behind the globe as it moves down. One should watch the eye movements and corneal light reflexes, checking for any asymmetry or double vision.

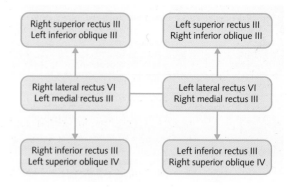

Fig. 14.20 Cardinal positions of gaze – paired extraocular muscles and their cranial nerve supply.

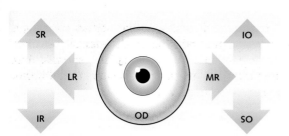

Fig. 14.18 Actions of the six extraocular muscles of the right eye. Do not confuse the direction of oblique muscle actions with their anatomical insertions.

**Eye movements**
*Unsure which eye has restricted or limited movement?* Cover one eye, then the other. Restricted or limited eye always sees the outside or peripheral image.
*Neurological or mechanical?* Does it fit a pattern consistent with a cranial nerve weakness?
*Watch for nystagmus*, but beware it can occur at extremes of gaze in a normal individual.

Fig. 14.19 Extraocular muscles, their action and cranial nerve supply

| Extraocular muscle | Action of exatrocular muscle | Cranial nerve supplying extraocular muscle |
|---|---|---|
| **SR** (superior rectus) | Elevation | |
| **IO** (inferior oblique) | Elevation and adduction | III |
| **MR** (medial rectus) | Adduction | |
| **IR** (inferior rectus) | Depression | |
| **SO** (superior oblique) | Depression and adduction | IV |
| **LR** (lateral rectus) | Abduction | VI |

A rash is an inflammatory process of the skin. It involves the dermis since this is where the blood vessels of skin are situated. There are also rashes that involve the epidermis, which give rise to particular surface changes. Therefore rashes can be grouped into those that only affect the dermis and those that affect the epidermis and dermis (Fig. 15.1). Rashes can be also divided to those that cover most of the body and those to just a localized area.

The key to making the correct diagnosis of a rash is describing and recognizing its typical features. It is also important to note the arrangement and distribution of the rash.

## DIFFERENTIAL DIAGNOSIS

### Rashes involving the epidermis

The distinguishing features of rashes that involve the epidermis are scaling, lichenification, vesicles and pustules, and alteration of pigmentation. The most well-known causes are eczema and psoriasis, and both conditions have typical characteristics, so a clinical diagnosis is relatively easy to make.

Other less common conditions that need to be considered include lichen planus, seborrhoeic dermatitis, pityriasis rosea and pityriasis vesicolor.

### Rashes involving only the dermis

A rash that only affects the dermis is identified by the lack of surface changes. The next step is to determine whether the rash is erythematous or purpuric. If the rash blanches and is palpable, then it is most likely a form of vasculitis. If, however, the rash is erythematous and generalized, the possible differential diagnoses would include drug eruptions or viral exanthems.

### Localized changes

There are many conditions that may just affect a specific part of the body. These include fungal infections, atopic eczema, contact dermatitis, psoriasis, fixed drug eruptions, and vasculitis, erythema multiforme and erythema nodosum.

### Generalized rashes

Numerous skin and systemic disorders present themselves as a generalized rash (Fig. 15.2). It is important to be able to distinguish which are benign from those that are life threatening.

Erythroderma is an example of a life-threatening condition. Although it is relatively easy to recognize, there several common causes that could have triggered the erythroderma and it is important to treat the underlying cause (Fig. 15.3).

Prompt treatment needs to be started with patients suffering from erythroderma, staphylococcal scalded skin syndrome, toxic epidermal necrolysis, severe erythema multiforme and Stevens–Johnson syndrome. These conditions can be life threatening.

**Fig. 15.1** Epidermal and dermal skin changes.

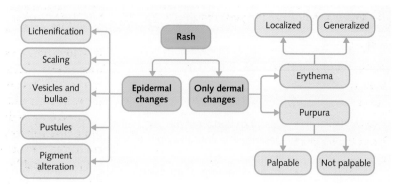

**Fig. 15.2** Characteristic features of generalized rashes

| Diagnosis | Clinical features |
|---|---|
| Erythroderma | Widespread, confluent erythema affecting over 90% of body surface area. Patient may be clinically unwell and have a pre-existing skin condition (causes listed in Fig. 15.3) |
| Staphylococcal scalded skin syndrome (SSSS) | Diffuse erythema and desquamating skin. Painful. Features most prominent around the mouth |
| Toxic epidermal necrolysis | Painful skin with at least two mucosal surfaces affected (oral, genital, or perianal) |
| Erythema multiforme and Stevens–Johnson syndrome (SJS) | Red targetoid lesions, which may be tender, and blister in the centre. When it affects the mucosal surfaces then it is known as SJS |
| Viral exanthems | Usually has a prodrome of non-specific symptoms. Rash is widespread, red and maculopapular. Often occurs in children |
| Bullous conditions | Numerous vesicles or bullae, which may be tense or flaccid. Check for mucosal involvement (see Chapter 24) |
| Urticaria | Pruritic erythematous papules/plaques – also known as wheals or hives. Lesions do not last for more than 24 hours. Tends to be recurrent |
| Psoriasis | Well-defined erythematous plaques of varying sizes. (See Chapter 23 for the different types of psoriasis) |
| Drug eruptions | Maculopapular, with a recent history of taking a new medication. The appearance of the rash very similar to viral exanthems |
| Pityriasis rosea | Herald patch, collarette of scale. Pink, oval macules/plaques. Self-limiting disease |
| Secondary syphilis | Copper, pink-coloured macules/papules. Non-itchy, symmetrical on trunk. Presence of a primary chancre |

## HISTORY

One of the most important symptoms to elicit is whether the rash itches. In eczema/dermatitis this is a prominent symptom; less so in psoriasis and other scaly rashes. If the itching also affects other members of the family or close friends, scabies needs to be considered, especially if the groin is also affected. However, pruritic conditions also occur in cutaneous T-cell lymphomas, and in pemphigus and pemphigoid.

**Fig. 15.3** Common causes of erythroderma

| |
|---|
| Psoriasis |
| Atopic dermatitis/eczema |
| Drug reaction |
| Lymphoma, leukaemia |
| Paraneoplastic |
| Pityriasis rubra pilaris |
| Unknown (20%) |

The possibility of contact dermatitis should be considered if localized areas are affected, especially if they have come in contact with chemicals during their work or hobbies. Thus it is important to obtain an occupational history and enquire about pastimes.

Drug eruptions tend to occur approximately 2 weeks after a new medication has been started but may occur at any time. Thus a thorough medication history should be obtained.

If the rash is exacerbated by sunlight, photosensitive rashes need to be considered, such as systemic lupus and discoid erythematous, photosensitive eczemas, and dermatomyositis. Associated symptoms should be also enquired about, such as proximal weakness (dermatomyositis), breathlessness and joint pains (dermatomyositis, SLE). Ask about blistering, which occurs in vesicobullous conditions. Prodromal symptoms may have heralded a viral exanthem.

It is also important to enquire for a personal history or family history of atopy, which is more common in eczema. Furthermore a family history of psoriasis predisposes an individual to this condition.

When taking the clinical history, it is important to establish if the rash itches, whether new medications have been taken recently, and the presence of prodromal, focal or systemic symptoms.

## EXAMINATION

It is important to start with the individual lesions. If they have surfaces changes such as scaling, lichenification, vesicles and pustules, then the rash involves the epidermis and the dermis.

The colour of the lesions is also important. In purpura, where there is extravasculization of blood, vasculitis needs to be considered, especially if the lesions are also palpable. Meningococcal septicaemia, and disseminated intravascular coagulation must also be considered.

Ample light is needed to examine the rash, preferably with natural sunlight. A magnifying glass is also very useful since it highlights detail that is not so readily seen with the naked eye.

## INVESTIGATIONS

In most cases, the diagnosis is made from the clinical history and the physical examination. However, there are several common investigations that can be performed to confirm the diagnosis (Fig. 15.4).

**Fig. 15.4** Common investigations to confirm the diagnosis in rash

| | |
|---|---|
| Blood tests | Full blood count – eosinophilia present in eczema, drug eruptions<br>Coagulation screen<br>Autoimmune screen |
| Scaling present | Skin scrapings for myocology, Wood's lamp |
| Skin biopsy | Needed when clinical features not characteristic |

# Blistering disorders

## Objectives

You should be able to:

- Investigate a bullous disorder.
- Give the causes of common blistering diseases.
- Understand how to manage bullous diseases.

There are many skin diseases that produce blistering in the form of vesicles and bullae. The clinical history and examination are important to help derive a diagnosis. A skin biopsy is also often performed to confirm the clinical diagnosis.

There are blistering conditions that are not immunologically driven. It is also important to consider infective and metabolite causes of blistering.

## DIFFERENTIAL DIAGNOSIS

In the differential diagnosis of blistering diseases they can be grouped by several criteria: aetiology (whether they are immunologically or non-immunologically driven); the level at which the blister is formed; and whether the blistering is generalized or localized.

The primary bullous disorders (those immunologically driven) include bullous pemphigoid, pemphigus vulgaris, dermatitis herpetiformis and linear IgA disease. These skin disorders tend to be generalized but have a predilection for certain age groups and areas of skin affected. These characteristics help to differentiate them clinically from each other (Fig. 16.1).

Several common viral infections can also cause blistering, such as herpes simplex, varicella, and herpes zoster. Bullous impetigo should be considered when there is associated crusting and rapidly developing erosions with yellow crusting (Fig. 16.2).

Other causes include drug eruptions, eczema, allergic reactions and insect bites, psoriasis and porphyria cutanea tarda. A life-threatening cause of blistering is staphylococcal scalded skin syndrome (SSSS).

## HISTORY

It is important to determine the age of the patient since certain bullous disorders are far more common in particular age groups. Pemphigus vulgaris, bullous pemphigoid, and porphyria cutanea tarda tend to affect those who are middle-aged or elderly, while chicken pox, dermatitis herpetiformis, bullous impetigo and SSSS tend to present in children or young adults.

### Site of blisters

The next question is to determine the location of the blisters. As shown in Fig. 16.1, several bullous diseases have a predilection for certain areas of the body. It is also important to elicit whether the mucous membranes are affected, which frequently occurs in pemphigus vulgaris.

### Depth of blisters

The ease with which the blisters break down provides a clue as to where the blister is formed – essentially the deeper the blister, the longer it will last. However, to confirm the level of the split, a skin biopsy needs

**Fig. 16.1** Differential diagnosis of immunological blistering disorders

| Diagnosis | Clinical features | Blister level (determined by histology) | Direct immunofluorescence |
|---|---|---|---|
| Bullous pemphigoid | Tense blisters on an erythematous base. Tends to affect older patients, and affect the limbs more than trunk. Mucosal surfaces less affected | Subepidermal | Linear IgG at basement membrane ± C3 |
| Pemphigus vulgaris | Flaccid blisters, widespread superficial erosions with oral involvement. Tends to affect younger age group compared to bullous pemphigoid. Trunk is affected more than limb | Suprabasal | Intercellular epidermal IgG |
| Dermatititis herpetiformis | Intense pruritus associated with erosions on extensor surfaces. Tends to be persistent | Subepidermal | Granular IgA at dermal papillae |
| Linear IgA bullous diseases | Tense blisters grouped around pre-existing lesions | Subepidermal | Linear IgA at the basement membrane |
| Pemphigoid gestationis | Associated with pregnancy. Tense blisters, with a centripetal distribution and tends to start in the abdomen | Subepidermal | Linear C3 at the basement membrane ± IgG |

to be performed. Blisters that last for several days to weeks without rupturing are likely to be subepidermal, such as in bullous pemphigoid. In contrast, blisters that easily rupture tend to be more superficial and are found in conditions such as pemphigus and bullous impetigo.

## Time-course of illness

The blisters of immunobullous disorders and porphyrias tend to develop over several weeks to months. This is in contrast to infections where blistering can occur over several hours to days.

**Fig. 16.2** Differential diagnosis of non-immunological bullous skin conditions

| Diagnosis | Clinical features |
|---|---|
| Bullous impetigo | Blisters that rapidly progressed to erosions covered with yellow-honey coloured crusting. Localized staphylococci and streptococci often isolated |
| Acute eczema | Intensely itchy, erythematous lesions with indistinct borders, weeping from vesicles. Need to also consider pompholyx eczema |
| Porphyria cutanea tarda | Rash in a photosensitive distribution – vesicles, bulla and erosions often found on the dorsa of hands. Associated with hypertrichosis, milia, and hyperpigmentation. Also consider variegate cutanea tarda |
| Erythema multiforme/ Stevens–Johnson syndrome (SJS) | Target-like lesions. SJS, the more severe form, associated with the mucous membrane affected. Often associated with herpes simplex |
| Drug eruptions | History of a new medication, and possibly taken in an overdose. Can produce widespread blisters. Rash can also be photosensitive |
| Toxic epidermal necrolysis | Flaccid blisters are large, and progress to sloughing of the skin. The skin is also painful |

## Other factors

It is important to elicit associated symptoms:

- Itching, which is present in pemphigus and pemphigoid, is more prominent in dermatitis herpetiformis, chicken pox and pompholyx eczema.
- Pain is commonly found in herpes zoster and eczema herpeticum.

A detailed drug history is essential since drugs can trigger erythema multiforme, toxic epidermal necrolysis and drug eruptions. Some skin conditions are associated with systemic disease, so a detailed past medical history needs to be obtained (Fig. 16.3).

## EXAMINATION

It is important to determine whether the blisters are tense or flaccid. If they are tense, one can deduce that they are from a subepidermal skin condition. However, if they are flaccid, the Nikolsky sign may be elicited by rubbing normal skin at the edge of the blister, which causes the superficial epidermis to slough off. This sign is found in pemphigus vulgaris and toxic epidermal necrolysis.

The location of the lesions needs also to be assessed:

- In bullous pemphoid the lesions are predominantly on the limbs.
- In pemphigus vulgaris the lesions are mostly on the trunk.
- Dermatitis herpetiformis are most notably on extensor surfaces, which have itchy blisters.
- Blisters in a dermatomal distribution are most likely to be from herpes zoster. Other localized and asymmetrical bullous conditions include herpes simplex, bullous impetigo, and cellulitus.

**Fig. 16.3** Association of systemic disorders with skin conditions

| Skin disease | Association |
| --- | --- |
| Dermatitis herpetiformis | Gluten-sensitive enteropathy (coeliac disease) |
| Porphyria cutanea tarda | Liver disease, e.g. hepatitis C, alcohol-induced liver disease |
| Dermatosis of pregnancy, pemphigoid gestationis | Pregnancy |
| Infections | Immunosuppression |

It is also important to examine the mucous membranes because several bullous skin diseases have a predilection to these areas, such as pemphigus vulgaris. Others include Stevens–Johnson syndrome and toxic epidermal necrolysis.

If blistering occurs in a photosensitive distribution (the areas of the skin exposed to the sun) porphyria, autoimmune diseases and drug eruptions should be considered as possible causes.

## INVESTIGATIONS

In most patients, the diagnosis can be derived from the clinical history and examination. There are numerous investigations that can be undertaken but specific tests should be chosen to confirm the diagnosis or to see if there is an associated condition.

The gold standard is the skin biopsy with direct immunofluorescence. Blood tests can also be performed to detect indirect immunofluorescence, which may be positive in some immunobullous disorders (see Chapter 24).

Immunofluorescence, which can be direct or indirect, is the key investigation in bullous disorders.

If porphyria is suspected it is important to test the urine, stool and blood for porphyrin metabolites. Anti-coelic antibodies need to be checked if dermatitis herpetiformis is suspected. Full blood count could also be assessed, as there is commonly an associated eosinophilia in drug eruptions.

If an infective aetiology seems likely, then skin swabs should be performed for bacterial and/or viral cultures. Where viral infection such as herpes simplex is suspected, electron microscopy could be performed.

**CBC**

- How would you investigate a bullous disorder?
- What are causes of immunological blistering diseases?
- Do the depth of the blister relate to its fragility?
- What systemic conditions can give rise to blistering?

Over recent years there has been a tremendous increase in public awareness of skin cancer. This has led to a rise in attendance at dermatology clinics with patients concerned about pigmented lesions. Most of these turn out to be benign, but it is important to be able to differentiate such benign lesions from the sinister ones such as a melanoma. The clinical history plays an important role in helping the clinician to know how urgently a pigmented lesion needs to be treated.

## DIFFERENTIAL DIAGNOSIS

A naevus is a benign proliferation of one or more type of normal cells found in the skin (Fig. 17.1). The commonest naevi are those derived from melanocytes (cells that produce melanin). Melanocytic naevi ('moles') are commonly found in Caucasians but less so in darker skinned races.

## HISTORY

In a pigmented lesion, an increase in size (especially if rapid), change in colour, an irregular shape, bleeding or crusting are reasons for concern. Benign lesions are unlikely to show these signs. It is also important to assess whether there was a pre-existing lesion. However, approximately 70% of melanomas occurs de novo (in previously normal looking skin).

Risk factors for melanoma should also be assessed, such as a family history of this condition, the presence of a large number of moles and a history of significant sun exposure.

## INVESTIGATIONS

If there has been no change in a pigmented lesion and it remains asymptomatic for a significant length of time, it is likely to be benign and best left alone with regular review by the patient.

If the pigmented lesion is associated with any sinister symptoms or looks clinically suspicious, it would be best to obtain a tissue diagnosis. This can be either in the form of an incisional biopsy (part of the lesion is removed) or excision biopsy (whole of the lesion removed). An incisional biopsy is chosen if the lesion is large and would require a significant surgical intervention – where it would be best to have a definite diagnosis before embarking on such a large procedure.

A photographs of a pigmented lesion provides a pictorial documentation which is useful when reviewing the lesion at a later date. If there has been no change in the lesion, then it is likely to be benign, and this 'watch and wait' approach would have prevented a surgical incision scar. However, if the presence of scar is not of major concern, it may be better to obtain a histological diagnosis.

### CBC

- Define a naevus?
- What are the different types of naevi?
- What features in the clinical history would make you think a mole could have malignant potential?
- How would you investigate a pigmented naevus?
- What are the risk factors for a melanoma?

If there is any doubt regarding the diagnosis of a pigmented lesion, a biopsy should be obtained. If the lesion is small, complete excision may be considered before a histological diagnosis is obtained.

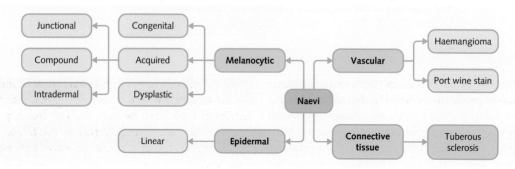

Fig. 17.1 Classification of naevi

# Lumps and bumps

## Objectives

You should be able to:

- Describe the clinical features of the common skin tumours.
- Name the skin lesions associated with trauma.
- Differentiate soft cutaneous nodules such as epidermal cysts and lipomas.

The majority of skin tumours are benign and many have distinctive features, which aids their diagnosis.

## DIFFERENTIAL DIAGNOSIS

Benign skin tumours can be classified by their site of origin, either epidermal or dermal.

*Benign epidermal tumours* include:

- Seborrhoeic keratoses (basal cell papilloma).
- Skin tags (fibroepithelial polyps).
- Epidermal cysts.

*Benign dermal tumours* include:

- Dermatofibroma (histiocytoma).
- Pyogenic granuloma.
- Keloid formation.

Fig. 18.1 shows the clinical features of these lesions.

Basal cell carcinoma, squamous cell carcinoma, keratocanthoma, and pyogenic granulomas are lesions that need to be reviewed in a dermatology clinic.

It is likely that if a swelling has occurred acutely (within 24–48 hours) and is painful, it is caused by trauma or infection. However, if it has occurred gradually, it could be either a benign or malignant tumour.

## HISTORY

Benign skin tumours often have a typical history. However, it is important to suspect a more sinister diagnosis if the lesion has not healed in several weeks or months. This should prompt consideration of a basal or squamous cell carcinoma, or even a melanoma.

Rapid growth of a lesion over several weeks is indicative of a pyogenic granuloma or keratocanthoma. The latter lesion can be very similar clinically and histopathologically to a squamous cell carcinoma.

It is important to enquire for associated symptoms, e.g.:

- Itching is often associated with seborrhoeic keratosis.
- Previous trauma, for example from insect bites, could have precipitated dermatofibromas or pyogenic granulomas.
- If there has been a rapid spread of similar lesions, this could be indicative of viral warts or seborrhoeic keratoses.
- The firmness of a lesion is also important, for example a skin tag is soft. In contrast, firm lesions may include a dermatofibroma, seborrhoeic wart, or keratocanthoma.

## EXAMINATION

The common lesions listed in Fig. 18.1 often have characteristic appearances, but some lesions can mimic others. For example, sebaceous hyperplasia can appear similar to a basal cell carcinoma; and an irritated seborrhoeic keratosis can look sinister.

Palpate the skin lesion to decide if it is soft or firm. This will help form your list of differential diagnoses for the lesion.

**Fig. 18.1** Common lumps and bumps

| Lesion | Clinical features |
|---|---|
| Seborrhoeic wart | Well-defined edge, warty and 'stuck on' appearance |
| Dermatofibroma | Firm, discrete nodule, mostly on lower legs. May have been on site of previous minor trauma |
| Syringoma | Small multiple skin nodules on face |
| Skin tag (fibroepithelial polyps) | Soft, pedunculated, often multiple, some pigmented |
| Epidermal cyst | Firm, mobile skin-coloured nodule with central punctum |
| Lipoma | Soft, mobile nodule, no central punctum |
| Campbell De Morgan spots | Bright-red papules, small, most often on front of trunk |
| Chondrodermatitis nodularis | Small, painful nodule on the edge of the helix of the pinna. Often seen in the elderly, especially in men |
| Basal cell carcinoma | Firm, 'pearly' translucent colour, rolled edge. May be pigmented and ulcerated |
| Squamous cell carcinoma | Hyperkeratotic papule/plaque, with elevated margin. Erythematous, and ulcerated |

## INVESTIGATIONS

See pigmented lesions (Chapter 17).

- If the clinical history and appearance of the skin lesion is characteristic of a benign lesion then no further action is needed.
- A skin biopsy is needed if the diagnosis of the lesion in unknown.

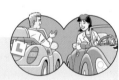

- What skin tumours grow relatively slowly?
- Describe the clinical features of the common skin tumours.
- How would you investigate a lump or a bump in the skin?
- What lesions are associated with a history of trauma?
- How can epidermal cysts be differentiated from lipomas?

# Hair and scalp problems

## Objectives

You should be able to:

- Understand the difference between non-scarring and scarring alopecia.
- Name several causes of alopecia.
- Explain what diseases are associated with alopecia areata.
- Appreciate the differences between hirsutism and hypertrichosis.
- Say which investigations are used to find the cause of alopecia and excess hair growth.

## TOO LITTLE HAIR (ALOPECIA)

A thorough history and clinical examination can often elicit the type of alopecia the patient is suffering from.

The causes of alopecia can be grouped into either scarring or non-scarring. They can also be grouped according to the extent of the body affected: either localized or generalized.

There is an underlying inflammatory process in scarring alopecia, which destroys the hair follicles. Subsequently, it is unlikely there will be significant amount of regrowth of hair.

### Differential diagnosis

The causes of alopecia can be categorized as shown in Fig. 19.1.

Alopecia can be either non-scarring or scarring. The presence of erythema and absence of hair follicles suggests scarring apolecia.

### History

It is important to assess the rate at which the hair is lost. Sudden hair loss suggests alopecia areata or anagen/telogen effluvium. In contrast, if the hair loss is gradual, it suggests male- or female-pattern alopecia.

Patients should be also asked how they handle their hair; this can make it more fragile and thereby increase the risk of breakage. This may occur with hair bleaching, hair straightening and pulling the hair tightly back, as with braiding.

An associated itch can caused by a fungal infection. With a rash present elsewhere, discoid or systemic lupus erythematous should be considered.

The patient's past medical history is also important since alopecia areata is associated with autoimmune disorders such as thyroid disease and pernicious anaemia. Anagen and telogen effluvium are associated with significant stress from systemic disease, medical treatment or psychological disorders, which often coexist.

A family history of alopecia, especially in males strongly suggests androgenetic alopecia.

### Examination

The areas where there is hair loss should be carefully examined for scarring, absence of hair follicles and erythema. This would be suggestive of scarring alopecia.

Hair loss from the temples and crown is characteristic of male-pattern alopecia. In contrast, traction alopecia is most prominent from the fronto-temporal hairline; it is caused by the constant tension of the hair being pulled back.

The presence of exclamation-mark hairs is diagnostic of alopecia areata. These are found especially around the periphery of patches of baldness on the scalp. If hair loss is from the whole scalp it is known as alopecia totalis and total body hair loss is indicative of alopecia universalis.

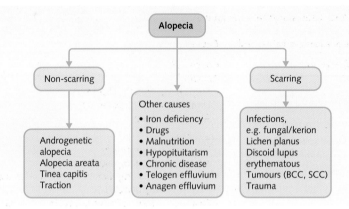

Fig. 19.1 Causes of alopecia.

Hair loss can occur else where on the body. The names of these conditions are according to the extend of hair loss.

A detailed physical examination should be performed to look for features suggestive of anaemia, thyroid disease and other autoimmune disease. Females with suspected excess androgen may show features of virilization, acne and hirsutism.

The nails will also provide diagnostic clues. Nail changes are often associated with systemic disease. In alopecia areata, the nails can be pitted and have a cracked appearance.

## Investigations

Blood tests are often performed to exclude coexistent systemic disease:

- FBC and haematinics, renal and liver function tests.
- Thyroid function.
- Auto-antibody tests.
- Hormone studies.

Fungal infection needs to be excluded if there is scaling present. Skin scrapings should be taken for microscopy and culture. Examination with Wood's light can be used, which will show green fluorescence in patches of infected skin.

A skin biopsy should be performed in cases of scarring alopecia.

## TOO MUCH HAIR (HIRSUTISM AND HYPERTRICHOSIS)

There are two types of excess hair growth, hirsutism and hypertrichosis, both of which tend to be more problematic for women: (Fig. 19.2).

- Hirsutism occurs when there is excess coarse terminal hair growth, in male-pattern distribution in a woman.
- Hypertrichosis occurs when there widespread hair growth.

## History

The distribution of abnormal hair growth will allow hirsutism to be distinguished from hypertrichosis.

Endocrine causes should be excluded. Any changes in the menstrual pattern are important; especially if there are associated features of virilization, such as androgenic alopecia, deepened voice, personality change, or acne.

In menopause, hirsutism can commonly occur. Women with a normal menstrual cycle and lack of features of polycystic ovary disease are unlikely to have a significant cause for their hirsutism.

Family history of hirsutism and racial background are important factors. Those from the Indian subcontinent and Mediterranean countries tend to be more commonly affected.

A history of the patient's medication is needed. Anabolic steroids should be considered in those do weight-training. Generalized hypertrichosis can be caused by phenytoin and minoxidil.

**Fig. 19.2** Causes of excess hair growth

| Type of excessive hair growth | Causes | |
|---|---|---|
| Hypertrichosis | *Congenital* | |
| | *Acquired* | |
| | – Porphyrias, hyperthyroidism | |
| | – Drugs (minoxidil, ciclosporin) | |
| | – Anorexia nervosa | |
| Hirsutism | *Endocrine* | |
| | – Pituitary | Acromegaly |
| | – Adrenal | Cushing's syndrome |
| | | Virilizing tumours, congenital adrenal hyperplasia |
| | – Ovarian | Polycystic ovaries, virilizing tumours |
| | *Drugs* | |
| | – Androgens | |
| | – Progestogens | |
| | – Corticosteroids | |

The psychological effects of excess hair growth can be devastating and the extent will vary from one person to the next.

## Examination

The location of the excess hair growth gives a clue to the cause:

- Androgen-dependent hair patterns include the face, chest, areolae, lower back, inner thigh, and external genitalia. If such a pattern is present, clinical signs of virilization should be searched for.
- In contrast, a uniform pattern of fine hair is unlikely to be androgen-sensitivity related.

There may also be features of a coexistent endocrine syndrome, such as Cushing's, which may include centripetal obesity, striae, and proximal muscle weakness.

## Investigations

If an endocrine cause is suspected, hormonal profiles should be performed. These tests would include:

- Thyroid function tests.
- Assessment of menstrual function with prolactin FSH, LH, total testerosterone and DHEA.

Hormonal blood tests are important blood investigations in hair growth disorders.

## Objectives

You should be able to:

- List the descriptive terms for the most common nail changes.
- Name diseases that are associated with nail changes.
- Describe the clinical features of nail fungal infections.

Inspection of the nails may produce an abundance of diagnostic clues, so it is important not to ignore them in the clinical examination. Nail changes may indicate systemic diseases or be the result of a local disorder. They can also be a manifestation of a skin disorder.

## DIFFERENTIAL DIAGNOSIS

The causes of nail problems can be placed in the following groups:

**Infections:**
- Onychomycosis.
- Paronychia – acute, chronic.
- Viral warts.

**Trauma**

**Tumours:**
- Periungual fibromas.
- Myxoid cysts.
- Melanoma.

**Skin diseases affecting the nail:**
- Psoriasis.
- Eczema.
- Lichen planus.
- Alopecia areata.

**Systemic diseases affecting the nail:**
- Chronic diseases.

## ASSESSMENT OF NAIL PROBLEMS

### History

The main areas to enquire about are:
- Any associated skin or systemic diseases, and
- Any previous trauma to the nails.

### Examination

Nail changes may be specific to another skin or systemic disorder (Figs 20.1–20.3).

### Investigations

In the majority of cases, nail changes are diagnosed clinically.

If fungal growth on the nails is suspected, they can be clipped and examined under a microscope for fungal hyphae and cultured in an appropriate medium. A skin biopsy could also be performed if there are surrounding skin lesions.

Do not ignore the nails when examining the skin. Changes in the nails can be the first manifestation of a systemic or skin disorder.

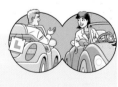

**CBC**
- Describe the main nail changes that can occur?
- What disorders are associated with nail changes?
- How can fungal infections affect the nails?

**Fig. 20.1** Specific nail changes and their associations

| Specific changes | Association |
| --- | --- |
| Pitting | Psoriasis<br>Alopecia areata<br>Lichen planus |
| Onycholysis | Psoriasis<br>Fungal infection<br>Trauma |
| Ridging | Transverse: Beau's lines<br>– Eczema<br>– Psoriasis<br>– Chronic paronychia<br>Longitudinal: lichen planus |
| Thickening | Psoriasis<br>Fungal |
| Colour changes | Yellow: fungal<br>– Psoriasis<br>– Jaundice<br>White: hypoalbuminaemia |

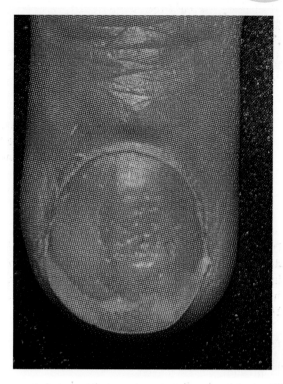

**Fig. 20.2** Nail pitting. (Reproduced with permission from J. Marks, J. Miller, *Lookingbill and Marks' Principles of Dermatology*, 4th edn, Saunders, Edinburgh.)

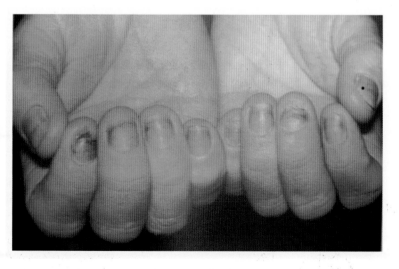

**Fig. 20.3** Yellow nail syndrome. (Reproduced with permission from C. M. Lawrence, N. H. Cox, *Physical Signs in Dermatology*, 2nd edn, 2002, Mosby, Edinburgh.)

## Objectives

You should be able to:

- List the different forms of eczema.
- Describe the clinical features of atopic eczema.
- Appreciate how acute and chronic forms of eczema be differentiated by histology.
- Describe the treatments for eczema.
- Understand the relationship between atopy and eczema.

The terms 'eczema' and 'dermatitis' are often used to describe the same skin disease. There are several stages of eczema, which have typical clinical characteristics:

- In the acute form, there are vesicles that weep, the skin is oedematous, and bullae may even be present.
- In the subacute form, the skin glistens with sebum and there is crusting.
- In the chronic form, the skin becomes thickened, dry and scaly.

Whatever the stage, the skin can be intensely pruritic, except in seborrhoeic eczema. It is also important to appreciate that acute and chronic forms of eczema also have characteristic histological features (Fig. 21.1A, B).

The main symptoms of eczema, with the exception of seborrhoeic eczema, is itch. This causes the patient to scratch, which damages the skin surface, thereby making it susceptible to infections.

Some clinicians use the term 'eczema' to indicate endogenous disease (disease originating within the body) such as atopic eczema, and 'contact dermatitis' to indicate exogenous disease (external aetiology). However, there are certain forms of eczema that do not satisfactorily fit into either category (Fig. 21.2). An alternative way of categorizing this condition is by its morphology and the sites affected.

## ATOPIC ECZEMA

### Clinical presentation

Atopic eczema is a common chronic pruritic skin condition. It is associated with numerous precipitating factors, which should emerge while taking the clinical history (Fig. 21.3).

Atopic eczema is associated with atopy – an increased tendency for asthma and rhinitis, as well as eczema. There is also usually a family history of atopy. Other symptoms and signs of atopy need to be sought; these symptoms include rhinorrhea, lacrimation, sneezing and wheezing.

Atopic eczema is associated with atopy, an increased tendency for hay fever and asthma.

The onset occurs within the first year of life in over 60% of cases. It is unusual to experience an exacerbation for the first time in an adult. The clinical appearance of the skin is dependent on the stage of the disease, acute or chronic. The distribution is always symmetrical and it has a predilection for the flexures (Fig. 21.4). When eczema is severe it becomes generalized.

### Acute form

In the acute form there are ill-defined erythematous areas, with vesicles and papules. There may be an element of scaling, and the skin is puffy and oedematous.

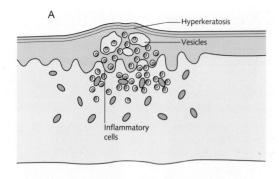

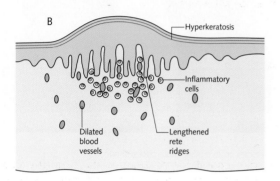

**Fig. 21.1** Histology of acute (A) and (B) chronic eczema. In the chronic form, the rete ridges are longer and there are no vesicles present. (Adapted with permission from D. J. Gawkrodger, *Dermatology: An Illustrated Colour Text*, 2nd edn, 1997, Churchill Livingstone, Edinburgh.)

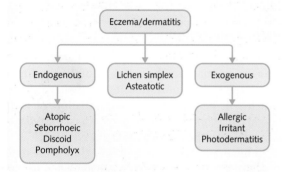

**Fig. 21.2** Types of eczema/dermatitis.

**Fig. 21.3** Exacerbating factors of atopic eczema

| Exacerbating factor | Comment |
|---|---|
| Stress | May result from the disease itself, or itself worsen the disease |
| Dry skin | Skin dehydration is caused by frequent washing, especially with soaps, and being in a warm, dry environment, such as rooms with central heating |
| Skin infection | This can be a consequence of the disease itself or may have occurred prior to the onset of the disease |
| Foods | Certain foods, such as eggs and milk |
| Change of climate | In winter, the condition seems to worsen, possibly owing to drying of skin from heaters. Summer is usually associated with an improvement |
| Skin irritation | Wool, in the form of either clothing or blankets. Even taking off clothing can cause an exacerbation |
| Hormones | Monthly exacerbations due to menstruation |

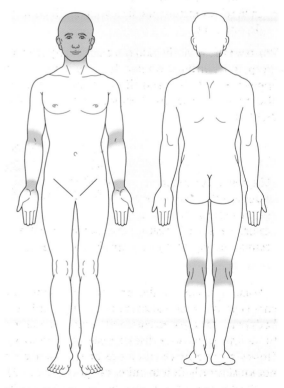

**Fig. 21.4** Sites of predilection. The flexural aspects of the limbs are particularly affected. (Areas affected are marked in darker green).

Repeated scratching causes excoriations, which may proceed into erosions which are then covered with crusting (Fig. 21.5).

## Chronic form

Repeated scratching and rubbing causes the skin to thicken with attenuation of the skin markings (lichenification). In darker skin types, lichenification may be localized around the follicles (follicular lichenificaton). Hyperpigmentation may also occur,

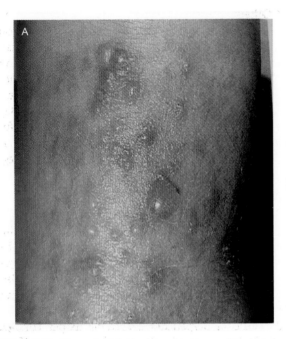
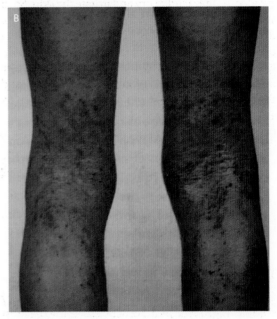

**Fig. 21.5** Atopic eczema. (A) Acute eczema shows an eruption of papules and vesicles on an erythematous background. (Adapted with permission from D. Gawkrodger, *Dermatology, An Illustrated Colour Text*, 2nd edn, 1997, Churchill Livingstone, Edinburgh.) (B) Eczema tends to be symmetrical and tends to affects the flexures. Note the excoriated skin and erythema.

particularly around the eyes (periorbital pigmentation), and repeated rubbing in this area may also cause loss of the lateral one-third of the eyebrows. The skin is generally dry, which may predate the onset of the acute form.

There is an increased risk of skin infections. Secondary bacterial infections are usually caused by *Staphylococcus aureus*. Viral infections include viral warts, herpes simplex (eczema herpeticum) and molluscum contagiosum. If the disease is severe in a child it may cause growth retardation.

### Diagnosis

Eczema is not difficult to diagnosis clinically, so investigations are not usually performed. The most useful investigation is a skin biopsy, which will exhibit features such as those described in Fig. 21.1. However, if there is a suspicion of coexistent skin infection, bacterial and/or viral skin swabs need to be performed.

### Treatment

The scratch–itch cycle in eczema needs to be broken since the continuous scratching damages the skin, thereby making it more susceptible to infection, which exacerbates the itch and perpetuates the cycle. The management of eczema is complex and needs to be approached on several fronts.

### Patient education

It is important to educate the patient that there is no cure for eczema since the aetiology of the condition is unknown. They must not neglect their skin care, which will help prevent an exacerbation of their eczema. If a child is too young to understand what is going on then the parents need to be educated.

In busy out-patient dermatology clinics, the time needed to explain the condition and its treatment may not be available, and therefore repetitive reinforcement may be needed. In some centres, a specialist dermatology nurse provides follow-up and reviews how well the patient is applying their treatment. The nurse may well be able to spend more time with the patient.

### Dry skin

Dry skin tends to be itchy and moisturising it often reduces the need to scratch. Aqueous cream and emulsifying ointment are examples of such treatment and they are simple and inexpensive. The use of conventional soaps and bubble baths should be avoided, as they tend to dry and irritate the skin. Soap substitutes and oily bath additives help to reduce the loss of moisture during washing. Emulsifying ointment can be used as a soap substitute – it lathers slightly, which will help wash the skin. There are many emollients and soap substitutes available, and the choice of preparation will depend on the preferences of the patient.

Emollients need to be continuously used even if the exacerbation of eczema has settled. This will help prevent further attacks.

## Topical treatments

Once eczema is active, it can be treated with a variety of topical agents. Topical corticosteroids are the most common by far.

### Topical glucocorticosteroids

Topical glucocorticosteroids are available with a range of potencies. The site on which they are to be used will determine the initial strength: the thicker the skin, the more potent a topical steroid is needed. For example, on the face a mild steroid is needed (e.g. 1% hydrocortisone), as the facial skin is relatively thin. In contrast, on the limbs, where the skin is thicker, a moderately potent or potent treatment is needed. The use of potent steroids may be initiated to obtain control of the eczema, and once this occurs, then the strength of it can be gradually reduced.

Topical steroids often come in two preparations: ointments and creams. Ointments are often preferred over creams because they are greasier, therefore moisturising the skin and more suited where it is dry. Creams can be used on weeping skin; however, they often cause irritation since they contain alcohol.

Care should be taken to prevent excessive topical steroid use, especially with potent ones. If the patient needs continuous use of topical steroids, tacrolimus or pimecrolimus could be considered.

### Others

Tacrolimus and coal tar are also important topical treatments. Tacrolimus is a relatively new topical treatment but it is expensive. It is often initiated by skin specialists as a steroid-sparing agent as it does not share the complications of excess topical steroid use.

Prior to the advent of topical steroids, the mainstay of treatment of eczema was coal tar. It is still a useful addition and comes in several different strengths. It can also be combined with topical steroids or impregnated into occlusive bandages.

## Infection

Repeated scratching and rubbing damages the skin, predisposing to infection which exacerbates the eczema. Bacterial infections may be treated with systemic antibiotics, such as flucloxacillin. There are also topical steroids combined with topical antibiotics but these are less effective than systemic antibiotics.

Eczema herpeticum caused by herpes simplex infections respond well to systemic aciclovir. If the infection is very severe with systemic complications, the drug should be given intravenously.

Eczema sufferers are prone to skin infections, which can exacerbate their eczema.

## Other systemic treatments

A sedative antihistamine may reduce the need to scratch, giving the patient much needed relief and allowing the skin to recover from such traumatic damage.

When the eczema is very severe and not controlled with topical treatments, phototherapy or ciclosporin may be tried.

## Prognosis

This condition resolves spontaneously in 40% of cases in young children. However, they may experience an occasional exacerbation during their adolescence or early adulthood. Nevertheless, many patients still suffer from eczema 15–20 years later, albeit less severe. Eczema can also have adult onset, which tends to be more severe than eczema that started during childhood.

## Objectives

You should be able to:

- List the diseases associated with seborrhoeic eczema.
- Describe the typical distributions of the different types of eczema.
- Appreciate that commonly used items can cause contact dermatitis.
- Understand how to perform a patch test.

## SEBORRHOEIC ECZEMA

### Clinical presentation

Seborrhoeic eczema (SE) is very common in adults, especially of those of Celtic descent. The main symptoms are dryness, flakiness and redness of the skin and the onset is gradual. Some also complain of pruritus but it is often not as pronounced as in atopic dermatitis.

There is an increased incidence of this condition in those with Parkinson's disease, and those on neuroleptic drugs. It is also associated with psoriasis, stress and anxiety, and immunosuppression from HIV and AIDS. Seasonal changes too have been implicated with this condition as some in patients it worsens during the winter where the environment indoors is dry and warm. The role of the commensal yeast *Pityrosporum ovale* is inconclusive at present, since an overgrowth of the yeast is not found in all cases of SE. Furthermore, eradication of this yeast does not cure SE.

SE is characterized by red, scaling, flaky patches on the skin. It has a predilection for the scalp, face, flexures and upper trunk. The classification of SE is based on the areas that it affects and the age of the patient.

### Scalp and face

This is the most common form of SE and tends to affect young adult males. It often has a symmetrical distribution with the areas of redness rather ill defined and predominantly affecting the nasolabial folds, scalp margins, eyebrows and ears. Significant dandruff may also be associated with this condition. When the scalp of an infant is affected, it is also known as cradle cap. Dandruff is a mild version of SE.

### Trunk

Relatively well defined patches, pink and scaly in nature, tend to affect the sternum and interscapular areas. It may be mistaken for pityriasis versicolor.

### Flexures

This form of SE commonly presents as a symmetrical, bright red/pink skin eruption, which is well marginated. The major flexural areas are affected – axillae, groins and sub-mammary regions. Secondary infection commonly occurs with *Candida albicans*. This is the least common form of SE and more often is found in the elderly.

### Diagnosis

The diagnosis is made on clinical findings.

Unlike other forms of dermatitis, seborrhoeic dermatitis tends not to be itchy.

### Treatment and prognosis

### Scalp

The scalp can be treated with medicated shampoos, which usually contain one of the following: tar, selenium sulphide or ketoconazole (Nizoral). If the SE is particularly severe, salicylic acid can be added, which may be left on for several hours – often overnight. A mild topical steroid can also be used, especially if there is erythema. Many of these shampoos can be purchased over the counter.

## Face, flexures, trunk

Topical steroids and ketoconazole shampoo can also be used to treat these areas. Hydrocortisone 1% is usually sufficient for the face; however, for the trunk a more potent steroid is needed. The steroids are often used in combination with a topical antibiotic. Lithium succinate has also been successfully used, although the mechanism of action has not been fully explained.

Phototherapy is effective for severe cases. Systemic antibiotics may be needed, especially if there is coexistent acne vulgaris, where the topical steroids will exacerbate the acne.

This condition tends to relapse and courses of the above medication can be tried again. Ketoconazole shampoo may be used 2–3 times a week to maintain a remission.

## DISCOID (NUMMULAR) ECZEMA

### Clinical presentation

Discoid eczema is characterized by very well-defined round lesions that are particularly itchy. The surface is red, scaly and dry, and has vesicles and papules on it. There may be similar lesions grouped closely together and they have a predilection for the limbs (Fig. 22.1) There may be crusting if the lesions become infected, often with staphylococci. This condition tends to affect either young adults or the elderly.

### Diagnosis

The diagnosis is made clinically. Tinea infection is a possible differential for this condition but tinea lesions tend to have an active margin. If in doubt, skin scrapings need to be taken. Psoriasis should also be considered, but the scaling is much thicker than that found in discoid eczema.

### Treatment and prognosis

The same treatments as for atopic eczema can used to treat this condition. It is typical that a relatively potent topical steroid is needed. If there is secondary infection, then the steroid could used in combination with a topical antibacterial.

This condition is chronic and may be difficult to control.

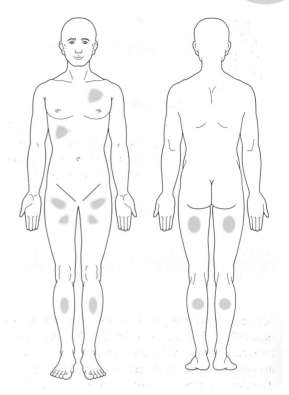

**Fig. 22.1** Distribution of discoid eczema.

## POMPHOLYX ECZEMA

### Clinical presentation

This is a common condition and is a special form of dermatitis that predominantly affects the hands and feet. Equal numbers of males and females are affected, and they tend to be aged under 40 years. They often complain of intensely itchy small vesicles breaking out on their palms or soles, and also the sides of their digits. These vesicles may then break and weep clear fluid. The skin may then become dry, cracked and fissured. The vesicles may even coalesce and form bullae.

The distribution is often symmetrical (Fig. 22.2). After chronic scratching, the skin becomes scaly, lichenified. There may also be a secondarily bacterial infection, as evidenced by crusting.

### Diagnosis

This is mainly a clinical diagnosis. However, there are two differential diagnoses that need to be considered: tinea and contact dermatitis. In tinea, the lesions tend to be asymmetrical, whereas contact dermatitis

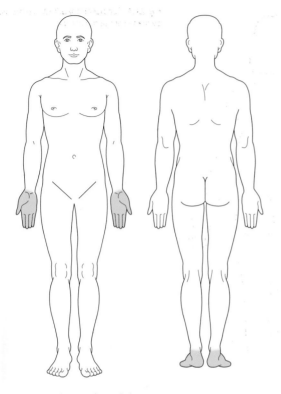

**Fig. 22.2** Distribution of pompholyx eczema.

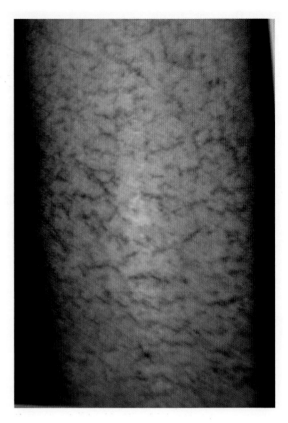

**Fig. 22.3** Asteatotic eczema. (Reproduced with permission from J. Marks, J. Miller, *Lookingbill and Makrs' Principles of Dermatology*, 4th edn, Saunders, Edinburgh.)

would be difficult to exclude until patch testing has been performed. Occasionally, pompholyx occurs as a secondary complication of tinea infection, so skin scrapings need to be taken from suspected areas.

## Treatment and prognosis

The first-line treatment is potent topical steroids, often used with polyethylene occlusive dressings. Potassium permanganate is useful following the rupture of the vesicles. Emollients and antihistamines are useful adjutants. Systemic antibiotics need to be considered if infection is suspected. If such treatments are not effective, then phototherapy is the next step.

It is usual for this condition to be chronic, with numerous relapses, but it is usually not disabling.

The treatment of pompholyx eczema is with potent topical steroids. Weaker preparations will not adequately penetrate the thick skin of the palms and soles.

## ASTEATOTIC ECZEMA

This is a common form of eczema that predominantly affects the limbs of the elderly. The lesions are dry, cracked, fissured skin and there is slight scaling on the surface. There is also a 'crazy paving' pattern with an erythematous base. It is associated with over-washing and a dry warm environment, both more common in institutions (Fig. 22.3). Diuretics may worsen drying of the skin. It is treated by reducing the dryness of the skin with repetitive use of emollients, bath oils and a mild to moderate potent topical steroid.

## LICHEN SIMPLEX CHRONICUS

This is a localized area of lichenification produced by repetitive rubbing of an area that is very pruritic. It may be stress related and there may be a psychological component to it as the repetitive rubbing often becomes a habit. These patches are often unilateral.

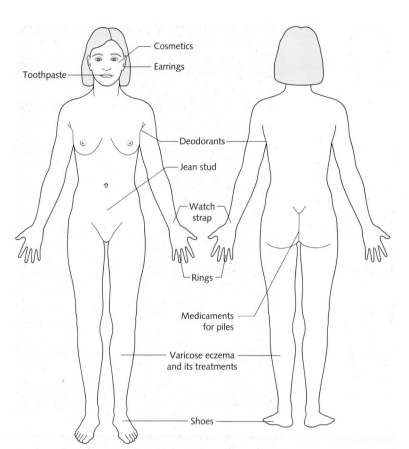

**Fig. 22.4** Contact dermatitis can be caused by many common materials.

Cosmetics

Earrings

Toothpaste

Deodorants

Jean stud

Watch strap

Rings

Medicaments for piles

Varicose eczema and its treatments

Shoes

This condition is often difficult to treat and it is important to break the scratch–itch cycle. Patients are told not to scratch the area but this advice is not easy to follow. Potent topical steroids and antihistamines can relieve the intense itch they may experience. Wet occlusive dressings containing zinc and/or tar may help.

## CONTACT DERMATITIS

When a chemical causes dermatitis it is known as contact dermatitis. This is due to the chemical penetrating the epidermis and causing an inflammatory response. The chemical may simply cause irritation of the skin, which is known as irritant contact dermatitis. If, however, it causes an allergic response, then it is known as allergic contact dermatitis.

### Clinical presentation

Both types of contact dermatitis have similar clinical presentations in that they both cause erythema in the acute stage and lichenification and excoriations in the chronic stage. However, in the irritant form there is less vesicle formation and greater scaling than in the allergic form. Also the irritant form may be so severe that it leads to necrosis or surface changes resembling a superficial burn. A chemical that causes irritant contact dermatitis tends to affect everyone who comes into contact with it. In contrast, an agent that causes allergic contact dermatitis will only affect those that are sensitive to it.

The affected area provides a clue to the source of the contact dermatitis (Figs 22.4, 22.5).

**Fig. 22.5** Common examples of allergens and irritants

| Allergens | Irritants |
|---|---|
| Nickel | Abrasives |
| Chromates | Solvents |
| Colophony (rosin) | Detergents |
| Fragrance | Oils |
| Preservatives | Water |

## Diagnosis

Patch testing is very useful in identifying the chemical that may be involved in contact dermatitis. Usually three separate visits to the clinic are needed during this investigation. The test materials are dilated and each material is placed in a small disc. The backs of these discs are attached on a sticky tape, which is then placed on the back of the patient. This allows the chemical to come in contact with the patient's back in a localized area and so it does not mix with the other chemicals that are tested. Patients return to clinic on the days 3 and 5 to have their backs examined to see whether the test materials have caused a reaction on the skin (Fig. 22.6).

## Treatment and prognosis

The best form of treatment in allergic and irritant dermatitis is to avoid contact with the offending chemical. However, it may be difficult to avoid the substance entirely, especially if it is essential to the patient's occupation. Wearing appropriate protection, such PVC gloves, can reduce the amount of exposure to the chemical.

**CCB**
- What conditions are associated with seborrhoeic eczema?
- What are the usual distributions of the different types of eczema?
- How strong do the topical steroids need to be when treating pomphylex eczema?
- What are the common possible house-hold products that can cause contact dermatitis?

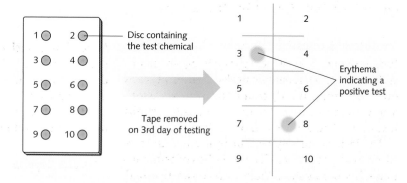

**Fig. 22.6** Patch testing.

## PSORIASIS

Psoriasis is a common chronic inflammatory skin condition typified by symmetrical, well-defined, erythematous plaques covered with thick silvery scale. It has several distinct variants, classified by the shape of the lesions and their location (see Figs 23.1–23.3).

### Clinical presentation

Pruritus is a common symptom, especially in the scalp, and it usually has an unsightly appearance. Joint pains may occur in psoriatic arthritis. There may be significant nail changes. Psoriasis may be precipitated by a number of factors, which should be sought for when taking the clinical history (Fig. 23.4).

### Psoriasis vulgaris (plaque variant)

Psoriasis vulgaris is the most common type of psoriasis (see Fig. 23.1). It has two peaks of onset: (1) early onset, occurring in early adulthood, which is associated with more severe disease and a positive family history; (2) late onset which occurs in middle-age.

The lesions are very well marginated with thick silvery-white scales, which rest on a bed of erythematous salmon-pink skin. When the scales are removed, fine blood points are produced, known as the Auspitz sign. The size of the plaques can range from several millimetres to several centimetres in length. The shape is very varied but is often annular. The plaques can affect anywhere on the body; however, the sites of predilection are on the scalp, the extensor surfaces of the limbs, the sacrum and the limbs themselves. The distribution is usually symmetrical (Fig. 23.5).

When the plaques are acute, they can be painful and tender to touch. Another difference from the chronic form is that they tend not to be scaly. Psoriasis vulgaris may spread rapidly and become erythodermic (see below).

### Guttate psoriasis

This form of psoriasis is more common in young adults. It may occur up to 4 weeks after a streptococcal sore throat. The onset is acute, and there is an eruption of 'drop-like' scaly papules (guttae), predominantly on the trunk and limbs. These lesions also have a silvery surface and do not exceed 1 cm in diameter (see Fig. 23.2).

### Flexural

Flexural areas include the axillae, groin and underneath the breasts, which are warm and moist. Due to this environment, psoriatic plaques in these areas are not usually scaly. They are often well-defined bright red plaques that are smooth. This type of psoriasis is more commonly found in the elderly.

### Palmo-plantar pustulosis

This is a localized form of psoriasis that only affects the hands and feet. It has a predilection for thenar and hypothenar areas, and the central and distal areas of the palms and soles. It is characterized by yellow sterile pustules, which evolve into dark red macules and crusts. There is also erythema, but the typical thick scaly psoriatic plaques may be absent (see Fig. 23.3).

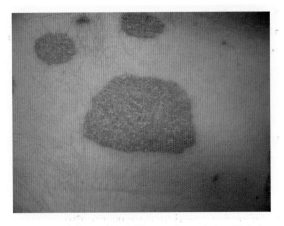

Fig. 23.1 Typical plaque psoriasis. There can be much more thick silvery scale present on the plaque.

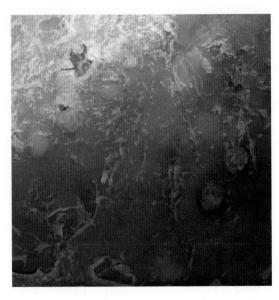

Fig. 23.3 Palmo-plantar pustulosis – the presence of sterile pustules.

Fig. 23.2 Guttate psoriasis – note the small, raindrop-like lesions.

**Fig. 23.4** Common trigger factors for psoriasis

| Trigger factor | Comment |
| --- | --- |
| Trauma | Rubbing and scratching can cause damage to the skin, thereby stimulating the formation of psoriatic plaques. This is known as Köbner's phenomenon. Plaques can form along surgical scars and scars from other sources of trauma |
| Stress | This is difficult to assess formally. Furthermore, psoriasis may be perpetuating the stress. |
| Alcohol | Stress may increase the intake of alcohol, thereby worsening the psoriasis. |
| Drugs | Lithium, beta-blockers, and antimalarials are commonly implicated in psoriatic exacerbations. They can also cause psoriasiform drug eruptions. Steroids can cause severe rebound reactions once they are stopped. |
| Infection | The guttate form of psoriasis is associated with streptococcal sore throats. Psoriasis is more common in those with HIV, and is often more severe and less likely to respond to treatment. |

## Arthropathy

Psoriatic joint pain is present in 5% of patients with psoriasis. There are four types:

- *Distal*: this is the commonest form of psoriatic arthropathy, which involves the distal inter-phalangeal joints of the hands and feet. This form is often asymmetrical.
- *Rheumatoid-like*: the clinical features are very similar to rheumatoid arthritis with a polyarthropathy. However, it is less symmetrical and the rheumatoid factor is negative. There are no rheumatoid nodules.
- *Ankylosing spondylitis*: there may be also peripheral involvement of the joints.
- *Mutilans arthritis*: this is a severe form of the arthropathy where there is joint erosion and osteolysis, culminating in ankylosis and destruction of the joints.

Nail changes and joint pains may be present without skin changes.

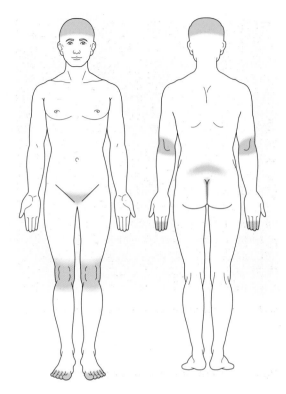

**Fig. 23.5** Common distribution of plaque psoriasis.

A variant of this pustolosis is acrodermatitis continua of Hallopeau, where it predominantly affects areas around the nails and fingertips with sterile pustules.

## ERYTHODERMA

Erythoderma is said to occur when at least 90% of the skin is red and inflamed. Psoriasis is one of the most common causes of erythroderma. It may develop without prior classical scaly lesions. In generalized acute pustular psoriasis, there are large areas of skin that are affected with pustules, which may coalesce.

## COMPLICATIONS

### Nails

Psoriasis affects the nails in over 25% of patients. The nails may be affected without the skin being involved, e.g. pitting and onycholysis (see Chapter 20). These nail changes usually remain despite resolution of the skin problems.

## DIAGNOSIS

In most cases, the variants of psoriasis are diagnosed clinically without too much difficulty. Nevertheless, there are dermatoses that appear similar to the different types of psoriasis, and if in doubt, appropriate investigations should be undertaken (Fig. 23.6).

**Fig. 23.6** The variants of psoriasis and their main differential diagnosis

| Variant of psoriasis | Differential diagnosis |
| --- | --- |
| Plaque | Tinea corporis, mycosis fungoides, lichen simplex |
| Guttate | Drug eruption, pityriasis rosea, tinea corporis, secondary syphilis |
| Flexural | Intertrigo, candidiasis, tinea curis, contact dermatitis |
| Palmoplantar pustulosis | Tinea manus, tinea pedis, pompholyx eczema |

## TREATMENT

The treatment of psoriasis is determined by several factors: the type of psoriasis, the site and extent of involvement, previous treatment and past medical history. First-line treatment usually involves topical agents. Such treatments can be applied at home, or in hospital – either on a day treatment ward or as an in-patient. Hospital supervision of treatment allows more potent topical treatments to be given and they can be closely monitored. Some patients find such an environment less stressful than being at home. Emollients should generally be used in conjunction with specific anti-psoriatic agents because they relieve itching and reduce the dryness of the skin (Fig. 23.7).

The treatment of psoriasis is performed according to the type and site involved and its severity. Systemic treatments are associated with significant side-effects.

## Topical treatments

### Coal tar preparations

Coal tar is usually safe and effective but its use is contraindicated in acute inflamed psoriasis where it may worsen the condition. Other disadvantages of this treatment are that it smells offensive, is messy to apply and can stain clothes. These problems have been largely avoided with the newer proprietary preparations, which come in the form of a cream, lotion, gel or shampoo. The potency of coal tar solution can be varied because it comes in a range of strengths (1% to 12%) and can be tailored to the patient's needs.

The effectiveness of tar is increased when combined with other treatments. If the plaques are thick, the penetration of tar is reduced. This may be counteracted with salicylic acid, which acts as a keratolytic – thereby removing the thick scales. The combination of a mild topical steroid with tar reduces the possibility of folliculitis due to the thickness of the tar preparation. Tar combined with UVB light treatment is known as the Goeckerman regimen, where tar acts as photosensitizer.

### Dithranol

The use of dithranol is generally declining but still has its place, especially when other topical treatments have

failed. It is very irritating to normal skin and cannot be used on the face, flexures and genitalia. It also stains the skin (temporarily) as well as clothes and baths.

Surrounding normal skin can be protected while using dithranol by applying a barrier, such as white soft paraffin – or the affected areas can be covered by tube-gauze. Short contact regimens are used where dithranol is left on for just 30 minutes. Adding dithranol in Lassar's paste (2% salicylic acid, 25% starch, 25% zinc oxide in white soft paraffin) is also useful, especially when it is less likely to spread to normal skin. The strength is steadily increased.

The Ingram regimen comprises dithranol combined with coal tar and phototherapy. It is suitable for stable plaque psoriasis. The majority of patients have a significant improvement within 3 weeks.

### Vitamin D analogues

Most patients prefer the use of vitamin D analogues because they do not stain and are less messy, although they can still cause irritation. Their effectiveness is comparable with dithranol and topical steroids. However, they may cause hypercalcaemia if applied to a large area of skin, and the amount that can be applied depends on the vitamin D analogue. The clinical improvement may plateau out with prolonged use, which is when other topical treatments are needed.

### Topical corticosteroids

Topical corticosteroids are generally well tolerated because they do not smell, are easy to use and non-irritant. Although they are very effective at removing the scaling, there is rapid rebound following cessation of use. Tachyphylaxis occurs with continued use (a decrease in benefit as use continues). Despite these complications, they can be used where there are few small psoriatic lesions, and in areas such as the scalp, flexures, palms and soles. Systemic steroids are best avoided due to the possibility of a severe rebound effect once they are stopped.

## Systemic treatments

The use of systemic treatments is indicated when the psoriasis fails to respond to topical treatments or phototherapy, when psoriasis is life threatening, or if the psoriasis disrupts the patient's activities of daily living. There are many systemic treatments but the most commonly used include methotrexate, ciclosporin and acitretin (Fig. 23.8). They are all associated with significant

**Fig. 23.7** Treatment of psoarisis

| Type of psoriasis | First-line treatments | Second line treatments |
|---|---|---|
| Mild to moderate plaque psoriasis | Coal tar<br>Vitamin D analogues ± topical steroids<br>Dithranol Emollients | UVB |
| Severe plaque psoriasis (>30% surface area) | As above<br>UVB, *PUVA* | Methotrexate<br>Ciclosporin A Acitretin |
| Widespread small plaques | Coal tar<br>UVB | |
| Guttate | Coal tar<br>UVB emollients | |
| Scalp | Coconut oil<br>Tar shampoo<br>Topical steroid lotions | Calcipotriol scalp lotion<br>Dithranol pomade |
| Flexural and genitalia | Topical mild/moderate steroids with antifungal | |
| Palmoplantar | Topical moderate/potent steroids | Acitretin<br>Local *PUVA* |
| Erythroderma from unstable or generalized psoriasis | In-patient: bed rest<br>Maintain temperature, fluid balance | Methotrexate<br>Acitretin<br>Ciclosporin |

**Fig. 23.8** Summary of the commonly used systemic treatments

| Drug | Dose | Monitoring | Side-effects |
|---|---|---|---|
| Methotrexate | Low test dose (2.5–5 mg) if tolerated typical weekly dose 7.5–20 mg | Initial test dose followed by FBC 7 days later<br>Regular liver function tests, including procollagen III (a specific marker for liver fibrosis) and FBC | Common: nausea – may be reduced by taking folic acid every day apart from the day of taking methotrexate<br>Rare: bone marrow suppression, liver damage<br>Caution in renal impairment |
| Ciclosporin | 2–5 mg/kg daily | Regular blood pressure monitoring and renal function | Hypertension, renal impairment, hirsuitism, gingival hypertrophy, muscular cramps |
| Acitretin | 10–30 mg daily | Liver function tests and cholesterol and triglyceride levels | Dryness and peeling of lips and skin<br>Increase of cholesterol and triglycerides<br>Teratogenic |

side-effects and need careful monitoring of various blood parameters, especially in the initial stages.

## Ultraviolet treatment (phototherapy)

When patients with psoriasis go to sunny climes, many notice improvement in their skin condition. The benefits of sunlight can be replicated artificially with ultraviolet lamps. UVB lamps can produce either broadband UVB (wavelength, 290–320 nm) or narrowband UVB (wavelength 311–313 nm). There is increasing use of narrowband UVB, produced by TL-01 lamps, because they cause less burning and have a greater therapeutic effect than broadband UVB. UVA light (wavelength 320–400 nm) can also be used but must be taken in combination with psoralen and this is known as PUVA. Broadband UVB can be combined with coal tar baths, and this is known as the Goeckerman regimen.

Phototherapy is best reserved for widespread guttate or thin plaque lesions. The main complications of this treatment include premature aging of the skin and increased risk of sun-related skin cancers.

You should be able to:

- Describe the clinical differences between bullous pemphigoid and pemphigus vulgaris.
- Appreciate the difference between direct and indirect immunofluorescence.
- Name other skin blistering disorders.
- Understand the systemic associations with dermatitis herpetiformis.

Blistering is seen in many common skin disorders, including herpes simplex, pompholyx, insect bites and bullous impetigo. It is also seen in trauma and burns. However, the primary blistering (bullous) skin conditions are less common and it is these disorders that will form the basis of this chapter. Immunofluorescence and histology are usually required to correctly diagnose a bullous disorder.

## Immunofluorescence

Immunofluorescence is important in the diagnosis of bullous conditions. There are two types: direct and indirect (Fig. 24.1).

# BULLOUS PEMPHIGOID

## Clinical presentation

This condition is a disease of the elderly, with the typical age of presentation between 60 and 80 years. The development of the blisters is rapid, and onset may have been preceded by the eruption of urticarial lesions over several weeks to months. Patients do not usually complain of systemic symptoms unless the disease is very widespread. The main symptom is pruritus, which can be very severe. Once the blisters rupture, there is tenderness in the affected areas.

Bullous pemphigoid is characterized by large, tense blisters, which may arise from normal or erythematous skin (Fig. 24.2). Bullae contain either serous or haemorrhagic fluid. The mucous membranes are less affected than in pemphigus and if they do become involved they are usually less painful and blisters do not rupture as easily. Bullae will eventually rupture and then be crusted over. The sites of predilection include limbs, trunk and flexures. Distribution is often symmetrical, and can occasionally be localized to an area of the body, usually part of the lower leg. The blisters tend not to scar, especially when treated early in the course of the disease.

## Diagnosis

The typical microscopic findings reveal intact subepidermal blisters (the top of the blisters is covered by the whole layer of the epidermis). Eosinophils are often found within the blisters and surrounding blood vessels in the dermis. Immunofluorescence highlights autoantibodies deposited on the basement membrane, the junction between the epidermis and dermis. These are typically IgG antibodies deposited in a linear fashion (Fig. 24.3).

Indirect immunofluorescence may detect anti-basement membrane antibodies in the serum in 70% of cases. However, levels of antibody do not correlate with disease activity. An eosinophilia may be found in pemphigoid.

## Treatment and prognosis

The first-line treatment for pemphigoid is oral prednisolone, with the usual starting dose of 30–60 mg a day. This initial high dose is continued until the emergence of new blisters is halted. The dose of prednisolone is then gradually reduced by 5 mg every 5–7 days. Potent topical steroids can be applied to the blisters, and are particularly useful in localized affected areas. Potassium permanganate can also be added to areas that are weeping.

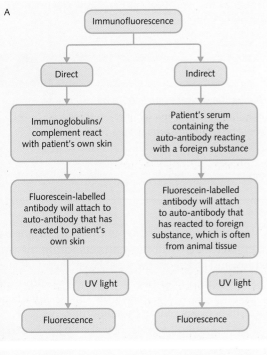

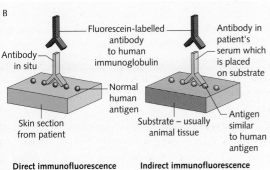

**Fig. 24.1** (A) Direct versus indirect immunofluorescence. (B) Pictorial representation of direct and indirect immunofluorescence.

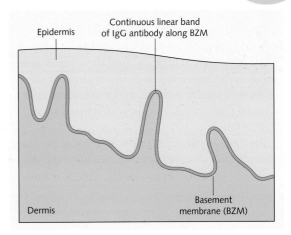

**Fig. 24.3** Fluorescein-labelled antibodies are deposited in the basement membrane, which is characteristic of bullous pemphigoid.

Azathioprine may also be prescribed as a steroid-sparing agent. However, this drug needs to be taken for several weeks before its full effect is appreciated. It is important to check the patient's level of the enzyme thiopurine methyltransferase (TPMT) before starting the drug. This enzyme is important in its metabolism, and patients with low levels are therefore at higher risk of accumulating azathioprine and suffering side-effects.

There is a tendency for this condition to recur, which may necessitate repeated courses of oral steroids and/or azathioprine.

## VARIANTS OF PEMPHIGOID

### Cicatricial pemphigoid

This is also a condition that mainly affects the elderly. It affects predominantly the mucous membranes, especially of the eyes and mouth. The blisters are easily ruptured and often heal with scarring. The main areas that are affected include the face and scalp. When the eyes are affected, it may result in an entropion, fibrosis, corneal ulceration and eventually blindness.

The management of this condition is similar to bullous pemphigoid but is generally less successful. Regular ophthalmological review is also needed when the eyes are involved.

### Pemphigoid gestationis

This is a rare bullous condition associated with pregnancy. It often occurs in the second trimester but can

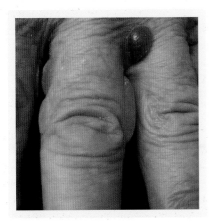

**Fig. 24.2** Blisters of bullous pemphigoid are intact and large.

present at any time during pregnancy and up to 1 week postpartum. Other associations include the oral contraceptive pill and choriocarcinoma.

The rash tends to begin around the umbilicus and spread to the rest of the body in a symmetrical fashion. It is intensely pruritic, and the lesions start as urticarial papules and wheals, which then proceed to tense bullae.

The disease will resolve after delivery of the baby; however, until then systemic steroids are required.

## PEMPHIGUS VULGARIS

### Clinical presentation

Pemphigus is often a more serious condition than pemphigoid and is much less common. It tends to affect those aged 40–60 years. There may be a history of localized oral blisters for several months before the onset of generalized cutaneous lesions. Patients do not complain of itching as in pemphigoid, but instead of burning and pain. If they have significant mouth involvement, the pain may be so intense it prevents adequate food intake, thereby causing weakness and poor wound healing.

The blisters, in contrast to pemphigoid, are flaccid and easily ruptured, and consequently often only erosions are seen (Fig. 24.4). These lesions are painful. The scalp and face are often affected. Other sites of predilection include the torso and flexures. Those bed-bound often have large areas of their back affected. It is important to examine the mouth for lesions.

The skin surrounding the bullae can be displaced by applying pressure to it with a finger; which is known as the Nikolsky sign and is a diagnostic feature of pemphigus.

During the clinical examination, the mouth should also be examined, as there could be significant erosions present.

### Diagnosis

A skin biopsy is needed to confirm the diagnosis. Light microscopy will show blisters within the epidermis, and just above the basal layer. There will also be acantholysis (separation of the cells within the epidermis) due to the loss of the intercellular connections between cells in the epidermis.

Direct immunofluorescence will stain IgG between the epidermal cells, producing a fine net-like pattern (Fig. 24.5). Indirect immunofluorescence will detect autoantibodies against the intercellular substance of the epidermis, which are found in the majority of patients. The antibody titres correlate relatively well with the activity of the disease. Patients also have an associated eosinophilia.

### Treatment and prognosis

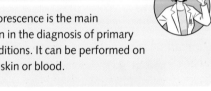

Immunofluorescence is the main investigation in the diagnosis of primary bullous conditions. It can be performed on a sample of skin or blood.

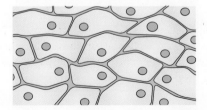

**Fig. 24.4** Blisters of pemphigus are usually not intact. They are more fragile than the blisters of bullous phemphigoid.

**Fig. 24.5** Fluorescein-labelled antibodies are deposited between epidermal cells, giving a 'chicken-wire' appearance. This is characteristic of pemphigus vulgaris.

If this disease is not appropriately treated it may lead to death. The mainstays of treatment are immuno-suppressants, which usually include prednisolone and azathioprine. High doses of prednisolone are given until emergence of new blisters ceases, at which point the dose can be gradually reduced. Steroids may be combined with other immunosuppresants. Pain from oral lesions may be relieved with a steroid-containing mouthwash.

Disease activity can be monitored by recording any new blister formation and laboratory measurement of pemphigus antibody titres. Complications of systemic steroids need to be diagnosed and treated appropriately.

High dose steroids are initially needed in bullous pemphigoid and pemphigus vulgaris to stop progression of the disease.

## VARIANTS OF PEMPHIGUS

### Pemphigus foliaceus

Pemphigus foliaceus is characterized by shallow erosions and crusting. Intact blisters are less often seen than in pemphigus vulgaris. The face, scalp and torso are affected, but oral lesions are often not observed. The target of the autoantibodies is slightly different to pemphigus vulgaris.

### Pemphigus vegetans

The typical features of pemphigus vegetans are pustular and vegetating lesions which mainly affect flexural areas such the groin and axillae. The mouth is also affected.

### Drug-induced pemphigus

The drugs that are most commonly associated in producing a pemphigus-like syndrome are penicillamine and captopril. The condition usually resolves once the drug is stopped.

## DERMATITIS HERPETIFORMIS

### Clinical presentation

Dermatitis herpetiformis is a chronic, intensely pruritic rash. It commonly affects the extensor aspect of the limbs, buttocks and trunk. The lesions are classically grouped urticarial vesicles and papules, in a symmetrical distribution. However, they are often excoriated because of the intense itching. When the lesions heal, they often leave post-inflammatory hyper- and hypopigmentation. The age group that is most commonly affected are those aged between 30 and 40 years.

This condition is associated with coeliac disease (gluten-sensitive enteropathy), so it is important to ask about the presence of bowel symptoms.

### Diagnosis

Although the clinical features are characteristic in this condition, a skin biopsy is performed to confirm the diagnosis. With direct immunofluorescence, deposits of IgA are detected at the dermal papillae, which is diagnostic of dermatitis herpetiformis. Tests for coeliac disease also need to be performed (Fig. 24.6)

### Treatment and prognosis

The pruritus may respond rapidly to dapsone, sometimes within hours. Prior to starting this drug, the level of glucose-6-phosphate dehydrogenase (G6PD) of the patient will need to be assessed. A deficiency of this enzyme is associated with severe haemolytic anaemia if the drug is ingested. While taking dapsone, regular full blood counts should be performed.

Patients should maintain a gluten-free diet, which may completely suppress the activity of the disease and/or allow a reduction of dapsone.

**Fig. 24.6** Investigations for coeliac disease

| |
|---|
| Autoantibodies: endomysial, tissue transglutaminase, gliadin |
| Small bowel biopsy: gold standard |
| Small bowel follow-through |
| Haematology: mild/moderate anaemia, B12 and folate deficiency |

# Lumps and bumps

## Objectives

You should be able to:

- Recognize common benign skin lesions.
- Recognize when seborrhoeic warts, actinic keratosis and epidermal cysts should be treated.
- Describe the differential diagnosis of a pyogenic granuloma.

The majority of skin tumours are benign and are mostly easily managed. The exception is malignant melanoma which if not treated at an early stage has a high mortality. This chapter concentrates on the common types of benign skin tumours – malignant melanoma is discussed in Chapter 26. It is important to distinguish benign tumours from sinister ones, especially with the increasing number of people seeking review of their skin 'lumps and bumps'.

## SEBORRHOEIC WARTS (BASAL CELL PAPILLOMA)

This is a common type of skin tumour, characterized by altered maturation of the epidermal basal cell.

### Clinical presentation

Seborrhoeic warts can differ widely in shape, size and pigmentation. The lesion is well-defined, with a warty papillary surface and a characteristic 'stuck on' appearance (Fig. 25.1). They occur most commonly on the trunk and the face, and generally affect the middle-aged and the elderly. Incidence increases with age, but it is also rising in young Caucasians owing to greater exposure to the sun. Although there is great variety in size, the warts are usually 0.5–4 cm. Seborrhoeic warts are usually asymptomatic but can cause irritation.

### Diagnosis

This skin lesion is usually diagnosed clinically. It may appear similar to a melanocytic naevus, actinic keratosis or malignant melanoma. If the diagnosis is in doubt then a skin biopsy needs to be performed, possibly as a shave biopsy.

## Treatment

Multiple lesions can be treated with liquid nitrogen cryotherapy. The disadvantage of this procedure is that histopathological examination of the lesion cannot be performed. Thicker lesions are best removed surgically, by either curettage or a shave excision. In both these situations, a local anaesthetic is given.

## SOLAR KERATOSIS (ACTINIC KERATOSIS)

### Clinical presentation

These skin lesions appear as adherent, dry, hyperkeratotic scale on sun-exposed areas. The common areas are the face, dorsum of the hands and the arms. In bald men they also develop on the scalp.

### Diagnosis

The diagnosis is usually made clinically. However, if there is associated inflammation, bleeding and pain the lesion would need a skin biopsy to exclude either an in situ or invasive squamous cell carcinoma.

### Treatment and prognosis

Cryotherapy may be lightly applied to a few lesions. However, if the lesions are extensive then a topical treatment is indicated, such as 5-fluorouracil cream 5% or diclofenac gel. Methyl-5-aminolevulinate cream followed by irradiation with red light may be used with thin solar keratosis.

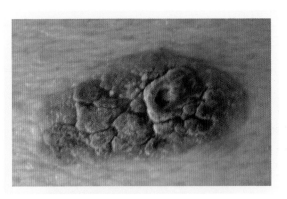

**Fig. 25.1** Seborrhoeic wart.

Solar keratosis may resolve spontaneously; however, lesions are likely to present for many years. Very rarely, they may progress to squamous cell carcinoma.

## SKIN TAGS (FIBROEPITHELIAL POLYPS)

### Clinical presentation

Skin tags are pedunculated papules that are small, soft and may be pigmented. They are common, particularly in the elderly or middle-aged, and have a predilection for the neck, axillae and groin. They are also more common in the obese.

### Diagnosis

Skin tags are often identified clinically. If they are pigmented, they can be confused with seborrhoeic keratosis or benign melanocytic naevi.

### Treatment and prognosis

Skin tags are often removed if they catch on items of clothing or if they look unsightly. It is a simple procedure of snipping the skin tag at its base with a pair of scissors, or by electrodesiccation. Patients should be warned they have a tendency to recur.

## MILIA

### Clinical presentation

Milia are small white keratin cysts (1–2 mm in diameter). They commonly occur on the face, particularly around the eyelids. They are associated with porphyria cutanea tarda, blistering skin diseases such as pemphigoid and following trauma.

### Diagnosis

A clinical diagnosis is made.

### Treatment

Removal of the contents of the cyst can be performed simply using a sterile needle. Cautery may also be used, even without local anaesthesia. Milia may spontaneously resolve after several months, especially in the young.

## EPIDERMAL CYSTS

### Clinical presentation

The cysts are smooth, firm, mobile and have a central punctum through which the cheese-like contents may be expressed. They range from 1 to 3 cm and are commonly distributed on the face or trunk. Epidermal cysts are usually asymptomatic, although they may be unsightly, especially on the face.

### Diagnosis

A clinical diagnosis is made. If the cyst wall ruptures inside the skin, the contents may induce an inflammatory response causing intense pain and the lesion will increase in size several times. When this occurs it is commonly misdiagnosed as infected.

### Treatment

Surgical excision is the treatment of choice and it is important to try to remove it without rupturing the cyst wall. The cyst should not be removed when inflammation is present.

## DERMATOFIBROMA

### Clinical presentation

A dermatofibroma is a firm nodule or papule with a smooth surface. It may be pigmented and can be very dark in colour (Fig. 25.2). Lesions can anywhere on the body but have a predilection for the lower legs. They may occur at previous sites of minor trauma, including insect bites. However, such a history is not often elicited.

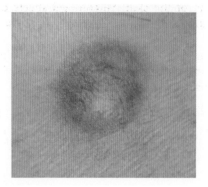

**Fig. 25.2** Dermatofibroma.

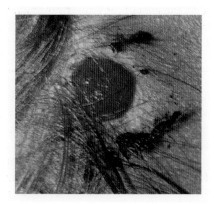

**Fig. 25.3** Pyogenic granuloma. (Reproduced with permission from S. Knight, *Crash Course: Muscle, Bones and Skin*, 2nd edn, 2003, Mosby, London.)

## Diagnosis

A dermatofibroma is relatively easy to diagnose clinically. The dimple sign is reasonably specific to this lesion – applying pressure to either side of the lesion with finger and thumb produces dimpling in the centre of it. Histological findings show a proliferation of fibroblasts, with dermal fibrosis.

## Treatment and prognosis

Excision of the lesion is indicated for diagnostic purposes or if it is symptomatic. Removal for cosmetic reasons should be considered with caution because the resultant scar may look worse than the actual lesion.

Dermatofibroma can persist for decades but may rarely resolve spontaneously.

## PYOGENIC GRANULOMAS

## Clinical presentation

Pyogenic granuloma is a lesion that enlarges rapidly over 2–3 weeks, often at sites of previous minor trauma such as an insect bite. The lesion is very vascular and bleeds easily. It is red, which can be bright to dusky in nature, and crusting may be present (Fig. 25.3). Fingers and lips are most commonly affected. The typical age of onset is under 30 years of age.

## Diagnosis

The diagnosis is confirmed histologically. An important differential diagnosis is amelanotic melanoma.

## Treatment and prognosis

This lesion may simply be removed by curettage and cautery. It is important to examine the specimen histologically to exclude a melanoma.

## LIPOMA

## Clinical presentation

Lipomas are large soft swellings that are freely mobile and made of adipose cells. They are flesh-coloured and usually found on the trunk, neck and upper arms. They are mostly asymptomatic, although they may be cosmetically unpleasing. Multiple lesions are common.

## Diagnosis

The lesion is diagnosed clinically.

## Treatment and prognosis

Surgical excision is often performed for cosmetic reasons. They may increase in size and number throughout life.

## HYPERTROPHIC SCARS AND KELOIDS

Hypertrophic scars and keloids occur due to excessive fibrous tissue forming on the scar at the site of skin trauma. Hypertrophic scars are those that remain confined to the area of the scar. In contrast, keloids are those that extend beyond the boundary of the original scar.

## Clinical presentation

Hypertrophic scars tend to be broad, raised, and have a shiny atrophic epidermis. Some exhibit telangiectasia. Keloids tend to be nodular and spread with claw-like extensions. Both types of scar are firm with smooth surfaces. The sites that are most commonly affected are the earlobes, shoulders and upper torso. They develop more often in Afro-Caribbean people. The age of highest incidence is between the 2nd and 4th decade.

## Diagnosis

These two types of scars are diagnosed clinically and are associated with a history of recent trauma at the site of the scar. A biopsy is not usually indicated in case of worsening of the scar.

## Treatment and prognosis

These scars are notoriously difficult to treat. Intralesional glucocorticoids are often used – usually injected on a monthly basis until the desired result is achieved or the case is complicated by thinning of the skin. Silicone gel sheets or tape impregnated with steroids may also be used (e.g. cica-gel preparations).

Hypertrophic scars tend to regress and become flatter and soft as time progresses. However, keloids can continue to increase in size.

## OTHER BENIGN TUMOURS

### Syringomas

Syringomas are single or multiple small, yellow-cream coloured papules. They mostly occur around the eyes, on the face, axilla and upper chest. They originate from eccrine ducts.

### Campbell De Morgan spots (cherry haemangioma, senile haemangioma)

Campbell-de-Morgan spots are small red/purple papules that can occur anywhere on the body but mostly occur on the back. They are asymptomatic but can be removed by hyfraction. They are benign capillary proliferations and do not signify a medical condition.

# Moles and melanomas

## Objectives

You should be able to:

- Describe the clinical features of benign melanocytic naevi.
- Recognize when a lentigo maligna becomes lentigo maligna melanoma.
- Understand how to manage a lesion that is suspicious of a malignant melanoma.
- Explain both the Clark method and the Breslow method of measuring the thickness of melanomas.

Moles are very common, especially in Caucasians. They are pigmented macules, papules or nodules derived from the proliferation of benign melanocytic cells. The location of these cells in the dermis determines the type of mole and its distinct clinical characteristics.

Some moles are present from birth and are known as congenital naevi, but most are acquired (that is, they develop after birth). The majority of moles present themselves during early childhood or adolescence. The numbers of moles on a person tends to stabilize by the time they reach their 30s and decreases by the time they reach their 40s.

There is an increased vigilance for malignant melanomas (MM) among the general public. As a consequence, there is a lower threshold for a medical opinion to be obtained on moles, and it is therefore important to be able to distinguish a benign mole from a MM, the latter needing specialist review.

## CONGENITAL AND ACQUIRED NAEVI

### Clinical presentation

#### Congenital naevi

Congenital naevi are present from birth and tend to be greater than 1 cm in diameter. The naevi often have two uniform shades of brown and have well-defined margins. They become hairy and protuberant as they mature. There is controversy as to whether these lesions are associated with an increased risk of malignancy, but it may be sensible to excise them if possible.

A variant of a congenital naevus is the bathing trunk or giant hairy pigmented naevus, so called

because it is a congenital naevus that covers a large confluent amount of skin (Fig. 26.1; it can literally cover a bathing trunk area and also it will be hairy). *This is associated with increased risk of malignant change.* Its complete excision is impractical, so careful follow-up is needed.

### Acquired naevi

There are three main types of moles and they are categorized according to where the clusters of melanocytes lie within the dermis (Fig. 26.2).

A benign melanocytic naevus can change its appearance throughout life, as it matures. Changes in the appearance of a mole do not necessarily mean malignant change.

### Other melanocytic naevi

#### Blue naevi
A blue naevus is a firm dark-blue to black papule or nodule that has a well-defined and irregular border. It consists of intensely pigmented melanocytes, which accounts for its dark colour.

#### Spitz naevi
A Spitz naevus is a firm dome-shaped papule/nodule which is uniform in colour, ranging from pink to dark brown. They characteristically grow rapidly and most commonly occur on the face and the neck. Histological examination shows the presence of spindle cells and other cells in abnormal patterns.

### Becker's naevi

This lesion consists of a localized area of brown pigmentation associated with excess hair growth from the lesion. It commonly occurs on the shoulders and upper torso.

### Lentigo maligna

A lentigo maligna (LM) is a flat lesion with marked variation of colour. It increases in size very slowly over the years. LM may eventually evolve into lentigo maligna melanoma, which occurs when the melanocytes breach the dermis. This stage may be identified by the focal appearance of nodules or papules, which suggest the vertical stage of melanoma growth (see melanoma section below).

## Diagnosis

The clinical features of moles are usually characteristic. However, if there is doubt regarding the diagnosis, the mole should be excised. Dermoscopy has improved the diagnostic accuracy of moles and avoids the need to remove them surgically.

If a Spitz naevus is suspected, histological confirmation is needed, despite a good clinical history and characteristic features.

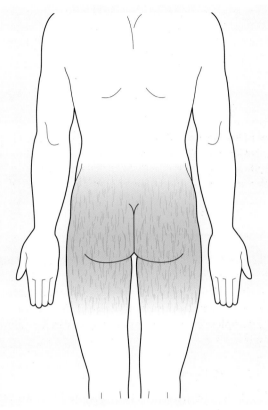

**Fig. 26.1** A possible distribution of a giant hairy pigmented naevus. It can literally cover the bathing trunk area and also it will be hairy.

### Halo naevi

A halo naevus consists of a rim of hypopigmentation surrounding a central pigmented melanocytic naevus (Fig. 26.3). The hypopigmentation is caused by an autoimmune destruction of the skin pigment. In time, the rest of the naevus will resolve. These lesions are associated with vitiligo.

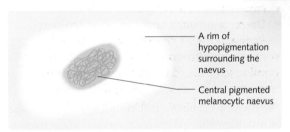

A rim of hypopigmentation surrounding the naevus

Central pigmented melanocytic naevus

**Fig. 26.3** Halo naevi.

**Fig. 26.2** Characteristics of benign melanocytic naevi

| Type of naevus | Clinical features | Histology |
|---|---|---|
| Junctional | Flat or slightly raised macules with a uniform, brown pigmentation. Also have well-defined, regular margins, and of 1 cm in diameter | Melanocytic cells proliferating at the dermal–epidermal junction above the basement membrane |
| Compound | Dark-brown to black papules or nodules. Smooth, dome-shaped, occasionally with hair growing out of them or with a papillomatous/warty surface. Tend to be less than 1 cm in diameter | Combination of melanocytic cells at the dermal–epidermal junction and in the dermis. The latter causes it to be raised |
| Intradermal | Smooth, round papule/nodule that is skin coloured or pigmented. Often occurs on the face | Melanocytic cells only in the dermis |

## Treatment and prognosis

Indications for the excision of a mole include:

- Diagnostic uncertainty.
- Recent changes, for example in size and colour.
- Cosmetic reasons.
- Irritation from recurrent trauma, such as catching on items of clothing.

Compound and intradermal naevi may be simply shaved off. However, patients must be warned about the risk of scarring, especially if the procedure is performed for cosmetic reasons.

## DYSPLASTIC NAEVI

Dysplastic naevi are derived from proliferation of melanocytes that have abnormal changes and may progress to a MM. They arise either from an existing mole or de novo.

## Clinical presentation

Dysplastic naevi have a different clinical appearance from other acquired moles:

- Larger size (diameter greater than 0.5 cm).
- Irregular and indistinct border.
- Asymmetrical.
- Deeply pigmented with variation of colour (variegation).
- Mostly found on trunk.

## Diagnosis

The diagnosis is often made clinically and confirmed by histology, following surgical excision of the naevus.

## Treatment and prognosis

Dysplastic naevi should be removed, especially if they are changing clinically.

In the dysplastic naevus syndrome, there are multiple dysplastic naevi, mainly occurring on the trunk and there is a much higher risk of developing MM. If there are at least two immediate relatives that have also developed MM, the risk of developing MM with this syndrome is nearly 100%.

## MALIGNANT MELANOMAS

MMs are invasive tumours derived from melanocytes, which usually arise in the epidermis. This form of skin cancer is associated with a high mortality, especially when it has metastasized. The incidence of MM has increased significantly over the last few years. In the UK the incidence is 5 new cases per 100 000.

Sun exposure is the most important risk-factor for developing MM. The disease is therefore most common in sunny countries (Australia has an incidence approximately 10 times that of the UK). Fair-skinned people and albinos have a higher risk of developing MM.

Malignant melanomas have a slow growing horizontal phase but a rapid vertical phase. They are best treated before they start their vertical phase.

## Clinical presentation

There are four variants of MM (see below).

### Superficial spreading malignant melanoma (SSMM)

This is the most common subtype of MM and accounts for approximately 50% of cases in the UK. Although it can occur anywhere on the body, in males, the usual site is on the back, whereas in females it is on the legs.

Patients often present with a mole that is increasing in size and changing colour. The lesion initially spreads in a horizontal fashion, known as the radial phase. This causes the margins to become irregular and indistinct. The colour varies from dark brown to black and there can be several different colours present. The lesion develops into a nodule or plaque which then begins to grow down into deeper layers. This is associated with a poor prognosis.

### Lentigo malignant melanoma

This type of melanoma arises from a lentigo maligna. They tend to occur in older people on sun-exposed areas of the skin, such as the face and arms. A lentigo maligna may develop into a lentigo malignant melanoma over many years. In the UK, 15% of melanomas are this particular type.

## Acral lentiginous malignant melanoma

Acral melanomas affect the palms, soles and nail beds. There is a significant variegation of colour. When it affects the nail beds it can cause destruction of the nail plate. Discolouration from trauma may mimic the lesion.

## Nodular malignant melanoma

Nodular malignant melanomas most commonly present on the trunk as a rapidly expanding darkly pigmented nodule (Fig. 26.4). Occasionally, the lesion may not be deeply pigmented, and is then known as amelanotic.

## Diagnosis

A MM should be suspected if there are changes in a pigmented lesion. Diagnosis is based on a seven-point checklist (Fig. 26.5). Lesions with any one of the major features or three minor ones could indicate a MM. They should be referred to a specialist as soon as possible.

Patients with a suspected MM should have a thorough physical examination, especially a search for enlarged lymph nodes. Enquires regarding systemic symptoms also need to be made.

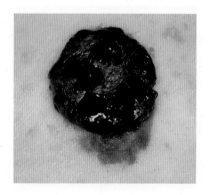

**Fig. 26.4** Nodular malignant melanoma. (Reproduced with permission from J.L. Bolognia et al., *Dermatology*, 2nd edn, 2008, Mosby, Edinburgh.)

**Fig. 26.5** Checklist to help suspect a melanoma

| Major features | Minor features |
| --- | --- |
| 1. Increase in size | 4. Diameter at least 7 mm |
| 2. Irregular shape | 5. Inflammation |
| 3. Irregular colour | 6. Oozing |
| | 7. Change in sensation |

## Treatment and prognosis

The mainstay of treatment is surgical excision. The amount of surrounding tissue that is also removed is proportional to the depth of the tumour. At present, there is no adjuvant treatment that is proven to be of benefit. There is controversy as to whether it is necessary to remove local lymph nodes as well, although this is normal practice in some centres. There are many clinical trials taking place in this field.

The prognosis of MM depends on how deeply it has invaded the tissues. This can be measured by the Clark or Breslow methods. In the Clark method, prognosis depends on the depth to which the melanoma has invaded into dermis. By contrast, the Breslow method records the depth of the tumour from the granular layer of the epidermis (Figs 26.6, 26.7).

The 5-year survival rate according to the Breslow method is generally grouped into three categories:

- Less than 1.5 mm    90% 5-year survival.
- 1.5–3.49 mm    75% 5-year survival.
- Greater than 3.5 mm    50% 5-year survival.

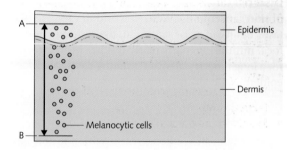

**Fig. 26.6** Breslow thickness. Measurement is performed from the granular layer of the epidermis to the bottom of the tumour (A–B).

**Fig. 26.7** Staging of melanomas

| Clark method | Breslow method |
| --- | --- |
| Level I<br>Melanoma cells within the epidermis | |
| Level II<br>Few melanoma cells within the dermal papillae | |
| Level III<br>Many melanoma cells occupying the dermal papillae | ≤0.75 mm |
| Level IV<br>Melanoma cells invading the reticular dermis | ≤1.5 mm |
| Level V<br>Invasion in the subcutaneous fat | ≥3 mm |

# Non-melanoma skin cancer

## Objectives

You should be able to:

- Describe the clinical features of basal and squamous cell carcinoma.
- Understand the different treatments of basal cell carcinomas.
- List the risk factors associated with squamous cell carcinomas.
- Describe the other types of non-melanoma skin cancers.

The most common skin cancers are basal and squamous cell carcinoma.

## BASAL CELL CARCINOMA

Basal cell carcinoma (BCC) is the commonest form of skin cancer in the Western world. It rarely metastases, but it can cause significant tissue destruction by local infiltration, particularly if it has been growing for a long time. It is derived from the basal cells of the epidermis.

### Clinical presentation

Patients with BCC often present with a lesion that does not heal and tends to bleed. It commonly affects the face and is often an incidental finding. Sun-exposed areas such as nose, ears and temples are most commonly affected. There are four types of BCC:

### Ulcerative

This is the commonest variant of BCC and is also known as a rodent ulcer. It is a papule or nodule that ulcerates in the centre. It may then be covered with an adherent crust. The edges are classically described as rolled-up and pearly in colour. Telangiectasia can be seen overlying the margins. They enlarge slowly.

### Nodular/cystic

These lesions are tense, with a pearly, translucent colour (Fig. 27.1). They do not ulcerate until late in the disease. They may also be covered with telangiectasia.

### Morphoeic

This type of BCC produces a morphoeic-like plaque. It has an ill-defined border and a whitish-yellow colour.

### Superficial

Superficial BCCs often occur on the trunk or limbs. These lesions appear as well-defined, scaly plaques. The margins are rolled and are pearly in nature. They also gradually thicken and ulcerate.

### Diagnosis

A skin biopsy of a suspected BCC is mandatory so that diagnosis can be confirmed histologically. This also provides information as to the extent of spread into the skin and the type of the lesion.

### Treatment and prognosis

Treatment of a BCC depends on the size, location, type of lesion and also the health of the patient. In most cases, simple surgical excision is indicated because it can completely remove the BCC and also confirm the diagnosis histologically.

Mohs micrographic surgery is a special technique that is useful if the BCC is infiltrating and does not have well-defined margins (e.g. the morphoeic type). It is also useful when the site would make simple excision technically difficult, for example the nasolabial folds, around the eyes and behind the ears, and when there have been recurrences after surgery.

Radiotherapy is indicated in those who are not fit for surgery. Large lesions can be shrunk with radiotherapy and when the BCC is smaller, surgery may be possible. However, radiotherapy is associated with the

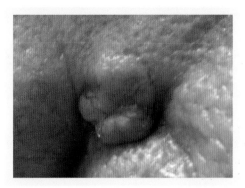

**Fig. 27.1** Basal cell carcinoma. (Reproduced with permission from S. Knight, *Crash Course: Muscle, Bones and Skin*, 2nd edn, 2003, Mosby, London.)

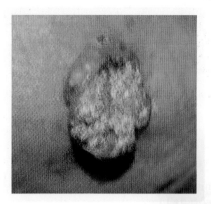

**Fig. 27.2** Squamous cell carcinoma. (Reproduced with permission from S. Knight, *Crash Course: Muscle, Bones and Skin*, 2nd edn, 2003, Mosby, London.)

development of skin cancer many years later and its use in younger people must be considered with caution.

Cryotherapy may be useful for superficial BCCs but a prolonged spray (30 seconds) is needed. Curettage and cautery can also be used for small BCCs (less than 1 cm) and for the superficial type. Newer topical treatments include 5-fluorouracil, imiquimod and photodynamic therapy. These topical treatments do not produce a scar so can produce a very good cosmetic result.

Despite these treatments 1–5% of BCCs do recur. Patients should be advised to avoid sun exposure and to use adequate sun protection.

> There are many ways of treating a basal cell carcinoma. The most appropriate method is dependant on its site, the type, and the fitness of the patient.

## SQUAMOUS CELL CARCINOMA

### Clinical presentation

Squamous cell carcinoma (SCC) often presents as a non-healing ulcer, most commonly in those over 55 years old. The ulcer usually has an everted margin with an irregular shape and enlarges rapidly. The base of the ulcer is often covered with crust. SCCs are often located in sun-exposed areas such as the face, ears, lower lip and on the limbs (Fig. 27.2).

There are several predisposing factors for SCCs:

- Chronic sun damage.
- Pre-existing lesion such as solar keratosis or Bowen's disease.
- Radiotherapy.
- Chronic ulceration and chronic scarring.
- Immunosuppression.

### Diagnosis

A diagnosis of SCC is confirmed by histology from a skin biopsy. Lesions that may look similar to SCC include keratoacanthoma, actinic keratosis and seborrhoeic keratosis.

### Treatment and prognosis

The treatment of choice is surgical excision. The appropriateness of surgery is determined by the size, location, nature of the SCC and the fitness of the patient. Radiotherapy may be a sensible alternative to surgery. Enlarged lymph nodes may suggest metastases, and these will need to be biopsied, as will any other suspected metastatic deposits.

## OTHER NON-MELANOMA SKIN CANCERS

### Kaposi's sarcoma

Kaposi's sarcoma is a form of skin cancer caused by the abnormal proliferation of the vascular parts of the skin. It presents with red–purple nodules or papules and can occur anywhere on the skin and also spread to other organs. Immunosuppression, such as from

HIV, is an important association. The diagnosis of this skin cancer should be confirmed by skin biopsy.

Treatment of individual lesions includes surgical excision, cryotherapy and radiotherapy. When AIDS is present, highly active antiretroviral therapy (HAART) may be given to control the underlying disease.

## Cutaneous T-cell lymphoma (mycosis fungoides)

The initial presentation of cutaneous T-cell lymphoma (CTCL) is with plaques that are similar to those found in eczema and psoriasis. The disease progresses very slowly, sometimes over many years, to thickened, erythematous, indurated plaques. The disease can remain in this phase or continue into a tumour phase, which involves ulceration of skin lesions and metastasis. When there is involvement of lymph nodes and other organs the prognosis is poor, with a mean survival of 2–3 years.

Sézary's syndrome is a rare variant of CTCL as defined by the presence of erythroderma, lymphadenopathy, increased white cell count (>20000/µl) with a significant proportion of abnormal white blood cells known as Sézary cells.

In the initial stages, potent topical steroids and ultraviolet B light may be effective in preventing disease progression. If these treatments fail, PUVA, photophoresis or electron-beam therapy may be tried.

## BOWEN'S DISEASE

Bowen's disease is a form of intraepidermal squamous cell carcinoma in situ. The risk of progression to squamous cell carcinoma is approximately 3%.

## Clinical presentation

Bowen's disease presents as a well-defined erythematous plaque with slight scaling. It may have been present for many years before it is brought to the attention of doctors as it is slow growing and asymptomatic.

In three-quarters of cases it occurs in women, mostly arising on the lower legs. Lesions usually occur singly, although in 10–20% of cases more than one lesion is found. Their appearance can be very similar to a patch of discoid eczema or a psoriatic plaque.

## Diagnosis

The diagnosis is often made clinically and confirmed by histology.

## Treatment and prognosis

Topical 5-fluorouracil can be applied to the lesion. Cryotherapy and curettage with electrocautery can also be tried. Photodynamic therapy has been used with success.

# Lichenoid skin conditions

### Objectives

You should be able to:

- Describe the clinical features of lichen planus and its variants.
- Understand how to manage lichen planus.
- List the conditions with similar characteristics to lichen planus.

Lichenoid eruptions are a collection of skin conditions, which all have a similar clinical appearance and look similar to lichen planus. Thus they all have shiny flat-topped papules.

## LICHEN PLANUS

Lichen planus (LP) is a common pruritic skin condition. It can affect the skin and mucosal membranes. The cause is unknown.

## Clinical presentation

LP often starts as an acute eruption of a very itchy rash. Despite this the patient remains clinically well. The rash is characterized by flat-topped, intensely pruritic, polygonal papules. Its colour ranges from pink to violaceous. The surface may show a network of fine white lines known as Wickham's striae (Fig. 28.1). The papules are often discreet but they can become confluent, which produces plaques and annular lesions. LP may also exhibit the Köbner phenomenon.

The eruption occurs in a symmetrical distribution. The sites of predilection include flexor aspects of the wrists, shins, scalp, mouth and the genital areas. In most cases the age of onset ranges from 30 to 60 years old. In approximately 10% of patients with LP there are also specific nail changes. These include pitting, longitudinal depressions along the nail plate and nail destruction.

There are several variants of LP:

- *Hypertrophic*: the lesions are large, thickened, well-defined purple plaques. They occur on the shins and are more common in black males. After the rash of LP has resolved, these plaques may still persist.

- *Annular*: these annular lesions are often few in number with a characteristic purple rim. They occur more commonly in the genital areas.
- *Follicular*: papules and plaques around the hair follicles. This can cause scarring alopecia.

The oral mucosa should be inspected in those suspected of lichen planus. A white net pattern or ulceration may be detected.

## Diagnosis

The clinical history and physical examination are often typical of LP. Clinical suspicions can be confirmed by histology. There are several skin conditions that have a similar clinical appearance and histology findings. The differential diagnosis for LP includes:

- Drug-related eruption.
- Graft vs host disease.
- Psoriasis.
- Lichen sclerosus.
- Lichen simplex.
- Pityriasis versicolor.

## Treatment and prognosis

The mainstay of treatment is potent topical steroids. Hypertrophic lesions may need the steroids to be applied under occlusion or into the lesion itself. Resistant cases often benefit from a short course of systemic steroids or PUVA. Other immunosuppressants have been reported to be successful, such as azathioprine and mycophenolate mofetil.

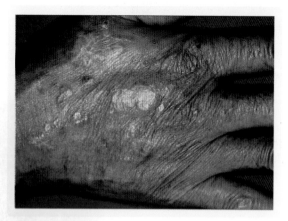

**Fig. 28.1** Lichen planus. (Reproduced with permission from J.L. Bolognia et al., *Dermatology*, 2nd edn, 2008, Mosby, Edinburgh.) The lesions are flat-topped and purple. Wickham's striae can be also seen.

In most cases, LP is a self-limiting condition which resolves within 9–18 months. The lesions heal with post-inflammatory hyperpigmentation and occasionally there may be residual atrophy of the skin. It is unusual for it to recur. Patients with oral LP have a small increase in the incidence of oral squamous cell carcinoma.

## OTHER LICHENOID SKIN CONDITIONS

### Lichenoid drug eruptions

Many drugs are associated with a LP-like drug eruption. The rash may resolve slowly after the cessation of the drug and will heal by post-inflammatory hyperpigmentation, especially in darker skins. Common drugs that can cause such a rash include: anti-inflammatory drugs, gold and penicillamine. The rash maybe associated with photosensitivity, especially with thiazides, quinine and lymecycline.

### Lichen nitidus

The individual lesions of lichen nitidus are very similar to LP but are of minute size, like pinpoints. They tend to be skin-coloured rather than purple. Histology is similar to that found in LP. Lichen nitidus is uncommon and the cause is also unknown. It is often asymptomatic, so treatment is unnecessary and may resolve spontaneously after a few weeks.

### Lichen sclerosus

Lichen sclerosus is a chronic atrophic disorder, commonly affecting the skin around the genital area, and is much more common in women. It is typified by well-defined white papules and indurated plaques. Hyperkeratosis, telangiectasia and purpura may also be present.

In genital areas, moderately potent topical steroids are normally used to treat affected areas. In non-genital areas, treatment is not often indicated.

This condition can be complicated by strictures in the genital area, which cause problems in urinary and sexual activity. These problems may be surgically corrected. There is an increased incidence of squamous cell carcinoma in areas of long-standing disease so it important to review these sites on a regular basis.

# Connective tissue disease

Connective tissue diseases may have skin manifestations and also affect other organs. In these diseases there is an abnormal immune response against normal cellular components, such as the nucleus. This is shown by the presence of autoantibodies that can be detected in the blood. This chapter will concentrate on the skin manifestations of these diseases.

## LUPUS ERYTHEMATOSUS

Lupus erythematosus (LE) may either affect the skin alone, when it is known as discoid lupus (DL), or it may affect the skin and other organs, when it is known as systemic lupus erythematosus (SLE).

## Systemic lupus erythematosus

### Clinical presentation

The most common age of presentation is around 30 years, and there is a strong predominance of females affected with a female to male ratio of approximately 8:1. The cutaneous manifestations of this disease are manifold and are found in 75% of cases (Fig. 29.1). Other systemic features include fatigue, joint pains and low-grade fever. When other organs are involved, such as the kidneys or lungs, specific symptoms relating to organ failure also appear.

### Diagnosis

The diagnosis of SLE can be made when at least four of the following 11 criteria are present:

1. Malar rash (Fig. 29.2).
2. Discoid rash.
3. Photosensitivity.
4. Oral ulcers.
5. Arthritis – non-erosive.
6. Serositis – pleuritis, pericarditis.
7. Renal involvement – proteinuria, cellular casts.
8. Neurological involvement – seizures, psychosis.
9. Haematological involvement – haemolytic anaemia, leukopenia, thrombocytopenia.
10. Immunologic involvement – anti-DNA, anti-Sm.
11. Antinuclear antibody – present in over 95% of patients.

## Discoid lupus

### Clinical presentation

The lesions of discoid lupus are oval, well-defined, erythematous, atrophic and scaly. They may be precipitated by sunlight, and therefore often appear on the face, scalp and hands. Scarring and hypopigmentation may follow resolution of these lesions, and if this occurs on the scalp, alopecia and follicular plugging follow.

### Diagnosis

The diagnosis of DL is often made clinically but skin biopsy with immunofluorescence is helpful if in doubt. Actinic keratosis and plaque psoriasis can exhibit similar lesions and should be considered in the differential diagnosis.

### Treatment and prognosis

If SLE is active, high doses of prednisolone are indicated. This may be combined with steroid sparing drugs such as azathioprine or cyclophosphamide.

**Fig. 29.1** Skin manifestations of SLE

- Butterfly rash – erythematous rash over the cheeks and bridge of the nose
- Photosensitive rash
- Vasculitis
- Alopecia – scarring/non-scarring
- Thrombophlebitis
- Blistering
- Raynaud's phenomenon
- Livedo reticularis
- Discoid LE (see text)

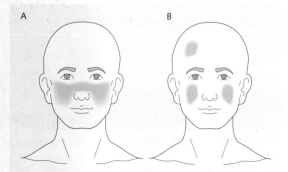

**Fig. 29.2** (A) SLE. Typical butterfly rash on the face. (B) DLE. Discrete discoid lesions on the face.

Antimalarials such as hydrochloroquine are useful for cutaneous lesions, particularly if they are widespread.

Discoid lesions may respond to potent topical corticosteroids. If this treatment fails, cosmetic camouflage can be applied. Simple measures, such as rest and sun avoidance with the use of sunscreens, are also helpful.

The prognosis of SLE depends on the specific organs affected; for example, renal failure presents the patient with a poor outlook. Approximately 5% of those with only discoid lupus develop into full-blown SLE.

## DERMATOMYOSITIS

Dermatomyositis is an autoimmune disorder causing inflammation of striated muscle. This results in proximal weakness and skin manifestations.

### Clinical presentation

The typical cutaneous manifestations include:

- Heliotrope rash, which characteristically occurs around the eyes.
- Gottron's papules – violaceous papules over the knuckles of the fingers (Fig. 29.3).

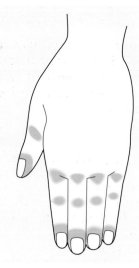

**Fig. 29.3** Dermatomyositis. The violet coloured plaques characteristically affect the knuckles of the hands and spare the rest of the fingers. In acute SLE, the knuckles are spared but the rest of the fingers are affected.

- Ragged cuticles, periungual erythema.
- Erythematous rash on the neck and upper chest, often in a V-shape.

### Diagnosis

When dermatomyositis is active, serum levels of creatine kinase are raised. Autoantibodies such as ANA and Jo-1 may also be increased. Muscle biopsies and electrophysiology studies will show characteristic changes indicative of dermatomyositis.

The diagnosis of dermatomyositis should be confirmed with immunological blood tests and skeletal muscle investigations.

### Treatment and prognosis

The usual treatment is high dose systemic corticosteroids, such as prednisolone. Alternatives include methotrexate and i.v. immunoglobulins.

Patients over 50 years old with dermatomyositis have a high risk of associated internal malignancy, and should be investigated appropriately. If the cancer is treated successfully, resolution of the skin lesions follows.

## SYSTEMIC SCLERODERMA

Systemic scleroderma is a rare multisystem disorder caused by deposition of excessive collagen in the skin and other organs, such as the heart, lung and gastrointestinal system. When it is limited to skin, this condition is known as morphoea.

### Clinical presentation

The common cutaneous features include:

- Raynaud's phenomenon.
- Non-pitting oedema of hands and feet.
- Thickening and tightening of the skin over fingers – sclerodactyly.
- Distal finger ulceration.
- Facial features include perioral furrowing, beak shape nose and telangiectasia (Fig. 29.4).
- Hyperpigmentation and hypopigmentation.
- Morphoea.

A clinical variant of this disorder is known as *CREST* syndrome (Calcinosis, Raynaud's phenomenon, oEsophageal dysfunction, Sclerodactyly and Telangiectasia).

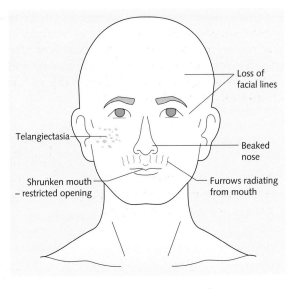

**Fig. 29.4** Scleroderma. Typical facial features.

Loss of facial lines

Telangiectasia

Beaked nose

Shrunken mouth – restricted opening

Furrows radiating from mouth

### Diagnosis

The diagnosis is made clinically. Autoantibody tests and skin biopsies can help confirm the diagnosis. Graft versus host disease produces a similar appearance but there will be a prior history of transplantation.

### Treatment and prognosis

Unfortunately there is no treatment that produces a consistent sustained improvement in this condition. Systemic steroids and numerous systemic immunosuppressants have been tried, as have γ-interferon and photophoresis. Thus treatment is mainly to control the complications resulting from this disorder.

## MORPHOEA

Morphoea is a localized form of scleroderma with no involvement of other organs.

### Clinical presentation

Morphoea consists of ill-defined, indurated plaques which can be oval or round. The surface is smooth and shiny. These lesions may be associated with purpura and telangiectasia. The edge of the lesions may be purple. If the scalp is involved, this results in scarring alopecia. Plaques are usually localized, but there is a generalized form of the disease.

### Diagnosis

The diagnosis is made clinically and confirmed by skin biopsy.

### Treatment and prognosis

There is no effective treatment for this condition. Topical and systemic steroids are often tried, as is PUVA. This condition can either spontaneously resolve or slowly progress.

You should be able to:

- List the common drugs that can cause a morbilliform rash.
- Name the conditions associated with erythema multiforme.
- Describe the management of toxic epidermal necrolysis.
- List the different skin conditions could mimic drug eruptions.
- Name the drugs that cause skin pigmentation.

Drug reactions are common and can occur with nearly any drug, although some cause a reaction more often than others. There are a number of types of drug reaction, the commonest being toxic erythema. Drugs may also stimulate skin disorders such as psoriasis, acne and lichen planus.

## TOXIC ERYTHEMA

Toxic erythema (TE) is the commonest type of skin reaction caused by drugs. It may also be caused by viral and bacterial infections. It is also known as a morbilliform or exanthematous drug reaction.

### Clinical presentation

TE is characterized by a generalized red maculopapular eruption on the skin. It is symmetrical and in some areas, confluent. During healing, there is often scaling and desquamation. There is usually associated pruritus. If the skin is tender, it may indicate a progression to toxic epidermal necrolysis.

Such drug eruptions can occur at any time from 1 day to 3 weeks after the offending drug has been administered. Patients who have previously become sensitized to a drug may develop a reaction within 2–3 days after re-administration. Sensitization may also occur during or after a course of the drug.

The most common drugs associated with TE include:

- *Antibiotics*: most notably penicillin derivatives (such as ampicillin, amoxicillin and flucloxacillin). Ampicillin and amoxicillin must be avoided if the patient has infectious mononucleosis because it causes a drug reaction in almost 100% of patients.
- *Non-steroidal anti-inflammatory drugs*: a drug reaction typically occurs 1–2 weeks after starting the drug and affects 1–3% of the population.
- *Barbiturates*.
- *Sulphonamides*: this is more common in patients affected with HIV.
- *Gold*.

A good history can help to distinguish the causes of a morbilliform rash. The differential diagnosis for such a rash would be drug-related and viral and bacterial infection.

### Diagnosis

The diagnosis of a drug reaction is usually made clinically, and there must be a history of a drug being administered. Blood tests may show an eosinophilia.

### Treatment and prognosis

Once the drug is discontinued, the rash will fade after a few days, but it can worsen before it improves. The pruritus may be controlled with antihistamines and calamine lotion. If the drug reaction is severe or it is not possible to omit the drug, oral steroids should be given. A 'Medic-Alert' bracelet can be worn to highlight the allergy.

## ERYTHEMA MULTIFORME

### Clinical presentation

This rash usually develops over several days and is asymptomatic. The lesions are red and round, with a paler centre, giving the appearance of a target. The sites of predilection are the hands, lower legs and face. However, the rash may be generalized. Blistering may occur at these lesions and in the oral mucosa. A very severe form of this condition is known as Stevens–Johnson syndrome (see below).

### Diagnosis

The typical appearance of the target lesions makes a clinical diagnosis relatively easy. It is also important to exclude other causes of erythema multiforme (EM), because it can be caused by infections such as:

- Herpes simplex – most common infective cause.
- Other viruses: infectious mononucleosis, orf, hepatitis B.
- Mycoplasma pneumoniae, histoplasmosis.

If blistering is present and the diagnosis is uncertain, a skin biopsy should be performed for immuno-fluoresence, which would be positive in a primary bullous condition but not in EM.

### Treatment and prognosis

Uncomplicated EM is self-limiting and usually resolves within 2–3 weeks. If there is an underlying infective cause, it should be treated.

## TOXIC EPIDERMAL NECROLYSIS AND STEVENS–JOHNSON SYNDROME

Toxic epidermal necrolysis (TEN) and Stevens–Johnson syndrome (SJS) are severe and life-threatening drug reactions. The difference between these two conditions is imprecise and they have very similar clinical features. In most cases, it takes 1–3 weeks for the skin condition to arise following the first administration of the offending drug.

> Toxic epidermal necrolysis and severe Stevens–Johnson syndrome are dermatological emergencies. Prompt supportive treatment is needed in both conditions.

### Clinical presentation

TEN and SJS often present with symptoms of flu-like illness and a maculopapular or erythema-multiforme-like rash. The skin then becomes tender, followed by fragile bulla formation and the sheeting of the skin. This exposes the underlying dermis, revealing a red, raw, oozing surface. The whole skin can be affected.

There are associated systemic features and there is a risk of multi-system failure. If the oral mucosa is affected it can make ingestion of food and fluids difficult.

### Diagnosis

The diagnosis is often made clinically. Immuno-fluorescence studies can help exclude a primary bullous condition.

### Treatment and prognosis

This is a life-threatening skin condition and requires treatment similar to that for major burns. The offending drug must be stopped immediately and careful supportive measures initiated to prevent other organ damage. The most common cause of mortality following TEN and SJS is sepsis.

## DRUG FIXED ERUPTION

This drug reaction is characterized by a well-defined, round erythematous plaques appearing after the offending drug has been taken. It recurs in the same place if the drug is taken again, usually within a few hours of its administration. The lesion may heal with blistering and post-inflammatory hyperpigmentation. These lesions can be numerous and cover large areas of the skin, especially if they become confluent. The most commonly implicated drugs include: antibiotics, NSAIDs, aspirin, quinine and sulphonamides.

## DRUG REACTIONS WHICH MIMIC OTHER SKIN CONDITIONS

Drugs reactions can mimic or aggravate other skin conditions are shown in Fig. 30.1.

## SKIN PIGMENTATION

Changes in the skin colour caused by drugs are relatively common and may cause cosmetic problems for the patient. Amiodarone and minocycline are two commonly used drugs that can cause hyperpigmentation.

- *Aminodarone*: causes a slate-grey pigmentation, often in a photosensitive distribution – face and hands. It is reversible but may take up to a year to resolve after the drug has been stopped.

- *Minocycline*: causes a blue-grey pigmentation. It should not be given to children under 12 years old since it can stain the teeth permanently. The discoloration takes several months to resolve after the drug has been discontinued.
- Numerous other drugs have been implicated in changing the skin colour. They include antimalarials, adrenocorticotrophic hormone, chlorpromazine and heavy metals.

## OTHER PATTERNS OF DRUG REACTIONS

Nail and hair changes can be caused by drugs (Fig. 30.2).

**Fig. 30.1** Drug reactions simulating other skin conditions

| Drug eruption | Comments | Typical implicated drugs |
|---|---|---|
| Acneiform | Papules and pustules are often seen but other features of acne vulgaris are not, such as comedones, cysts and scars | Topical and systemic steroids, oral contraceptives |
| Bullous | Blisters can develop in those who take overdoses of barbiturates and can generally occur as part of another pattern of drug reaction | |
| | A pemphigus-like reaction can also occur | Penicillamine, captopril |
| Eczematous | Topically applied treatments can cause a contact dermatitis. An eczematous reaction caused by systemic ingestion is rare | |
| Lichenoid | Improvement after cessation of the drug may be slow. There may be an element of photosensitivity and the oral mucosa may also be affected | Gold, chloroquine, phenothiazine, penicillamine |
| Lupus | A systemic lupus erythematous-like disease can be caused by certain drugs. The renal and central nervous system is not usually affected. Also the anti-DNA antibodies levels are normal but the anti-histone antibodies are increased | Penicillamine, anticonvulsants, hydralazine, minocylcine |
| Psoriasiform | Drugs can provoke a psoriasis-like eruption or exacerbate existing psoriasis | Beta-blockers, gold, methyldopa |
| Pityriasiform | A rash like pityriasis | Gold, captopril |
| Vasculitis | This is due to an immune-deposition | Allopurinol, captopril, penicillins |

**Fig. 30.2** Other drug changes

| Drug eruption | Comment | Typical implicated drugs |
|---|---|---|
| Hair changes | Alopecia can be caused by telogen or anagen effluvium (see Chapter 37) | Anticoagulants, chemotherapy |
| Nail changes | See Chapter 20 | |
| Necrosis | Skin necrosis can be caused by drugs taken orally or at sites of injection | Warfarin |

# Bacterial infections

## Objectives

You should be able to:

- List the typical clinical features of a bacterial skin infection.
- Treat a superficial bacterial skin infection.
- Name the causes the staphylococcal scalded skin syndrome.
- Understand the features of erythrasma.

The skin acts as an important barrier to infection. This function is reduced when it is damaged, for example by an underlying skin disorder such as eczema. Numerous micro-organisms live on the skin without causing any problems. They mostly reside on the stratum corneum or around the hair follicles. The specific type and the numbers of various bacteria vary according the site and age of the person. The most common bacteria naturally found on the skin are staphylococci, corynebacteria and propionibacteria. If a bacterial infection occurs the typical symptoms are redness, swelling, warmth and tenderness. Types of bacterial infections can be categorized by the type of bacteria that causes the infection or how deep the infection penetrates into the skin.

## IMPETIGO

Impetigo occurs when the epidermis is infected, most commonly with *Staphylococcus aureus* and *Streptococcus pyogenes*.

## Clinical presentation

Impetigo often first presents with blisters that may have a purulent exudate. When they rupture it forms a yellow-golden hard crust, which is typical of impetigo. This condition is very contagious and can spread rapidly to other parts of the body. The condition usually progresses over days to weeks. Infection usually starts when the surface of the skin is broken, such as from minor trauma or from an underlying skin disorder. It is common in active eczema owing to the skin being damaged from repeated scratching.

## Diagnosis

The diagnosis is made clinically. Bacterial skin swabs should be performed prior to commencing treatment.

## Treatment and prognosis

Treatment is usually a short course of systemic antibiotics (usually flucloxacillin or erythromycin). Topical antibiotics can be applied to localized infected areas. It is important to remove the crust before applying the topical treatment. This may be done by soaking the crust in water.

If the condition is left untreated, it may progress to ecthyma. An underlying dermatosis can lead to a recurrence of the infection.

Disturbing the surface integrity of the skin predisposes it to infection. This may occur in the presence of an underlying dermatosis.

## ECTHYMA

Ecthyma is a superficial infection that extends into the dermis. It can be caused by the same bacteria that cause impetigo. The typical lesions are well-defined crusted ulcers. They are often signs of neglect as they tend to take weeks to months to develop. Scarring occurs following resolution of these lesions. Treatment is with systemic and topical antibiotics. It is also important to remove the crust.

## FOLLICULITIS

Folliculitis occurs when the hair follicles become infected. It often presents as tender, small round lesions on the limbs. The lesions are yellow pustules that are surrounded by erythema. Hair protruding from them may also be seen. The lesions are usually grouped. Crusting often follows the rupture of the pustules. Although *Staph. aureus* is often the offending organism, it is important to perform a bacterial swab on the affected areas. Acute staphylococcal infection can be treated with a systemic antibiotic such as flucoxacillin. The use of antibacterial soap may prevent further attacks.

## LOCALIZED BACTERIAL INFECTION

### Clinical presentation

#### Abscess

An abscess is a well-defined collection of pus. It may arise in any level of the skin and often presents as a tender, erythematous nodule. Its centre is often fluctuant.

#### Furuncle

A furuncle is an abscess next to a hair follicle. It presents as a tender, red nodule which has a necrotic centre. They often arise in the beard areas, occipital scalp, axillae and buttocks.

#### Carbuncle

A carbuncle is a deep abscess that is formed from several interconnecting abscesses, usually originating from a group of hair follicles. They often form several furuncles and are very painful. These lesions may cause systemic symptoms.

### Diagnosis

A diagnosis is usually made clinically. Bacterial swabs and culture help to confirm the diagnosis.

### Treatment and prognosis

Treatment is usually with systemic antibiotics. However, when the infection is deep, antibiotics may not be able to penetrate significantly. This is an indication for excision and drainage.

A deep sited skin infection may need excision and drainage, and also systemic antibiotics.

Courses of systemic antibiotics may be given on a regular basis, for example every month, to prevent recurrent infections. The use of an antiseptic soap may also be helpful.

Obese patients or patients with diabetes are more prone to such infections. It is important to resolve these underlying problems to reduce the risk of further infections.

## STAPHYLOCOCCAL SCALDED SKIN SYNDROME

This is a serious condition where there is widespread shedding of the skin. It is often caused the release of a toxin from a staphylococcal infection, although other types of bacterial infections have been implicated. The patient usually suffers from a fever and there may also be hypotension and multi-organ failure. There is often a good prognosis, especially if prompt systemic antibiotics are given, such as flucloxacillin.

## NECROTIZING FASCIITIS

Necrotizing fasciitis is an infection of the soft tissue underneath the skin. It can progress rapidly and be fatal. There is usually an ill-defined area of erythema and oedema, which then becomes necrotic. There is often a pyrexia and other systemic features of compromise such as collapse and hypotension. Early surgical debridement and systemic antibiotics are the treatments of choice. Many organisms have been implicated in this condition. Diabetics and the immunocompromised are more susceptible to this infection.

## ERYSIPELAS

Erysipelas is an acute infection of the dermis by *Strep. pyogenes* but other organisms have also been implicated. It presents with a well-defined area of erythema with oedema and tenderness. The face and legs are usually the areas affected. Septicaemia may also be present. A penicillin is often the treatment of choice. However, if there is a penicillin allergy, erythromycin may be given as an alternative. A site of entry for the organism should be determined.

## CELLULITIS

Cellulitis is the infection of the subcutaneous tissue and is often caused by *Strep. pyogenes*. Clinically, it presents in a similar way to erysipelas and it may be difficult to differentiate between them clini-

cally. However, the borders of cellulites are less well defined than erysipelas.

## ERYTHRASMA

Erythrasma is a skin infection that occurs between two adjacent skin folds, such as the groin, axillae or under the breast. It is caused by *Corynebacterium minutissimum*. The area of skin affected is a well-defined brown patch and the surface may be scaly. If it occurs between the toes it may be macerated, thereby making difficult to differentiate it from tinea. Prior to starting antibiotics, a bacterial swab is indicated. The affected area may fluorescence under a Wood's lamp producing a pink colour.

**Objectives**

You should be able to:

- Describe the clinical characteristics of the common generalized viral rashes.
- Discuss the virus that causes both chicken pox and shingles.

## GENERALIZED ERYTHEMATOUS VIRAL RASHES

There are several viral skin infections that have a similar clinical appearance (Fig. 32.1). Measles and rubella occur less frequently than before due immunization programmes in many countries. Many of these viral diseases have prodromal symptoms of fever, malaise and coryzal symptoms. These rashes tend to affect young children. Diagnoses are usually made clinically and can be confirmed by serology. The disorders tend to be self-resolving and usually only supportive treatments are indicated.

Vaccination against a virus does not always offer 100% immunity against it.

## MOLLUSCUM CONTAGIOSUM

Molluscum contagiosum is a very common rash that mainly occurs in children. When it is severe in adults, it may indicate an underlying immunodeficiency. The lesions are flesh-coloured papules that have umbilicated centres. The lesions are usually 1–2 mm in diameter. They can occur singly, which may be confused with a viral wart. These lesions are also pruritic. It may take up to 6 months for the rash to spontaneously resolve. Eczematous eruptions may occur around the papules. No specific treatment is indicated for this rash.

## ORF

An orf is a rapidly enlarging papule with a central pustule. It develops into a bullous lesion which ruptures and ulcerates and is also surrounded by erythema. The sites that are commonly affected are the face, hands, arms and legs. It tends to infect people that come into contact with sheep. The lesions spontaneously heal without scarring and may take several weeks for this to occur. No specific treatment is indicated for the infection.

## HERPES SIMPLEX

Herpes simplex is a common viral skin infection and there are two types: type I tends to affect the face, type II the genital areas. However, both can be found elsewhere on the body. The typical lesions are painful crops of vesicles that occurred suddenly. The vesicles rupture and form crusts. Enlarged local lymph nodes may also be present. Tingling can occur before the appearance of the skin eruption.

The diagnosis is made clinically. It can be confirmed by taking viral swabs from ruptured vesicles. Systemic aciclovir is the treatment of choice when the rash is severe. Topical aciclovir is only useful before the occurrence of the skin lesions. This virus can lie dormant and be reactivated, causing recurrent herpes simplex infection. Recurrent infections may be precipitated by stress and other illnesses. Prophylactic aciclovir is useful to prevent further attacks.

**Fig. 32.1** Clinical characteristics of viral rashes

| Disease | Incubation period | Clinical features |
|---|---|---|
| Measles | 10–12 days | Often starts as a maculopapular rash on the face and within 3–4 days spreads to the rest of the body to produce a morbilliform rash. Inside the mouth, Koplik's spots (white spots surrounded by erythema) may be present. A prodrome is usually present |
| Rubella, German measles | 14–21 days | A pink maculopapular rash starts on the face. It spreads to the rest of the body within the first day. By the third day the rash may have completely resolved, and for this reason, the rash is also known as the '3-day rash'. It is associated with petechiae on the soft palate (Forchheimer's sign) and cervical lymphadenopathy. Peri-auricular lymphadenopathy is a specific feature of this condition. Prodromal symptoms are often absent |
| Chicken pox (varicella) | 14–21 days | This rash is characterized by many localized collections of pruritic vesicles that evolve into pustules and crusts. The initial vesicles of the rash are classically described as 'dewdrops in a rose petal'. It takes 1–3 weeks for the rash to resolve. However, it may cause residual scarring. There is often a mild prodrome. When it occurs in adults, it could be complicated by pneumonitis and encephalitis |
| Fifth disease (erythema infectiosum) | 4–14 days | The rash starts as erythematous, confluent plaques on both cheeks, which gives a 'slapped-cheek' appearance. It progresses to the rest of the body over the next few days and forms a maculopapular eruption. A mild fever and malaise may occur 2 days prior to the initial rash |
| Hand, foot and mouth disease | 7 days | There are multiple superficial ulcers in the mouth and vesicular lesions on the hands and feet. This combination is very characteristic for this disease. Within a week the rash fades and heals with no residual scarring. This rash tends to occur in epidemics |
| Roseola infantum | 7–14 days | There is a preceding high pyrexia and when it falls a pink blanchable maculopapular rash appears on the neck and trunk. It resolves within a few days. The age of onset is less than 24 months |
| Gianotti–Crosti syndrome | Unknown | The rash consists of small erythematous lichenoid papules on the face and limbs. It can be caused by several viruses such as hepatitis B virus. The lesions gradually resolve over 2–3 weeks |

## HERPES ZOSTER

The same virus is responsible for both chicken pox and herpes zoster (shingles). After the resolution of chicken pox, the virus can lie dormant in the ganglia of nerves. When it is reactivated it can cause a localized eruption of erythematous papules. After 1–2 weeks, they evolve into pustules and then become haemorrhagic and form scabs. The distribution is unilateral and dermatonal.

The rash resolves in 2–3 weeks. It can cause residual pain known as post-herpetic neuralgia and nerve paralysis. Systemic aciclovir is often given for the skin eruption to reduce the risk of it becoming severe.

## VIRAL WARTS

Viral warts are caused by the human papilloma virus. There are several distinct clinical variants.

### Clinical features

- *Common warts.* Common warts are firm hyperkeratotic papules that occur commonly on the face and fingers. They have red/black spots on the surface which are characteristic of these warts. They correspond to thrombosed capillary blood vessels. Some have a filiformatous (finger-like) surface. If they occur on the palmar aspect of the fingers they can interfere with the person's normal fingerprints.

- *Planar warts.* Planar warts have a flatter and shinier surface than common warts but tend to be coloured light brown. They are also hyperkeratotic papules and often affect the hands.
- *Plantar warts.* Plantar warts develop on the soles of the feet. They grow inwards due to the pressure from weight-bearing. The lesions are painful and can form large plaques from multiple hyperkeratotic papules.

## Diagnosis

The diagnosis is usually made clinically. A callus may have a similar clinical appearance to a plantar wart. Removal of the top layer of the lesion will reveal thrombosed blood vessels if it is a viral wart. This is a simple method which helps differentiates the two lesions. If there is still doubt, a skin biopsy would be indicated.

## Treatment and prognosis

No single treatment has been found to be completely effective. It may be sensible to leave them alone since the majority they will spontaneously regress (60–70% after 3 months).

Indications for treatment include pain and to improve appearance. Topical salicylic acid combined with daily filing is commonly used. However, salicylic acid should not be used on the face. Curettage and cautery is also used widely, as well as cryotherapy. Lasers and photodynamic therapy have also been used.

If viral warts are asymptomatic, they can be left alone without treatment. They usually spontaneously resolve eventually.

## PITYRIASIS ROSEA

The aetiology of pityriasis rosea is still unknown but it is thought to be caused by a viral infection, hence its inclusion in this chapter.

There are numerous erythematous scaling papules which are mainly found on the trunk and upper parts of the limbs. They follow the direction of the ribs, going away from the spine, giving a similar appearance to the branches of a Christmas tree. Preceding the rash, there may be a large erythematous patch, known as the herald patch, which has the characteristic collarette scaling. The rash will spontaneously resolve within 12 weeks. The rash may be itching; this can be improved with anti-histamines and topical steroids.

# Fungal infections

You should be able to:

- Appreciate the differences between dermatophytes and yeasts.
- Describe the clinical features of the different types of tinea.
- Give an account of the investigations used to detect fungal infection.
- Understand the iatrogenic nature of topical steroids and tinea incognito.
- Describe the clinical presentation of candida infection.

## DERMATOPHYTE INFECTIONS

Dermatophyte infections are caused by the fungal species of *Microsporum*, *Trichophyton* and *Epidermophyton*. They produce hyphae, which are thread-like filaments composed of cells joined together in a linear fashion. They colonize keratin on the skin, nails and hair. However, they do not penetrate into living cells.

### Clinical presentation

These infections, also known as tinea, are described in Fig. 33.1.

### Tinea incognito

This type of infection occurs when systemic or topical steroids have altered the usual appearance of the fungal infection. The areas affected are usually asymptomatic and tend to be persistent. Pustules and vesicles may also be present.

### Diagnosis

The diagnosis of tinea is best determined by direct microscopy, which is when the hyphae are seen under a microscope. Samples are obtained by scraping the skin at the margin of the lesion by using a scalpel blade. It is collected either on a piece of card or directly on to a glass slide. Potassium hydroxide is the added to the sample and it is gently heated. The prepared sample is then reviewed under a microscope. Some of the skin scrapings are sent for culture.

Nails and hair can also be collected and prepared in a similar way for microscopy. A skin biopsy is rarely required.

The Wood's lamp will fluorescence a green colour for dermatophyte infection of the hair.

### Treatment and prognosis

Topical antifungals, such as terbinafine, can be used for localized infected areas. Systemic treatments are indicated for scalp, nail and severe skin infections. Griseofulvin, itraconazole and terbinafine are commonly used systemic antifungals. For nail infections, a prolonged course is often necessary and may lasts for months. Fungal infection has a tendency to recur, especially if there are predisposing factors present; these include diabetes, excessive sweating, wearing tight clothing and the prolonged use of a topical steroid.

## YEAST INFECTIONS

Yeasts are single cell organisms that reproduce by budding (the cells separate after cell replication). There are two common yeast infections: candidiasis and pityriasis vesicolor.

### Candidiasis

*Candida albicans* is a commensal organism that found in the mouth, gastrointestinal tract and vagina in the majority of normal individuals. However, it is not often found on the skin. Predisposing factors that encourage its growth are: moisture, humidity,

173

**Fig. 33.1** Clinical characteristics of tinea infections

| Site of infection | Name | Clinical features |
|---|---|---|
| Feet | Tinea pedis | When the infection occurs between the toes, the skin can become macerated with fissuring and erythema. This is known as the wet type. There may just be dry scaling, known as the dry type<br>A dry, scaly erythematous rash can involve the soles and the sides of the feet. This is known as the 'moccasin distribution' – the area that a moccasin shoe would cover. Vesicles and bullae may also occur with this infection |
| Hands | Tinea manuum | There is erythema and scaling which usually affects the dominant hand. The scaling edge is well defined. Tinea pedis may also be present, and both feet are usually affected – sometimes this is known as the 'two feet, one hand' distribution |
| Groin | Tinea cruris | The groin is affected by large erythematous plaques. The edge is raised and well defined and there may be vesicles or bullae present. There is often central area clearing. Post-inflammatory hyperpigmentation may be present |
| Trunk/limbs | Tinea corporis | The appearance of the lesions is similar to those described for tinea cruris. They can, however, be of varying sizes and shapes |
| Face | Tinea facialis | |
| Scalp | Tinea capitis | This infection is mainly found in children. It can affect the hair shaft and result in localized areas of hair loss. An inflammatory mass known as a kerion may develop. Yellow crusting may also form. |
| Nails | Tinea unguium | The nails are thickened, discoloured and fragile. This may be precipitated by trauma and is more common in diabetics. The infection is often found in association with tinea pedis. Paronychia can complicate the infection |

damaged skin, immunosuppression, immobility, diabetes mellitus, use of antibiotics and steroids. Two opposing skin surfaces (intertrigo), such as underneath the breasts and in flexures, increases the temperature and local moisture, making a good environment for *C. albicans* to thrive.

## Clinical presentation

The clinical appearance of *C. albicans* depends on the area that it is affected.

- *Mouth*. White plaques on the oral mucosa which can be scraped off with a blunt instrument. This reveals a raw surface that has a tendency to bleed.
- *Genital*. When the vagina and vulva are affected they become red and itchy. There is also a thick yellow-creamy discharge. The penis can be affected in a similar way.
- *Intertrigo*. There is a pustular erythematous rash on the skin, which may become macerated. It has a tendency to affect the groin, the axillae and beneath the breasts. When hands are not properly dried, intertrigo can develop between the finger webs.

- *Paronychia*. The nailfold becomes boggy and inflamed. Pus may be extruded by light pressure in this area. The nail plate may become thicken and discolored. When there is coexisting bacterial infection, the nail plate may become green.

Intertrigo can be very similar clinically to erythrasma. A Wood's lamp could be used to help differentiate between the two conditions. Skin scrapings should be taken before treatment is started.

## Diagnosis

Skin scrapings and a skin swab should be performed. The diagnosis can be confirmed following microscopy and culture.

## Treatment and prognosis

The main treatment of candida skin infection is topical or systemic antifungals, similar to those used to treat dermatophyte infection. It is important to pay attention to body folds and hands to prevent recurrent infections. This can be helped by applying a drying powder in these areas to reduce the moisture.

Oral candida infection can also be treated with anti-candida drugs that come in a number of forms to help oral intake. Oral hygiene is important to reduce the risk of further infections.

## Pityriasis versicolor

Pityriasis versicolor is a common yeast infection, and is caused by the commensal *Pityrosporum orbiculare/Malassezia furfur*. It is usually asymptomatic and affects the trunks and limbs of young adults. The lesions are well-defined macules of varying sizes, which may coalescence to form large patches. There is superficial scaling on these lesions. Hypopigmentation may complicate resolution of the rash.

Diagnosis is made clinically and may be confirmed by examining and culturing part of the skin scrapings. A Wood's lamp may produce a blue–green fluorescence if the infection is present.

The initial treatment is topical antifungals, which can be in a lotion form such as selenium and ketoconazole. If the fungus is not eradicated with topical treatments or is recurrent, systemic treatment is indicated, for example ketoconazole tablets.

Objectives

You should be able to:

- Name the risk factors for a scabies infection.
- Describe the treatment of scabies.
- List the different types of lice.

## SCABIES

### Clinical presentation

Scabies is a common infestation that causes an intensely pruritic eruption all over the body, but usually spares the face (Fig. 34.1). People who have a close physical relationship with the patient also have similar symptoms. The pruritus tends to be worse at night but can be severe throughout the day. Predisposing factors include residing in a nursing home or being immunocompromised.

Burrows can be found in this condition; these are linear skin-coloured ridges, usually about 0.5–1 cm long. An erythematous papular rash can develop on the trunk and between the finger webs. Inflammatory nodules and scaling can also be found. When the disease is very severe, it is known as Norwegian scabies. Crusting may develop from a secondary bacterial infection.

### Diagnosis

The diagnosis is made clinically and can be confirmed by visualizing a mite under a microscope. A mite can be obtained by scraping a burrow with a scalpel blade. The scrapings are then placed on a glass slide with a few drops of potassium hydroxide, ready to be examined with a microscope.

### Treatment and prognosis

The usual treatment is repeated applications of topical permethrin or malathion. Each dose needs to be left on the body for several hours and needs repeating. If the infestation is severe, ivermectin can be used and is given as a single dose. It is also important to treat close relatives, especially if they are symptomatic, at the same time, in order to prevent each from reinfecting the others. Bed linen and clothing should be washed at 60°C or above.

Pruritis may persist for several weeks after treatment and does not necessarily indicate failure. Sedative antihistamines can be helpful to relieve such symptoms. Secondary bacterial infections will need antibiotics. Hygiene and eradication of the mite from the patient's surroundings is important to prevent reinfection.

## PEDICULOSIS (LICE INFESTATION)

Pediculosis/lice are blood-sucking wingless insects (Fig. 34.2). There are two variants of the louse: the pubic louse (*Pthirus pubis*), which only affects the pubic region, and *Pediculus humanus*. The latter louse may just affect the head (pediculosis capitis) or the body (pediculosis corporis).

Lice infestations are intensely itching. There are usually numerous excoriation marks; this may result in secondary eczema and bacterial infections. The lice and their eggs (nits) can be seen with the naked eye.

Malathion can be used to treat the lice in all areas. When lice are present in the hair, a fine-tooth comb can be used to remove them. It is important to treat those who come in close contact with the patient otherwise there is a risk of reinfection.

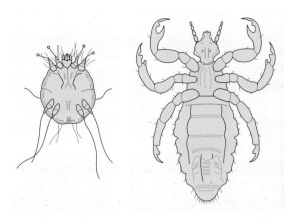

**Fig. 34.1** Scabies mite.　　**Fig. 34.2** Louse.

# Reactive skin disorders

**Objectives**

You should be able to:

- Describe the typical lesions of urticaria.
- Appreciate the different types of urticaria.
- Name the causes of vasculitis.
- Understand how to investigate a patient with vasculitis.
- List the systemic disorders associated with pyoderma gangrenosum.

## URTICARIA AND ANGIOEDEMA

Urticaria is a common skin disorder which is caused by the release of histamine and other vasoactive substances from blood cells. They cause skin lesions commonly known as 'hives' or 'nettle rash'. These are transient, red and itchy swellings. Angioedema is a severe form of urticaria in which the subcutaneous tissues are affected; the mucous membranes may also be involved.

## Clinical presentation

Patients often complain of numerous soft, itchy red swellings. The lesions can vary in size from tiny papules to wheals and plaques of a few centimetres. They tend to last for a few hours but not more than 24 hours and resolve completely, leaving no residual marks. There is also often central pallor. The sites of predilection include areas where the clothing is tight and exposed areas of the skin. In angioedema there is often swelling of eyelids, lips and tongue.

## Diagnosis

Patients often have no skin lesions to see by the time they are reviewed by a doctor. However, the clinical history is very characteristic, thereby making diagnosis relatively straightforward.

Urticaria is often categorized into three main groups: acute, chronic or physical.

## Acute urticaria

In acute urticaria there is a sudden eruption of urticarial skin lesions which occurs soon after contact with an offending allergern. Foods such as seafood, strawberries, eggs and peanuts are often implicated.

Gastrointestinal symptoms often coexist if the trigger is a food. Certain drugs, which include aspirin and antiobiotics, can also cause this form of urticaria.

Rechallenge of a suspected substance will reproduce the clinical features. However, this should be avoided because there is a risk of anaphylaxis.

## Physical urticaria

Physical urticaria can be precipitated by dermographism, pressure, changes to temperature, water, and a cholingeric response.

### Demographism

This is an exaggerated response to minor trauma, including scratching or direct pressure. This can be demonstrated by firmly stroking the skin – after a few minutes a linear urticarial lesion appears that fades within 30 minutes. This response is found in approximately 5% of the normal population.

### Pressure urticaria

Pressure urticaria occurs where there is a sustained pressure to an area of skin. This can occur by wearing tight clothing; standing will affect the soles of the feet, and sitting will cause lesions to erupt on the buttocks. These lesions last for several hours.

### Cholinergic urticaria

This form of urticaria produces numerous small intensely pruritic papules. It tends to occur in young people and be precipitated by sweat brought on by exercise, spicy foods, heat and emotions. The eruption often resolves within an hour.

### Other forms of urticaria

Heat and cold urticaria are caused by temperature changes. Sun exposure can also precipitate urticaria.

Cold urticaria can be diagnosed by applying a cold substance on the skin, such as an ice cube. Drinking cold water may cause swelling of lips, tongue and pharynx.

## Chronic urticaria

This form of urticaria can be defined as one lasting more than 30 days, for which no cause has been found (idiopathic). It usually occurs most days and may last for years. Stress is suspected to be an exacerbating factor.

Urticaria may rarely occur as part of a systemic disorder such as a vasculitis, connective tissue disease and primary bullous conditions. Thus it is important to perform baseline blood tests including full blood count, renal and liver function tests and an auto-immune screen.

### Treatment and prognosis

The main treatment is antihistamines, which specifically block the $H_1$ receptors. Factors that precipitate urticaria should be avoided. In a third of cases, salicylates were found to exacerbate urticaria. Subsequently, foods that contain salicylates should be avoided and dietary advice may be useful.

If the airway is affected adrenaline and systemic steroids are indicated. However, steroids take several hours before the full effect occurs.

The prognosis in the majority of urticaria is good, apart from hereditary angioedema. However, it can cause considerable distress if intense itching arises. One study found that 50% of patients still had wheals 5 years after first presentation. Therefore it is important to warn patients that there may not be complete remission.

## HEREDITARY ANGIOEDEMA

Herediatory angioedema is a rare autosomal-dominant condition that is potentially fatal. It causes transient swelling of the face, larynx and the gastrointestinal tract. Urticarial lesions are not usually found in this condition. It is caused by a C1-esterase inhibitor deficiency. This causes the complement system to over-activate, resulting in excessive accumulation of vasoactive substances, including histamine. Acute attacks can be treated with fresh frozen plasma and danzol can help prevent attacks.

## VASCULITIS

Vasculitis is inflammation of the blood vessels. There are many causes of vasculitis; however, in approximately 50% of cases it is idiopathic (Fig. 35.1).

**Fig. 35.1** Causes of vasculitis.

| Cause | Examples |
| --- | --- |
| Drugs | Sulphonamides, penicillins, phenothiazines |
| Connective tissue disorders | Systemic lupus erythematosus, rheumatoid arthritis, Wegener's, polyarteritis nodosa |
| Infection | Streptococcal, viral hepatitis |
| Neoplasias | Leukaemia, lymphomas |
| Dysproteinaemias | Cryoglobulinaemias |

## Clinical presentation

The typical feature of vasculitis is palpable purpura. These lesions are well-defined erythematous papules, sometimes with a haemorrhagic centre. The purpuric lesions do not blanch. They can be singular or confluent. The lower third of legs and the ankles are often affected first and then the lesions become widespread.

Focal symptoms occur when other organs are affected so it is important to perform a thorough systemic enquiry during the clinical history. Systemic symptoms and signs may appear if there is renal, joint or gastrointestinal involvement. There may also be pruritus, burning, lethargy and myalgia.

## Diagnosis

Patients with vasculitis need to undergo numerous blood tests and a skin biopsy. Full blood count and renal function tests help to determine the function of the bone marrow and the kidneys respectively. Several immunological blood tests are performed, which include antinuclear factor, rheumatoid factor, antineutrophil cytoplasmic autoantibodies (ANCA), complement and immunoglobin levels. Viral hepatitis antibodies titres and possibly bacterial cultures help to determine a possible infective cause.

## Treatment and prognosis

If there is an underlying cause for the vasculitis, this needs to be treated. The mainstay of treatment is systemic steroids, especially in moderate to severe disease. Immunosuppressants such as azathioprine and cyclosphosphamide have also been used. The prognosis of this disease depends on the underlying condition, which may be poor. If it is idiopathic, several attacks of vasculitis may occur over the years.

## HENOCH–SCHÖNLEIN PURPURA

Henoch–Schönlein purpura is a specific form of vasculitis that mainly affects children. It is often preceded by an upper respiratory tract infection. There are vasculitic lesions mostly on the legs and buttocks, although the abdomen and arms may also be affected. It is usually self-limiting and takes 3–4 weeks to resolve. However, if the kidneys or the bowels are affected the prognosis can be poor.

## LIVEDO RETICULARIS

Livedo reticularis is bluish-red net-like pattern that occurs on the skin. It can be reversible and tends to occur when it is cold. However, when it is permanent it may be caused by a vasculitis.

## ERYTHEMA AB IGNE

Erythema ab igne may have a similar appearance to livedo reticularis since it also has a net-like appearance. However, the pattern lines are coarser and usually described as reticulate. It is commonly found where there has been prolonged contact with a hot object, for example the shins of elderly people who regularly sit in front of a fire. This condition can be associated with an underlying vasculitis.

## ERYTHEMA NODOSUM

Erythema nodosum is caused by the inflammation of subcutaneous fat. It tends to affect women, especially in the lower legs. There are many causes of this condition but in approximately 20% it is idiopathic (Fig. 35.2).

### Clinical presentation

Erythema nodosum often presents with crops of tender and red nodules, usually on the lower legs. They are ill-defined and can become indurated. The lesions vary in size and range from 2 to 4 cm in diameter. Malaise, arthralgia and fever also tend to accompany them. There may also be a history of a systemic disorder.

### Diagnosis

The history and physical characteristics of these lesions make a clinical diagnosis relatively uncom-

**Fig. 35.2** Causes of erythema nodosum.

| Cause | Examples |
|---|---|
| Drugs | Sulphonamides, oral contraceptives |
| Bacterial infections | Streptococci, mycoplasma, tuberculosis, leprosy |
| Viral infections | Infectious mononucleosis, cat-scratch fever |
| Fungal infections | Coccidioidomycosis |
| Systemic disorders | Crohn's disease Ulcerative colitis Sarcoidosis Behçet's disease Lymphoma |

plicated. A coexistent condition should be sought by performing a series of basic investigations. These include full blood count, chest X-ray, ASO titres and a Mantoux test. Inflammatory bowel disease should be suspected if there are bowel symptoms present.

### Treatment and prognosis

Non-steroidal anti-inflammatory drugs are useful in controlling the pain from the nodules. Active treatment of them is not usually indicated because they resolve within 6 weeks, without scarring. However, if the symptoms are very severe and an infectious cause is excluded, systemic steroids may be tried. If an underlying cause is present, this needs to be treated.

## PYODERMA GANGRENOSUM

Pyoderma gangrenosum is a rapidly expanding ulcer that is associated with significant morbidity. It is classically described as an ulcer with an overlying bluish-purple edge. The base may be necrotic or covered with granulation tissue. It commonly attacks the lower legs and the buttocks. It is associated with systemic disease in 50% of cases. These conditions include inflammatory bowel disease, Behçet's disease, myeloma, chronic hepatitis and rheumatoid arthritis. A skin biopsy is not diagnostic but is often helpful to exclude other causes of ulcers. If there is an underlying condition, this needs to be treated first. High-dose systemic steroids are often indicated; however, an infective cause should be excluded before starting steroids. The clinical course can last for years if left untreated.

You should be able to:

- List the causes of hypopigmentation.
- Describe the clinical features of vitiligo.
- Give an account of the causes of hyperpigmentation.

There are three main colours of the skin: white, brown and black. These colours vary in the amount of melanin that is present. Carotenoids and oxyhaemoglobin also contribute to skin colour. However, colour changes of the skin mostly involve the melanocytes that produce melanin.

## HYPOPIGMENTATION

The causes of hypopigmentation can be separated into two groups: genetic and acquired (Fig. 36.1). Genetic causes tend to cause generalized hypopigmentaton; in contrast, acquired causes are more localized.

### Albinism

Albinism is an autosomal recessive condition which causes the melanocytes not to synthesize melanin properly in the skin, hair and eyes. This causes loss of pigmentation in these structures. Its variants are based on the extent of the function of the melanocytes. The skin can be white or yellow and the hair is white. Albinos also have poor eyesight, nystagmus and photophobia. Skin cancers and premalignant skin lesions are more common. There is no specific treatment for this condition. It is important to provide advice on sun protection and regularly review their skin for cancerous changes.

Albinos are at higher risk of developing skin cancers so it is important to advise them to protect themselves from the sun as much as possible.

### Phenylketonuria

Phenylketonuria is an autosomal recessive disorder caused by deficiency of phenylalanine hydroxylase. This enzyme converts phenylalanine to tyrosine, which is important in the production of melanin. There is an accumulation of phenylalanine in the body and this can cause brain damage and epilepsy. The patient's skin is often fair and they have blonde hair and blue eyes. Photosensitivity may also be associated with this condition.

In the UK there is routine screening for this condition soon after a baby is born. The condition is treated by dietary restriction of phenylalanine, which will prevent permanent neurological damage. This highlights the importance of detecting this condition early.

### Vitiligo

#### Clinical presentation

Vitiligo causes localized patches of hypopigmentation, which can occur throughout the body. It is more noticeable in people with darker skins and can cause significant morbidity from an unsightly appearance.

The patches of depigmentation are well defined and have a hyperpigmented border. It is completely white. The distribution is often symmetrical and the sites of predilection are around the mouth and eyes, neck, axillae and bony protuberances. Skin associations with this disorder include alopecia areata, halo naevi and white hair. It is also associated with autoimmune disorders.

#### Diagnosis

The diagnosis is made clinically. If there is any doubt, a skin biopsy should be performed.

Fig. 36.1 Causes of hypopigmentation.

Hypopigmentation

Genetic → Albinism, Phenylketonuria

Acquired → Vitiligo, Post-inflammatory

## Treatment and prognosis

This condition is difficult to treat but potent topical steroids are often tried. It is also important to emphasize the need for photoprotection since darkening of the skin highlights the depigmented area. Cosmetic camouflage can help hide the lesions. PUVA has also been tried but a lengthy course over weeks to months is required.

The extent of recovery is difficult to predict. Although spontaneous recovery does occur in a few areas, it is often insufficient for the patient to be satisfied with the cosmetic appearance. There is often a lengthy period of stability during the course of the disease.

## Post-inflammatory hypopigmentation

Common causes of post-inflammatory hypopigmentation are pityriasis alba, eczema, pityriasis versicolor and leprosy. The depigmentation is incomplete so the areas that are affected are lighter than the surrounding skin rather than white, as in vitiligo. There is no treatment indicated other that treating the underlying cause.

## HYPERPIGMENTATION

In the majority of cases, darkening of the skin is caused by excess melanin deposition. Other causes include excess iron in the skin from haemochromatosis, drugs and carotenaemia. (The last can be caused by eating too many carrots.) The causes of hyperpigmentation can be categorized into those that are generalized and those that are local (Fig. 36.2).

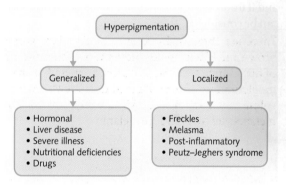

Fig. 36.2 Causes of hyperpigmentation.

Hyperpigmentation

Generalized
- Hormonal
- Liver disease
- Severe illness
- Nutritional deficiencies
- Drugs

Localized
- Freckles
- Melasma
- Post-inflammatory
- Peutz–Jeghers syndrome

## Generalized hyperpigmentation

Certain hormones can increase melanocyte activity, thereby increasing melanin deposition. This occurs most noticeably in Addison's disease, which is the overproduction of the hormone ATCH. In this disorder, the skin creases, buccal mucosa, scars and areas prone to pressure are prone to darken. Similar changes can occur in Cushing's syndrome, hyperthyroidism and acromegaly.

Nutritional deficiencies such as pellagra and scurvy also cause increased skin pigmentation. Malabsorption syndromes can lead to such deficiencies.

Drugs can also cause such skin changes by simulating melanocytes or have been deposited in the skin. Certain drugs can interact with sunlight to darken the skin, e.g. chlorpromazine.

## Melasma

Melasma is a localized patch of light or dark brown hyperpigmentation with ill-defined margins. It tends to occur on the face and in young adult women. It is associated with pregnancy and the oral contraceptive pill. A strong sun cream should be used. The pigmenatation can be lightened by the use of a bleaching cream such as topical hydroquinine. The melasma may resolve spontaneously after several months or improve after pregnancy.

## Post-inflammatory

The areas of the skin damaged by previous inflammation can leave residual hyperpigmentation. Such examples include lichen planus, lupus, acne and eczema. Treatment of this condition is not indicated and if troubling for the patient, cosmetic camouflage can be considered.

Numerous skin dermatoses can cause post-inflammatory changes such as skin infections, eczema, psoriasis and acne.

## Peutz–Jeghers syndrome

Peutz–Jeghers syndrome is a rare autosomal dominant condition which is associated with brown macules on the lips and oral mucosa. It is associated with gastrointestinal bleeding from polyps in the bowel.

# Disorders of sebaceous and apocrine glands

## Objectives

You should be able to:

- Describe the mechanism of acne formation.
- Understand the different types of acne treatment.
- List the key clinical features of rosacea and acne.
- Understand how perioral dermatitis can be formed.
- Appreciate the limiting effects of hidradenitis suppurativa on the patient's quality of life.

## ACNE VULGARIS

Acne is a very common condition that mainly affects those in adolescence. It is a chronic inflammatory disorder of the pilosebaceous units on the face and the upper body. The sebaceous unit is sensitive to the hormone androgen, which causes it produce more sebum. Androgen becomes more abundant during puberty, subsequently causing the sebaceous unit to become overactive and more prone to blockage. This is important in the aetiology of acne.

## Clinical presentation

There are different typical lesions in acne. Comedones are small keratin plugs that can be either open (black heads) or closed (whiteheads; Fig. 37.1A) Small papules and pustules can also be present, which can be associated with inflammation (Fig. 37.1B). Numerous nodules or large cysts indicate severe acne (Fig. 37.1C). Resolution of lesions may be complicated by scarring, keloids and post-inflammatory hyperpigmentation. The surface of the skin is also greasy. These lesions mainly occur on the face and the back.

## Diagnosis

The diagnosis is made clinically. The variants of acne include:

- *Infantile acne (milk spots)*. Within the first months of a baby's life, localized areas of acne spots may occur, mainly on the cheeks. They usually resolve spontaneously.

- *Acne conglobata*. This is a severe form of acne with numerous nodulocystic lesions. It may result in significant scarring. If there are systemic symptoms such as fever and malaise it is known as *acne fulminans*.

Topical and systemic steroids can induce the formation of acne so it important to obtain a drug history.

## Treatment and prognosis

Acne often resolves spontaneously by the time patients are in their early 20s. It can, however, persist into the 40s. Many people find the appearance of acne lesions unacceptable and seek treatment.

### Mild acne

Mild acne can be treated with the many types of topical therapy available. Benzoyl peroxide is commonly used and can be combined with antibiotics, salicylic acid or sulphur to increase its effectiveness. However, some find benzoyl peroxide irritating to the skin and it can bleach clothes. Topical retinoids are particularly effective for acne when the main lesions are comedones or papulopustules. Topical antibiotics commonly used are clindamycin and erythromycin.

### Moderate acne

When topical treatment has failed or if there is moderately severe acne, systemic treatment is needed. Oral antibiotics are usually considered and the commonest ones used are oxytetracycline and minocycline. Patients should take antibiotics for at least 4 months.

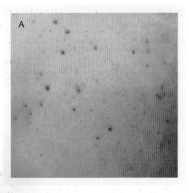
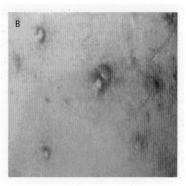
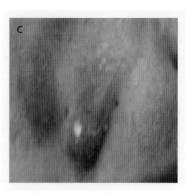

**Fig. 37.1** (A) Comedones. (B) Pustules. (C) Cysts. Courtesy of Stiefel Laboratories (UK).

Co-cyprindiol (Dianette) can be considered for females. It contains an anti-androgen, cyproterone acetate. It can also be used as a contraceptive. Its efficacy is similar to systemic antibiotics.

Prolonged use of Dianette is associated with an increased risk of thromboembolic disease. It should not be prescribed solely as contraception.

### Severe acne

Isotretinoin (Roaccutane) has dramatically improved the management of acne. It is used for severe acne, acne that is refractory to the above-mentioned treatment, or when it leaves residual scarring. The drug is usually taken for 4–6 months.

Many on isotretinoin experience dry lips and are more prone to nose bleeds. In some it causes night blindness. It is important not to become pregnant while taking this drug because it is associated with teratogenicity. The need for adequate contraception needs to be emphasized while taking it, and for up to 1 month after its cessation. Rarely, it can also cause hepatotoxicity.

Intralesional steroids such as triamcinolone can be used to reduce the inflammation from large nodular lesions.

The use of isotretinoin has revolutionized the treatment of acne. Currently the threshold for its use has lowered but it is important regularly to monitor its use because it can cause significant complications.

## ROSACEA

In rosacea there is sebaceous gland hyperplasia and dilated blood vessels. In contrast to acne, sebum production is normal. It is a common condition which affects people in their 40s and 50s.

### Clinical presentation

A common complaint is flushing of the face. Lesions that are seen include telangiectasia, small red papules, and at the top of these papules yellow pustules can occur. However, there are no comedonal lesions. The distribution is symmetrical. Lymphoedema can occur around the eyes and the nose may enlarge, known as rhinophyma. Alcohol, hot drinks, topical steroids and sunlight can worsen the condition. This condition can cause red, gritty eyes.

## Diagnosis

The diagnosis is made clinically. It can be confused with acne but the age of the patient and the absence of comedones helps distinguish it from acne.

## Treatment and prognosis

Rosaeca is often remediable to medical treatment but it tends to relapse.

Factors that precipitate the condition, such as alcohol and hot drinks, should be avoided. The papulopustular lesions can be controlled with oral antibiotics such as tetracyclines or erythromycin. The improvement often occurs within a few days of taking the antibiotic. A low-dose antibiotic can be used to prevent recurrences. Topical metronidazole is also useful. If these treatments fail, isotretinoin can be used. The telangiectasia can be treated with laser therapy.

## PERIORAL DERMATITIS

Perioral dermatitis occurs following the use of topical steroids around the mouth. There is a papulopustular eruption on an erythematous background. Scaling can be present but comedones are not. The condition can be treated with oxytetracycline and cessation of the topical steroids. Periorbital dermatitis is a similar condition which can affect the area around the eyes.

## HIDRADENITIS SUPPURATIVA

Hidradenitis suppurativa is a chronic disorder of the apocrine glands. It produces inflamed, tender pustules and nodules which regularly produce purulent discharge. There may also be sinuses and abscesses. The sites of predilection are the axilla and groin and have a symmetrical distribution. Healing can be complicated by significant scarring.

Large inflamed and tender nodules can be treated with intralesional steroids. Oral antibiotics are given for chronic disease. Systemic steroids and isotretinoin have also been tried. Abscesses can be surgically drained. Very extensive disease may need skin grafts.

You should be able to:

- Describe the difference between telogen and anagen effluvium.
- List the causes of telogen and anagen effluvium.
- Explain the clinical features of alopecia areata and idiopathic hirsutism.
- List the skin disorders that can cause scarring alopecia.

Hair problems can be categorized into too little or too much hair, or by its structural integrity.

## HAIR LOSS

### Telogen effluvium and anagen effluvium

Hair growth is separated into three phases:

- *Anagen phase*: this is the growing phase, which lasts for 4–5 years
- *Catagen phase*: during this phase, the hair follicle regresses and involution occurs. It lasts for a few days to weeks.
- *Telogen phase*: this is the resting phase during which hair is shed. It lasts for approximately 3 months.

Each hair grows according to its own growth cycle, which repeats itself. However, the normal hair cycle can be interrupted.

### Telogen effluvium

Telogen effluvium causes transient generalized hair loss on the scalp. All the hair is in the telogen phase and is shed prematurely when it converts into the anagen phase. It occurs after a few weeks up to 4 months following a precipitating event such as a severe illness, surgery or delivery of a baby. Certain drugs can also cause this condition; they include heparin, warfarin, carbimazole and excess vitamin A. The hair may be lost in several localized areas to begin with. Beau lines may be found in the nails,

which signifies a previous illness. Hair regrowth will occur after several months. Treatment is not required.

### Anagen effluvium

In anagen effluvium, growth of all the hair follicles on the scalp suddenly stops. This causes loss of hair in a similar pattern to telogen effluvium but the hair loss is much quicker. It is most commonly caused by chemotherapy. Hair regrowth occurs once there is cessation of the cause.

### Male pattern baldness (androgenic alopecia)

Male pattern baldness often starts after puberty and is complete by the 40s. There is a genetic component to this condition. It can also occur in women but tends to begin later in life, in or after the 7th decade.

The baldness often starts at the front, followed by the top of the head, leaving the sides of the head with hair. These areas can also become affected and approximately 15% of men lose all their hair on their scalp this way (Fig. 38.1).

There is no successful treatment for baldness. Topical minoxidil and oral finasteride have been tried with limited improvement in some. Hair transplants can also be used, but this is more common in America. This treatment is also associated with only limited success in some.

### Alopecia areata

*Alopecia areata* is a common cause of localized hair loss on the scalp. However, hair can be lost from other parts of the body. If the hair from both the scalp

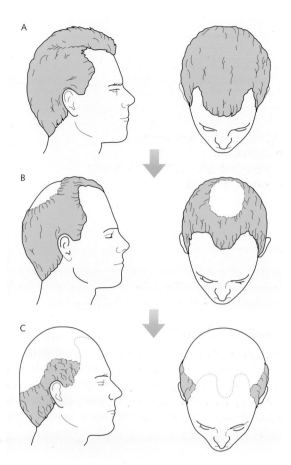

**Fig. 38.1** Male pattern baldness. (Reproduced with permission from D. Gawkrodger, *Dermatology: An Illustrated Colour Text*, 2nd edn, 2002, Churchill Livingstone, Edinburgh.)

and the eyebrows is lost, then the condition is known as *alopecia totalis*. When there is complete hair loss from the body, it is known as *alopecia universalis*.

## Clinical features

There is usually a well-defined patch of hair loss on the scalp but several areas can be affected. The hair loss in the patch is complete and there are no clinically detectable changes on the skin. Short, broken hairs may be found in these patches, known as 'exclamation hairs', which indicate active disease and are diagnostic for this condition.

The hair loss occurs gradually over weeks to months. The scalp is not painful or itching. It is also associated with nail pitting. There be may also be association with autoimmune disease such as vitiligo and myasthenia gravis.

## Diagnosis

A clinical diagnosis is made. The lack of symptoms and skin changes allow the diagnosis to be made easily.

## Treatment and prognosis

In most cases regrowth of the hair occurs spontaneously within a year. However, recurrences occur frequently. Poor prognostic signs for recovery include numerous patches of alopecia, large areas affected, childhood onset and other areas of the body affected.

Treatment is difficult to assess owing the spontaneously recovery of this condition. Topical and intralesional steroids are most commonly used. Dinitrochlorobenzene and dithranol can cause significant irritation and are unacceptable in some. Phototherapy has also been tried.

## Other causes of hair loss

Hair loss can be due to physical means such as trauma or burns. Lichen planus and lupus erythematosus can also cause alopecia and they have been discussed in the relevant chapters. However, in these conditions there is scarring and atrophy where the hair loss occurs and this is known as scarring alopecia. In contrast, telogen and anagen effluvium, alopecia areata and male pattern baldness are known as non-scarring alopecia as no skin changes are detectable. Tinea capitis can result in scarring alopecia.

## IDIOPATHIC HIRSUTISM

Idiopathic hirsutism is largely determined by race. Asian women are far more commonly affected than those of Anglo-Saxon and Chinese decent. The hairs are fine and dark and tend to grow above the upper lip, forming a moustache, around the nipples and on the upper limbs. These hairs are usually removed by physical means such shaving, plucking, electrolysis, lasering and waxing. The colour of the hairs can be lightened by bleaching.

## STRUCTURAL DEFECTS

Abnormalities affecting the hair shafts are rare and are usually inherited in nature. They cause the hair to be thin and weak, which allows it to be broken easily.

**Objectives**

You should be able to:

- Name the causes of leg ulcers.
- Understand how to investigate a patient with a leg ulcer.
- Distinguish the clinical features of a venous leg ulcer from an arterial one.
- List the conditions that can cause a neuropathic leg ulcer.

Chronic leg ulceration affects approximately 1% of the population and 3–5% of those over 65 affected. The incidence of leg ulcers is increasing owing to an aging population. Most leg ulcers are caused by venous or arterial diseases. Other causes are shown in Fig. 39.1.

## VENOUS INSUFFICIENCY

An increase in pressure in the venous system in the leg can lead to ulceration. This is most often caused by deficiency of the valves of the deep veins in the legs. However, the complete mechanism leading to valve insufficiency has not been completely elucidated.

### Clinical presentation

The clinical features of venous disease usually start in middle age and are progressive (Fig. 39.2). Risk factors for venous insufficiency are varicose veins, obesity, immobility and previous venous thrombosis in the leg.

### Diagnosis

A complete clinical history and examination needs to be performed to identify the risk factors for venous insufficiency. The ankle brachial pressure index is assessed with a Doppler to exclude arterial disease (ankle brachial pressure index >0.9) and to assess superficial venous reflux.

### Treatment and prognosis

Patients are best managed in the community, where they can maintain their independence and mobility,

which is especially important in the elderly population. In addition, the sheer number of patients involved would overwhelm hospital services.

The treatment of these leg ulcers is often long term because improvement is slow. The presence of risk factors for venous insufficiency, such as obesity, should be improved,. Simple measures include leg elevation and improving mobility. The mainstay of treatment is compression bandaging, which helps control the oedema of the leg. Venous eczema should be treated with regular emollients and a mild to moderate potency topical steroid could also be used.

A small proportion of patients with venous disease may be suitable for surgical intervention. Venous surgery involves superficial incompetent veins being tied off and removed. Skin grafting to repair the ulcer can be also be used in selected patients.

## ATHEROSCLEROTIC DISEASE

The risk factors for peripheral vascular disease are smoking, diabetes, hyperlipaemia, hypertension, obesity and age. These factors are often found in the presence of a leg ulcer caused by arterial disease.

### Clinical presentation

The clinical features of arterial compromised leg are a cold, hairless leg with dystrophic toenails. The skin is cyanotic and there are symptoms of claudication. The ulcer typically occurs on the mid-shin and is painful, often at night. The ulcer is also deep-seated.

**Fig. 39.1** Causes of leg ulcers

| |
|---|
| Venous insufficiency |
| Peripheral arterial disease |
| Diabetes |
| Infection |
| Vasculitis |
| Neoplastic, e.g. squamous cell carcinoma, melanoma |
| Trauma |
| Pyoderma gangrenosum |

## Diagnosis

The location of the ulcer and the presence of pain help to differentiate it from a venous ulcer; however, both types of leg ulcers can coexist. Foot pulses are often impalpable. Doppler studies and contrast angiography are used to locate the site of obstruction.

## Treatment and prognosis

Initial treatment is to control the risk factors for atherosclerotic disease. Surgical intervention can be used to relieve the atherosclerotic obstruction in amenable patients. If their risk factors are not controlled adequately, then their leg ulcer will enlarge.

The presence of arterial disease prevents the use of compression bandaging.

Venous leg ulcers usually occur on the medial or lateral malleolus. Arterial leg ulcers are often painful and are located on weight-bearing areas of the leg.

## OTHER LEG ULCERS

### Neuropathic ulcers

Neuropathic ulcers are usually caused by diabetes. The foot has altered or even absent sensation, and is warm, with palpable pulses. The ulcers are located in high-pressure areas such the soles, metatarsal joints and heel. In diabetes there is usually atherosclerotic disease.

### Vasculitis (see Chapter 35, p. 178)

Leg ulcers caused by a vasculitic process will also have other cutaneous vasculitic changes, such as palpable purpura and petechiae. The ulcers become neurotic and punched out.

**Fig. 39.2** Clinical features of venous insufficiency

| | |
|---|---|
| • Leg feeling heavy and swelling | |
| • Hyperpigmentation | Brown stippled pattern – from haemosiderin deposition Telangiectasia Atrophie blanche – white lacy scarring |
| • Eczema | Can be complicated by contact and allergic dermatitis |
| • Lipodermatosclerosis | Fibrosis around the ankle causing to be indurated with oedema above and below the induration. The leg may give the appearance of an 'inverted champagne bottle' |
| • Ulceration | This may occur after minor trauma. The medial malleolus is often affected. The ulcer may enlarge if left untreated |

# History taking in the dermatology patient

40

## Objectives

You should be able to:

- Understand the key aspects that should be elicited when taking a clinical history from a dermatology patient.
- Give examples of cutaneous manifestations of systemic disorders.

It is possible to make a spot diagnosis with many skin disorders, but it is still necessary to obtain a history of the condition. The length of time spent on taking a clinical history depends on the skin complaint; a severe or complex problem will need a more involved history than a mild condition that has arisen only recently.

As with taking a history from a general medical patient, the process is divided into five main sections:

- Presenting complaint.
- Past medical history.
- Medication history.
- Social and family history.
- Systemic enquiry, including the impact of disease on the patient.

Taking a clinical history of a skin disorder follows a standard format of history taking that can be applied to any body system. History taking remains very important in dermatology.

## PRESENTING COMPLAINT

The purpose of this section is to elicit when and where the skin problems started, and if the skin lesions have changed over a period of time. It is also important to know the speed of onset, and whether the condition improves but relapses. You should enquire about any exacerbating factors, such as sunlight and stress.

Check for other symptoms associated with the skin condition, such as pruritus, pain and burning.

## PAST MEDICAL HISTORY

A previous history of a skin disorder is important since there will be a tendency for it to recur. For example, childhood eczema may recur even in adult life. There may be an associated history of atopy (increased propensity for asthma and hay fever).

A recent illness may predate the onset of a skin disorder, such as a streptococcal sore throat occurring prior to the start of guttate psoriasis.

Systemic diseases may have cutaneous manifestations. Examples include paraneoplastic syndromes and autoimmune diseases. Furthermore, the medication the patient takes for these conditions may actually be the culprit in causing their skin problem. Those who are immunocompromised are predisposed to infections (e.g. candida), and some skin cancers.

## MEDICATION HISTORY

Many skin disorders are iatrogenic – that is, they are caused by treatment the patient is receiving. Therefore, a comprehensive drug history is vital, and it is important not to forget 'over-the counter' medications. Cosmetics and moisturizing creams can cause local irritation and dermatitis.

40

## SOCIAL AND FAMILY HISTORY

Genetic factors are involved in many skin disorders, such as psoriasis and eczema. However, the extent to which inheritance determines the clinical course will vary between patients.

Environmental factors are also important:

- *Occupational exposure.* If the skin disorder improves during weekends and holidays, this may suggest exposure to contact allergens at work.
- *Weather* is another important environmental factor. For example, exposure to the sun during a vacation may improve psoriasis. A change in weather may precipitate eczema and urticaria.

## SYSTEMIC ENQUIRY

A cutaneous lesion may even be the first sign of a systemic disorder (Fig. 40.1).

**Fig. 40.1** Examples of systemic disorders with skin signs

| Systemic disorder | Skin manifestations |
|---|---|
| Diabetes mellitus | Granuloma annulare |
|  | Necrobiosis lipoidica |
|  | Recurrent skin infections |
|  | Xanthomas |
| Inflammatory bowel disease | Erythema nodosum |
|  | Pyoderma gangrenosum |
| Nutritional deficiencies | |
|    Scurvy | Perifollicular pupura |
|  | Corkscrew hairs |
|    Pellagra | Dermatitis |
|  | Hyperpigmentation |
| Renal insufficiency | Generalized pruritis |
|  | White nails |
|  | Pigmentation |

## QUALITY OF LIFE

It is important to discover the impact that the skin complaint has on the patient's way of life. This will give you a guide to the strength and speed of treatment that needs to be given.

# Examination of the dermatology patient

## Objectives

You should be able to:

- Use dermatological terminology to describe a skin lesion.
- List the terms used to describe secondary skin changes.

The essence of examining the skin is to expose as much of it as possible under good lighting – ideally with natural light. A magnifying glass is a useful aid and may detect features of a skin lesion that are not visible to the naked eye. Once the skin lesion is examined, it must be described.

## DESCRIBING SKIN LESIONS

Dermatology is a visual medical specialty and uses descriptive terms that have precise meanings. The correct use of this terminology will allow you to describe skin lesions succinctly and enable clinicians to visualize what you are seeing. The description of a singular lesion is less complicated than describing a rash. In this section, a structured approach to describe any skin lesion is presented.

To describe a singular lesion, start by stating its location. Palpation of the lesion will identify if it is raised. Closer examination will note secondary changes on the surface of the lesion (Fig. 41.1).

## Morphology (Fig. 41.2)

Fig. 41.2 represents some of the descriptive terms used in dermatology.

## Flat lesions

### Macule (A)

A macule is a flat well-circumscribed area of less than 1 cm in diameter that has changed (Fig. 41.3).

### Patch

A patch is essentially a large macule with a diameter of greater than 1 cm. The colour changes are the same as those found in macules.

### Telangiectasia

Telangiectasia describes dilatation of the dermal capillaries, giving the appearance of fine red/pink linear streaks across the skin.

## Solid raised lesions

### Papule (B)

A papule is a well-defined area of skin of less than 1 cm in diameter (some restrict it to a diameter of less than 0.5 cm). The origin of the elevation may be epidermal or dermal. It may have a top that is flat, dome-shaped or have a warty appearance.

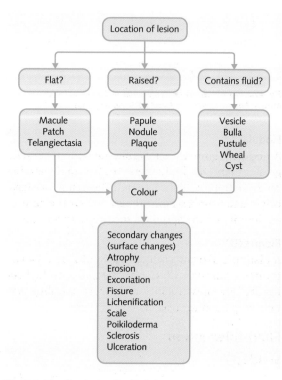

**Fig. 41.1** Algorithm to describe skin lesions.

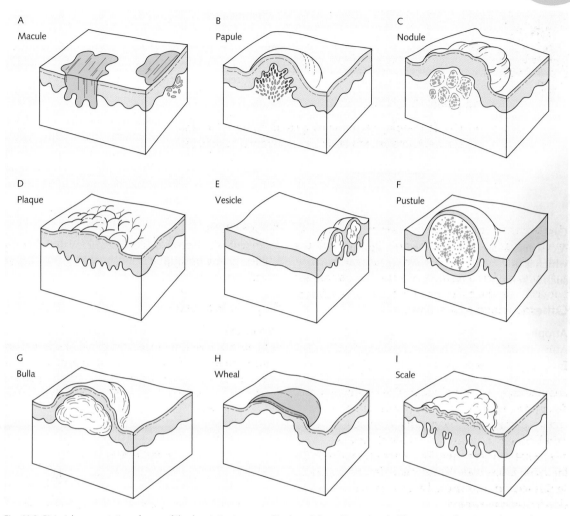

**Fig. 41.2** Pictorial representation of some of the descriptive terms used in dermatology. (Reproduced with permission from S. Knight, *Crash Course: Muscle, Bones and Skin*, 2nd edn, 2003, Mosby, London.)

## Nodule (C)

A nodule is similar to a papule but with a diameter greater than 1 cm in diameter (or 0.5 cm depending on the definition of the papule). The lesion may have originated from a papule. It may involve the dermis, epidermis and the dermis or the subcutaneous fat.

## Plaque (D)

A plaque is plateau-like raised area of skin. It can be formed from the coalescence of papules or thickening of a local area of skin. The presence of scaling may help with the diagnosis, as with psoriasis.

## Fluid-filled lesions

### Vesicle (E)

A vesicle is a raised lesion which is filled with clear fluid and with a diameter of less than 0.5 cm.

## Pustule (F)

A pustule is a raised lesion containing purulent green–yellow fluid. It may be sterile, as in psoriasis, or caused by an infection.

### Bulla (G)

A bulla is similar to a vesicle but with a diameter greater than 0.5 cm. The lesion may be situated within the epidermis or below it, in the dermis. Bullous pemphigoid and pemphigus vulgaris are such examples. Insect bites are one of the commonest causes of bulla.

### Wheal (H)

A wheal is a pruritic, transient, pink, oedematous swelling of the skin. It is often associated with a pale centre and can occur at any site on the body. The shapes of these lesions are variable and do not last for more than 24 hours. Wheals are the characteristic finding in urticaria.

**Fig. 41.3** Different colour macules and possible causes

| Colour change | Causes |
|---|---|
| White | Vitiligo, post-inflammatory changes (less white than in vitiligo) |
| Brown, blue, black | Melanocytic naevi. The actual colour depends on the concentration and depth of the pigment |
| Red/pink – erythema | Vasodilatation and inflammatory changes |

## Cyst

A cyst has a closed cavity with an epithelial lining which is filled with either fluid or semi-solid matter, such as keratin. A sebaceous cyst is such an example.

## Other terms: surface changes

### Atrophy

Atrophy occurs when there is a reduction of epidermis, dermis or subcutaneous fat. If the epidermis becomes thin, then there is fine wrinkling, loss of skin markings, hypopigmentation and translucency. Blood vessels may become visible.

### Erosion

An erosion occurs when there is superficial loss of the epidermis, and often heals without scarring.

### Excoriation

An excoriation is the loss of part or all of the epidermis as a consequence of scratching. Such lesions are usually linear or discrete circles, and may be shallow or deep. They tend to occur in pruritic skin conditions such as eczema.

### Fissure

This is an exaggerated linear split in the skin surface.

### Lichenification

In lichenification there is thickening of the skin, with attenuation of skin markings. It occurs due to chronic rubbing of the affected area, which may be the result of pruritis secondary to eczema.

### Scale (I)

Scaling of the skin causes it to be dry and flaky. It is the accumulation of keratinocytes, which readily detach from the surface of the epidermis. This is often an indication of inflammation and thickening of the epidermis. Scaling may be fine, as in pityriasis, or thick, as in psoriasis.

### Poikiloderma

Poikiloderma is said to occur when there is a combination of hyperpigmentation, skin atrophy and telangiectasia in a skin disorder.

### Sclerosis

In sclerosis, a localized area of skin has hardened or become indurated. This occurs as a result of infiltration, collagen proliferation, or dermal or subcutaneous oedema.

### Ulceration

An ulcer occurs when the full thickness of the epidermis is lost and some of the dermis. Ulcers are often well circumscribed and they heal with scarring. The surface may be covered with crusts or discharge exudate (serum, pus or slough).

Once the shape and the surface of the skin lesion have been assessed, then the margin and its consistency need to be described. If there are numerous lesions, their arrangement and symmetry should be described.

## Margin

Certain lesions have characteristic skin margins (Fig. 41.4).

**Fig. 41.4** The significance of lesion margins

| Margin | Description | Examples |
|---|---|---|
| Well defined/discrete | The lesion is clearly defined from the surrounding area | Psoriasis |
| Poorly defined/indistinct | The border merges with the surrounding skin | Eczema |
| Active edge | The edge may be raised, with relative clearing in the centre | Ringworm Annular lichen planus |
| Rolled | The border is raised and rolled up | Basal cell carcinoma |

# Common investigations in the dermatology patient

**Objectives**

You should be able to:

- Understand how to perform skin scrapings to detect a fungal skin infection.
- Appreciate how the Wood's lamp can be used be used in skin investigations.
- Understand the principle of dermatoscopy.

The diagnosis of skin disorders can usually be made clinically. However, there are occasions where dermatologists will use investigations to confirm their clinical suspicions and to detect any associated pathology.

## PHOTOGRAPHY

Skin lesions are often photographed, especially if they are unusual or when the diagnosis is not obvious. The hospital's medical illustration department usually takes the photographs.

## MICROBIOLOGY

### Cultures

Skin swabs can be taken for bacterial growth from ulcers or erosions. Virology cultures are usually requested to identify a member of the herpes virus. Electron microscopy can also be used to detect the herpes virus.

### Skin scrapings

Skin scrapings are performed if the diagnosis of a scaling rash is unknown (see Chapter 33, p. 173, diagnosis of tinea).

### Microscopy in the clinic

The microscope is a very useful yet simple piece of equipment. It can be used to detect hyphae from suspected skin fungal infections, or for the presence of mites and eggs.

### Wood's light

The Wood's light is an ultraviolet lamp and emits radiation with a wavelength of 360 nm. It will cause the skin to fluoresce in different colours in the presence of certain skin conditions (Fig. 42.1).

### Dermatoscopy

Dermatoscopy is a diagnostic technique that is used in the diagnosis of numerous skin lesions, in particular pigmented ones. It is essentially a hand-held magnifier which needs immersion oil to be applied on the surface of the skin lesion. The oil reduces the amount of light scattering at the skin's surface. This allows the epidermis and the junction between the epidermis and the dermis to be examined in detail.

### Skin biopsy

Different skin lesions may have similar appearances; a skin biopsy will help to determine the nature and severity of a condition. A biopsy can be examined under increasing magnification under a microscope and stained with various histological stains. It is important to include a clinical differential diagnosis on the request form, as it will help the histopathologist.

**Fig. 42.1** Different fluorescences that can be obtained from a Wood's lamp.

| Sample | Fluorescence colour | Diagnosis |
| --- | --- | --- |
| Hair | Green | Scalp ringworm infections |
| Skin | Yellow | Pityriasis vesicolor |
| Skin | Coral pink | Erythrasma |
| Urine and faeces | Bright pink | Porphyria cutanea tarda |

### Objectives

You should be able to:

- Understand the difference between sensorineural and conductive hearing losses, and list the more common causes of each.
- Say which parts of the history and examination are important.
- Describe bedside clinical hearing tests (tuning fork tests).
- Enumerate other useful hearing tests.
- Recognize when further investigation of hearing loss is required.

Patients commonly request advice from specialists and general practitioners regarding hearing loss. Loss may be unilateral or bilateral, of acute or chronic duration, and associated with other otological symptoms.

## DIFFERENTIAL DIAGNOSIS OF HEARING LOSS

The first decision to make is whether the hearing loss is caused by problems in the vibratory mechanism of the outer or middle ear (conductive loss), or is due to loss of transmission in the pathways of the eighth nerve (sensorineural loss) (Fig, 43.1).

### Causes of conductive hearing loss

- *External ear* or ear canal, e.g. congenital atresia, wax, foreign body, infection (otitis externa).
- *Tympanic membrane*, e.g. perforation.
- *Middle ear*, e.g. fixation of the ossicles (otosclerosis), glue ear (otitis media with effusion), acute otitis media.
- *Eustachian tube* dysfunction, with or without middle ear effusion, e.g. allergic rhinitis, tumours of the nasopharynx (nasopharyngeal carcinoma).

### Causes of sensorineural hearing loss (SNHL)

- *Congenital and intrauterine* causes, e.g. associated with congenital inner ear abnormalities or

with prematurity, low birth weight, jaundice, intrauterine infections.
- *Noise induced.*
- *Traumatic.*
- *Toxic*, e.g. aminoglycoside toxicity or following acute middle ear infection.
- *Autoimmune.*
- *Age-related* (presbyacusis).
- *Cerebellopontine angle tumours*, e.g. vestibular schwannoma (used to be called acoustic neuroma).
- *Sudden onset* SNHL. A separate entity thought to be a herpes simplex mononeuritis.
- *Ménière's disease.*

## HISTORY TO FOCUS ON IN HEARING LOSS

### Unilateral or bilateral

Hearing loss that affects one ear only is more worrying than if it affects both.

This is because unilateral conductive losses may be caused by pathology of the Eustachian tube orifice, e.g. a nasopharyngeal carcinoma. Unilateral sensorineural losses may be the presenting symptom of a vestibular schwannoma.

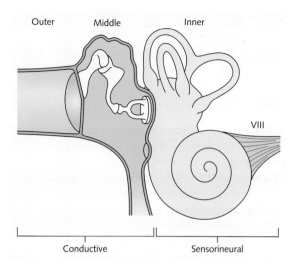

Outer    Middle    Inner

VIII

Conductive          Sensorineural

**Fig. 43.1** Conductive versus sensorineural hearing loss.

## Time of onset

Other family members are often the best judges of gradually worsening hearing. Acute onset of hearing loss is associated with otitis externa, otitis media, and toxic, traumatic and infective causes of SNHL. It may occasionally be seen as a result of compression by vestibular schwannomas. A more chronic course is typically seen with age-related SNHL and noise-related losses. Hearing loss that fluctuates is usually seen with middle ear effusions and also in Ménière's disease.

## Ear discharge

Otitis externa is typically associated with a mild discharge; more copious discharges suggest middle ear infection with a perforated tympanic membrane. Cholesteatoma, a chronic middle ear infection, produces persistent, foul-smelling discharge.

## Other otological symptoms

Ear pain (otalgia) is seen in acute infections of the external and middle ear, but is otherwise uncommon. Tinnitus and vertigo may be seen with middle and external ear infections, but are more commonly an indicator of inner ear pathology, e.g. Ménière's, schwannoma, ototoxicity, etc.

## Birth and pregnancy history

In cases of congenital deafness it important to ask about factors such as prematurity, birthweight, NICU stays, neonatal jaundice and other congenital abnormalities.

## Family history

Otosclerosis is an inherited form of conductive hearing loss and is transmitted as autosomal dominant manner with incomplete penetrance. Other forms of congenital hearing loss are caused by specific inheritable abnormalities or may be sporadic.

## Drug history

It is important to note that the use of aminoglycosides, aspirin, loop diuretics and many of the anti-neoplastic agents among others can cause a sensorineural deafness.

## Occupational history

Both acute and chronic noise exposure at work, recreationally or accidentally, can result in noise induced hearing loss.

> Noise exposure that leaves ringing in the ears afterwards is loud enough to permanently damage hearing, so ask about hobbies such as shooting, DJing, headphone use, etc.

## EXAMINATION OF THE PATIENT WITH HEARING LOSS

### Test the hearing clinically (see Chapter 65, p. 304)

- Do you have to raise your voice to make the patient hear you?
- Ask the patient to repeat two-syllable words, both when whispered and when spoken, e.g. cowboy.
- Perform tuning fork tests. (Weber's and Rinne's.)

### Examine the external ear and ear canal using an otoscope

Look for wax, swelling of the ear canal (otitis externa or exostoses).

It sounds obvious, but if you can see all or part of the tympanic membrane then the cause of the hearing loss is not in the external ear.

## Examine the tympanic membrane

(Fig. 43.2)

- Are there any perforations?
- Is it bulging (middle ear fluid), or retracted/ sucked in (Eustachian tube dysfunction)?
- Is the colour normal (pinky-white and slightly translucent)?
- Is there evidence of inflammation (red), or middle ear effusion (yellowish and serous, greyish in glue ear)?
- Light reflex. Greatly over-rated and mostly ignored by specialists.

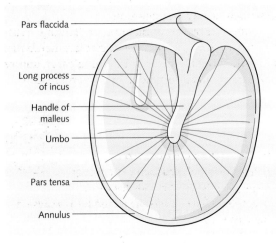

Pars flaccida

Long process of incus

Handle of malleus

Umbo

Pars tensa

Annulus

**Fig. 43.2** The normal tympanic membrane (right ear).

## INVESTIGATION OF THE PATIENT WITH HEARING LOSS

### Hearing tests (see Chapter 65)

Commonly used tests include:

- Pure tone audiogram – standard test of patient responses to tones of varying frequency and intensity.
- Other tests may be necessary where the patient cannot cooperate with testing, e.g. oto-acoustic emission testing (OAEs), brain stem evoked response audiometry (BERA).
- Tympanometry.

### Imaging

Most patients require no further imaging. There are some situations where further information is required:

- Unilateral SNHL. A gadolinium-enhanced MRI scan of the internal auditory meatus is performed to exclude a vestibular schwannoma.
- Hearing loss associated with malformations of the external ear, acute trauma or chronic middle ear infections in adults (cholesteatoma) where a fine section CT of the temporal bones may be invaluable.

### Other tests

The vast majority of patients will require no further investigation than careful examination and standard audiological testing (PTAs and tympanometry). However, some patients with SNHL may warrant further investigations to find out the cause of their disability; these may include an autoantibody screen and specialist genetic testing.

Vertigo is the erroneous impression of movement. Few things can be as unpleasant as vertigo, as anyone who has suffered from seasickness will testify. Patients readily volunteer that they 'wanted to die' during acute attacks. Similar feelings may overtake medical students confronted with this troubling symptom.

## DIFFERENTIAL DIAGNOSIS OF VERTIGO

### Central causes

- Cerebrovascular disease.
- Migraine (common cause in children).
- Multiple sclerosis.
- Vertebrobasilar insufficiency.
- Cervical vertigo (degeneration causing altered proprioceptive input).
- Drug induced (aminoglycosides, alcohol, etc.).

### Peripheral causes

There are three common pathologies:

- Benign paroxysmal positional vertigo (BPPV).
- Ménière's disease.
- Acute vestibulitis.

More rarely …

- Vestibular schwannoma.
- Suppurative middle ear disease affecting the inner ear (acute suppurative otitis media or cholesteatoma).

## HISTORY TO FOCUS ON IN VERTIGO

### Is this true vertigo?

The first step in wading through the mire that is 'dizziness' is to establish if the symptoms are due to an abnormality in the vestibular system. The hallmark of vestibular dysfunction is rotatory vertigo, often described as the room spinning.

Other causes of imbalance or 'feeling lightheaded' or 'funny turns' may be cardiac, metabolic, musculoskeletal, ocular or neurological in nature and can usually be excluded by a careful history.

Vestibular dysfunction does not cause collapse or loss of consciousness, although many patients wish it would! Beware of hyperventilation or cardiac abnormalities as a cause in these patients.

### Duration

Possibly the easiest way to discriminate between the common causes of vertigo is to ask how long each attack lasts: vertigo lasting for seconds is benign paroxysmal positional vertigo; minutes to hours suggests Ménière's disease, and days to weeks, vestibulitis.

## Position

BPPV is a momentary vertiginous sensation associated with sudden changes in head position, typically rolling over in bed.

## Other otological symptoms

Ménière's disease comprises episodic vertigo, often preceded by a feeling of aural fullness, tinnitus and a fluctuating hearing loss. With each attack hearing tends to deteriorate.

Ear discharge associated with vertigo suggests that spread of suppurative middle ear disease to the inner ear may have occurred. *This is an emergency* and requires prompt investigation and treatment before intracranial spread of infection occurs. Acute vestibulitis often follows an upper respiratory tract infection (URTI) and produces severe vertigo sometimes lasting many days. If the hearing is also affected then the term labyrinthitis may be used.

## EXAMINATION OF PATIENTS WITH VERTIGO

### Otological examination

Look for signs of suppurative middle ear disease, e.g. ear discharge and a perforation. Test hearing clinically and perform Weber's and Rinne's tests.

### Neurological examination

Perform cranial nerve examination, looking especially for nystagmus.

Nystagmus is involuntary rhythmic pendular movement of the eyes. Physiologic nystagmus may be seen at extremes of gaze in normal individuals. Pathological nystagmus can occur with visual impairment, central disease or vestibular dysfunction.

Cerebellar signs may also be sought if indicated.

### Special tests

- Gait assessment.
- Romberg's test. If there is a vestibular lesion the patient will tend to fall to that side.
- Unterberger's test. The patient walks on the spot with the eyes closed for 30 seconds. Rotation greater than 30° in either direction suggests vestibular pathology.

### Medical examination

Simple medical examination, such as checking the pulse and performing sitting and standing blood pressure measurement, can be invaluable in identifying non-vestibular causes of imbalance.

## SPECIAL INVESTIGATIONS IN THE PATIENT WITH VERTIGO

### Vestibular function testing

The Dix–Hallpike test is the diagnostic test for BPPV and aims to replicate the symptoms of dizziness and signs of nystagmus by a rapid change in head position.

Further tests are used to assess both vestibulo-ocular and vestibulo-spinal reflex arcs. The former include electro-nystagmography (ENG), caloric testing and visual pursuit, the latter postureography.

### Imaging

In cases where the diagnosis is not clear, or if there is a suspicion of central pathology, i.e. vertigo with hearing loss or other cranial nerve pathology, then a gadolinium enhanced MRI scan is invaluable. CT scanning is performed if there is any suspicion of middle ear infection.

Ear discharge, or otorrhoea, is most often a product of inflammation of the outer or middle ear. More rarely it may be due to CSF leakage following a head injury.

## DIFFERENTIAL DIAGNOSIS OF EAR DISCHARGE

- Otitis externa.
- Perforated acute otitis media (children).
- Chronic suppurative otitis media.
- Trauma to external canal or tympanic membrane (TM).
- CSF otorrhoea.
- Rarities, e.g. tumours of external or middle ear.

## HISTORY TO FOCUS ON IN EAR DISCHARGE

### Nature of the discharge

The external ear is lined with skin and does not contain mucous glands, therefore otitis externa tends to produce scanty serous discharge or makes the ear feel 'wet'. There are lots of mucous glands in the middle ear and a discharge originating here is more profuse and often mucoid in nature. Blood-staining is not uncommon in discharge from the middle ear because of the friability of inflamed middle ear mucosa. A more serosanguinous discharge may be seen with carcinomas of the external or middle ear. Cholesteatoma is an accumulation of keratin within the middle ear cleft. If infected it produces a chronic foul-smelling mucopurulent discharge.

## Otalgia (ear pain)

Most episodes of ear discharge are pain free; however, pain may be present in a number of situations. In children pain may be a consequence of acute otitis media; it precedes the ear discharge and rapidly settles following perforation. Pain is not uncommon in otitis externa and is often worsened by movement of the external ear or otoscopic examination. Deep-seated and intractable pain with ear discharge suggests 'malignant' otitis externa or true malignancy.

Pain (otalgia) occurs with ear discharge in:
Acute otitis externa (especially with a furuncle).
Acute otitis media.
Complicated chronic suppurative otitis media, e.g. mastoiditis.
'Malignant' otitis externa.
Malignancy of the external ear canal.

### Trauma

A history of head injury (or neurosurgery) preceding the ear discharge should alert you to the possibility of CSF otorrhoea.

## EXAMINATION OF PATIENTS WITH EAR DISCHARGE

### External ear

Look for signs of acute otitis externa (i.e. cellulitis of the pinna may spread to surrounding skin), or chronic otitis externa (i.e. eczematous change).

## Ear canal

Oedema and tenderness of the canal and visible keratinous debris suggests otitis externa. Pigmented fungal spores and material like 'wet paper' are often seen in fungal otitis externa. This condition is often intensely itchy. Vesicles may occur in the ear canal with varicella zoster infection and may precede facial palsy (Ramsay Hunt syndrome). Ulceration or exposure of bone may occur in malignancy and 'malignant' otitis externa.

## Tympanic membrane

It is an obvious point but middle ear discharge can only occur in the presence of a perforated TM. So look for perforations. Also remember to look for ventilation tubes (grommets). Do not forget to look up in the Attic for signs of cholesteatoma (see p. 231). Polyps visible in the external canal usually originate as a result of inflamed middle ear mucosa pushing through a perforation.

## INVESTIGATION OF A PATIENT WITH AN EAR DISCHARGE

## Hearing tests

Audiometry and tympanometry may show the presence of a conductive hearing loss. This occurs often in chronic suppurative otitis media, invariably in cholesteatoma and occasionally in otitis externa.

## Imaging

High resolution CT scanning is used to look for disease of the middle ear and mastoid and to help in the diagnosis and staging of suspected malignancy.

## Microbiology

Ear swabs are useful to guide antibiotic choice and may identify a fungal otitis externa. They are ideally performed in all patients with an ear discharge.

## Tests for CSF

B2 transferrin is found only in CSF and endolymph. Modern tests are extremely sensitive and require less than 0.3 ml of fluid for analysis.

### Objectives

You should:

- Know the different causes of otalgia.
- Know about the importance of referred otalgia.
- Know what to look for in the examination of a patient with otalgia.
- Know which investigations to perform.

Due to the complexity of their development, the structures of the ear derive sensory innervation from a number of different cranial and spinal nerves (Fig. 46.1). Otalgia, or the feeling of pain in the ear, can be caused by disease within the ear itself, by pain from surrounding structures, or, alternatively, by pain referred from the more distant reaches of these sensory nerve branches.

## DIFFERENTIAL DIAGNOSIS OF OTALGIA

### Pain from ear disease

#### Disease of the external ear

- Wax impaction.
- Otitis externa.
- Furuncle.
- Malignant otitis externa.
- Malignancy of external canal.

#### Disease of the middle ear

- Otitis media with effusion (glue ear).
- Eustachian tube dysfunction.
- Acute otitis media and mastoiditis.
- Complications of chronic suppurative otitis media.

### Pain from surrounding structures

- Disorders of the temporomandibular joint.
- Periauricular lymphadenopathy.

### Referred otalgia – from any of the nerves with a sensory input to the ear

- *Facial nerve*. Bell's palsy, Ramsay Hunt syndrome.
- *Trigeminal nerve*. Nasal and paranasal sinus malignancy, oral cavity lesions, dental pain.
- *Glossopharyngeal nerve*. Tongue base, tonsil malignancy, tonsillitis, especially quinsy, glossopharyngeal neuralgia.
- *Vagus nerve*. Laryngeal, pharyngeal or oesophageal pathology.
- *Cervical plexus*. C2, C3 root lesions.

## HISTORY IN THE PATIENT WITH OTALGIA

### Pain history

It is important to take a comprehensive pain history. Dull, mild pain which lasts only a short time may be seen in otitis media with effusion and Eustachian tube dysfunction. Deep-seated severe unremitting pain suggests malignancy or malignant otitis externa. Neuralgic pain, as seen in glossopharyngeal neuralgia, is unilateral, extremely severe and lancinating (stabbing) in nature.

Pain from inflammation of the external ear tends to be worse with movement of the ear and occasionally with chewing. However, pain that is provoked by chewing or wide mouth opening often has its origin in the temporomandibular joint or its surrounding muscles.

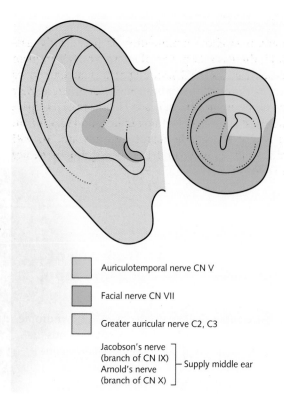

Auriculotemporal nerve CN V

Facial nerve CN VII

Greater auricular nerve C2, C3

Jacobson's nerve
(branch of CN IX)
Arnold's nerve        } — Supply middle ear
(branch of CN X)

**Fig. 46.1** The nerves responsible for referred otalgia.

Obviously when trying to establish the origin of ear pain it is important to enquire about other ear symptoms. Hearing loss, tinnitus, ear discharge and vertigo all suggest ear disease as a cause for the pain. On the other hand, in the absence of ear symptoms it is worthwhile enquiring about other upper aero–digestive tract symptoms such as hoarseness or dysphagia.

## EXAMINATION OF THE PATIENT WITH OTALGIA

### Examine the ear

Using an otoscope carefully examine the ear. Examine the pinna and external ear canal looking for oedema, erythema, furuncles, herpetic vesicles, canal polyps and ulceration with bone exposure. Then examine the tympanic membrane, noting the presence of bulging or erythema, perforations and middle ear discharge. Palpate over the mastoid process for tenderness.

## Examine the temporomandibular joint (TMJ)

Ask the patient to open and close their mouth. Look for limitation of movement and ask about pain on mouth opening. Palpate the joint feeling for crepitus. Tenderness at the condylar neck and in the muscles of mastication is seen in TMJ dysfunction.

Temporomandibular joint dysfunction is a very common cause of 'ear' pain. It may be bilateral and is usually worse with chewing. It usually responds to non-steroidal anti-inflammatory drugs and a soft diet. A special dental appliance may also be helpful.

If the examination of these structures is normal, and especially if this is combined with normal audiograms and tympanometry, then the cause of the pain may be referred otalgia. It is then necessary to examine the nose, nasopharynx, oral cavity and teeth, larynx and pharynx to rule out disease here. The easiest way to do this is with a flexible naso-endoscope.

If a patient has normal ears and TMJs but still has ear pain, be very suspicious that this may be referred otalgia. Be especially wary if the patient is a smoker or has any other symptoms suggestive of an upper aero–digestive tract cancer, e.g. voice changes, dysphagia, weight loss. Have a very low threshold for investigating these patients further using either CT imaging of the upper aero–digestive tract and/or endoscopy.

## INVESTIGATION OF THE PATIENT WITH OTALGIA (Fig. 46.2)

### Audiometry and tympanometry

Normal results from these tests combined with normal otoscopy findings increase the possibility that the cause of the otalgia lies outside the ear.

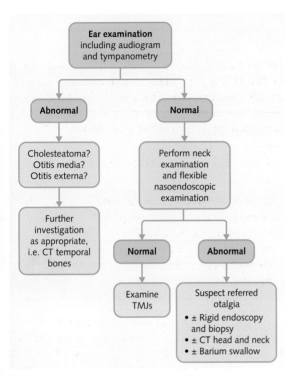

**Fig. 46.2** Algorithm for the investigation of otalgia.

## Imaging

Barium swallow examination is particularly useful if there is a suspicion of referred otalgia from an oesophageal site. CT scanning of the temporal bones and occasionally other head and neck structures may be useful in the difficult case. Finally, in cases where no satisfactory explanation can be found for ear pain it is wise to exclude neurological disease. An MRI scan of the brain is often the investigation of choice in these cases.

# Nasal blockage

**Objectives**

You should be able to:

- Describe the differential diagnosis of nasal blockage.
- Ask the appropriate questions in the history.
- List the appropriate investigations to perform in a patient with nasal blockage.

The paired nasal cavities act together to prepare inspired air for delivery to the lower respiratory tract and as the sites of the organs of olfaction. The presence of a rich and variable blood supply allows warming, humidification and the filtering of particles to occur speedily and efficiently.

The physiological nasal cycle is the result of the alternating engorgement of the nasal mucosa in each side of the nose. It is under the regulation of the autonomic nervous system. The result is increased nasal blockage which changes sides every 3–6 hours. It may be misinterpreted as a symptom of nasal disease.

## DIFFERENTIAL DIAGNOSIS OF NASAL BLOCKAGE

- Physiological – nasal cycle.
- Congenital, e.g. choanal atresia.
- Traumatic, e.g. septal deformity.
- Rhinitis, which may be:
  - Infective (usually viral)
  - Allergic (seasonal or perennial)
  - Non-allergic, e.g. Wegener's, sarcoid.
- Nasal polyps, which may be:
  - Isolated
  - Associated with respiratory disease.
- Adenoidal hypertrophy (children).
- Malignancy of nose, sinus or postnasal space.

Nasal blockage may follow trauma, especially where the nasal bones or septum have become deformed. It is important to find out if the blockage happens only in specific situations. An example of this is the patient with perennial allergic rhinitis attributable to house dust mite allergy whose nose becomes blocked when in bed. If the patient has seasonal allergic rhinitis (hay fever) then blockage may only occur in spring and summer. Nasal polyposis causes persistent blockage that may be made worse with alcohol.

In children, adenoidal hypertrophy, peaks at around 4–6 years, and may cause nasal blockage and mouth breathing, often with a mucopurulent nasal discharge.

## HISTORY TO FOCUS ON IN NASAL BLOCKAGE

### Timing and nature of the blockage

A variable blockage that switches from side to side may represent the normal physiological nasal cycle.

### Associated nasal symptoms

Itchy eyes, nose and throat, sneezing and nasal discharge often accompany nasal blockage in allergic rhinitis and acute viral rhinitis. The itching and sneezing are less common in non-allergic rhinitis where blockage is mainly accompanied by watery nasal discharge.

## Associated respiratory symptoms

There are important associations between allergic rhinitis and asthma, and between nasal polyposis and ciliary dysfunction or cystic fibrosis. There may also be nasal manifestations in sarcoidosis and Wegener's granulomatosis. In the absence of such diagnoses all patients with nasal blockage should be asked about respiratory symptoms, especially shortness of breath, cough and wheeze.

## EXAMINATION OF PATIENTS WITH NASAL BLOCKAGE

See also Chapter 65, p. 309, and Fig. 47.1.

## General

Look for signs of atopy, e.g. eczema, and chronic chest disease, e.g. hyperinflation.

## Examination of the nose

Look for obvious external nasal deformity. Assess each side of the nasal airway.

Look at the nose from below for a septal deviation. From the front look for septal deformity, inferior turbinate hypertrophy, rhinitis, nasal polyps, foreign bodies, etc.

### Rhinoscopy

If a rigid naso-endoscope (Fig. 47.2) is available it should be possible to examine the entire nasal cavity back to the nasopharynx. This allows the identification of crusting, rhinitis (characteristically pale, wet and oedematous mucosa), nasal polyps (white, translucent and grape-like) and pus originating from the sinus ostia in sinusitis. A flexible naso-endoscope may also be employed to examine the nasopharynx and Eustachian tube orifices looking for swelling or adenoidal enlargement.

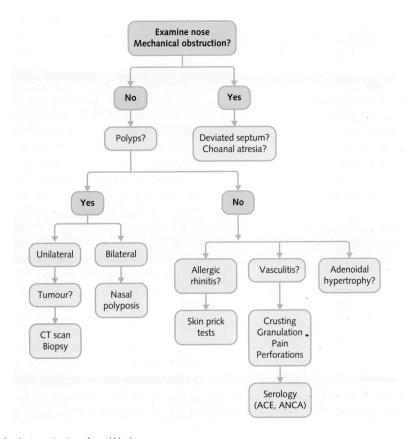

**Fig. 47.1** Algorithm for the investigation of nasal blockage.

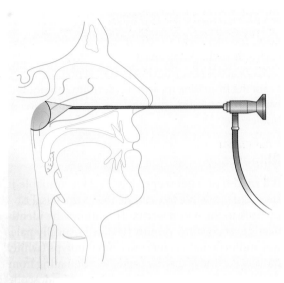

**Fig. 47.2** A rigid naso-endoscope. (Reproduced with permission from R.S. Dhillon, C.A. East, *Ear, Nose and Throat and Head and Neck Surgery: An Illustrated Colour Text*, 9th edn, 2006, Elsevier, Edinburgh.)

## INVESTIGATION OF THE PATIENT WITH NASAL BLOCKAGE

See p. 310.

Most diagnoses can made based on a thorough history and examination.

### Specialist rhinological investigations

These are used to quantify nasal blockage (nasal inspiratory peak flow and acoustic rhinometry) and to measure disease activity within the nose (nitric oxide measurement and tests of mucociliary transport).

Allergic rhinitis is one of the most common causes of nasal blockage. The assessment of coexistent allergy by skin prick testing is particularly useful.

### Respiratory investigations

Respiratory diseases frequently affect the nose, and so examination of the respiratory system, assessment of pulmonary function and special tests, e.g. ESR, serum ACE, ANCA and immunoglobulin assessment, are sometimes required.

### Imaging

Most patients do not require imaging. In patients with nasal polyps, fine-cut CT scans of the nose and paranasal sinuses are requested prior to surgery and also to exclude rarer pathology such as inverted papilloma. If malignancy is suspected then CT scans are used for diagnosis and staging.

Beware the patient with unilateral nasal polyps. Inflammatory polyps are by their nature generally bilateral. Patients with unilateral polyps require careful examination, a CT scan of the sinuses, and often a biopsy to exclude a neoplasm such as an inverted papilloma (see Chapter 56) or a sinonasal malignancy.

The role of the nasal mucosa as both humidifier and warmer of inspired air demands a copious blood flow. A disadvantage of this, however, is the propensity of the nasal mucosa to bleed (see Chapter 56).

## DIFFERENTIAL DIAGNOSIS IN EPISTAXIS

### Local factors

- External trauma.
- Nose picking.
- Drying of mucosa – nasal O2, septal spurs.
- Effects of ageing on blood vessels.
- Septal perforation.
- Tumours.

### Systemic factors

- Platelet factors.
  - Thrombocytopenia ( many causes).
  - 'Anti-platelet' medications, e.g. aspirin.
- Clotting abnormalities.
  - Inherited, e.g. haemophilia , von Willebrand's disease.
  - Acquired, e.g. liver disease, anticoagulants.
- Vessel wall abnormalities.
  - Hereditary haemorrhagic telangiectasia.

For many patients there are, however, no identifiable risk factors. Many healthy people suffer from epistaxis. While it has been noted that many patients with an active nose bleed are hypertensive at the time of bleeding, no causative association has been proven.

## HISTORY TO FOCUS ON IN EPISTAXIS

It is important to note the duration of any bleeds, their site, and whether they are unilateral or bilateral. Anterior bleeding presents most often as unilateral epistaxis; bleeding originating more posteriorly may present with bleeding from both sides or may even be spat from the mouth. Nasal blockage, facial pain and unilateral deafness may suggest tumour as a cause for epistaxis. Other important things to note are whether the patient is hypertensive or has an abnormal bleeding tendency, as a result of either disease or anti-platelet or anticoagulant medication.

A good screening question for platelet and clotting abnormalities is 'Have you had problems with bleeding when you have had teeth extracted?'. It is likely that anyone with a marked bleeding diathesis would have suffered considerable post-extraction haemorrhage.

## EXAMINATION OF THE PATIENT WITH EPISTAXIS

### General examination

- Vital signs and the recognition of shock.
- Mucosal lesions associated with hereditary haemorrhagic telangiectasia may be visible on the skin or lips.

## Nasal examination

Try to identify the site of the bleeding within the nose. This can be done with a head-light and Thudicum's speculum or a fibreoptic endoscope. Pay particular attention to Little's area and examine the nasopharynx for pathology.

## INVESTIGATION OF THE PATIENT WITH EPISTAXIS

## Haematological investigations

Full blood count, crossmatch, group and save, clotting (liver disease and anticoagulants).

## Imaging

A CT scan is ordered later if there is any suggestion of neoplasia. Angiography is occasionally required if therapeutic embolization is considered.

## MANAGEMENT OF THE PATIENT WITH EPISTAXIS

An algorithm for the management of epistaxis is shown in Fig. 48.1.

**Fig. 48.1** Algorithm for the management of epistaxis.

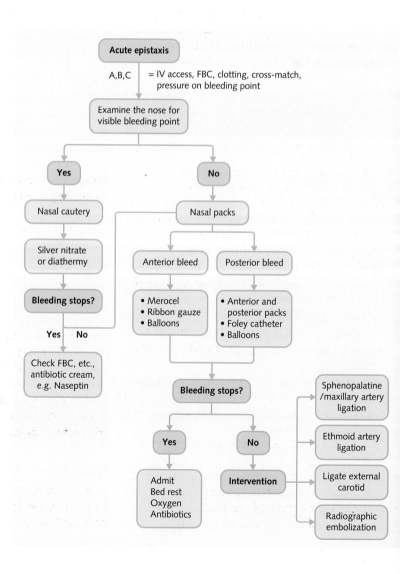

### Objectives

You should be able to:

- Give an account of the differential diagnosis of a neck lump.
- Understand what questions to ask in the history, especially to elicit a diagnosis of malignancy.
- Describe a neck lump (site, size, etc.).
- Say which further investigations are appropriate for a patient with a neck lump.

The complex anatomical arrangement of the neck means that pathology of many different tissues can present as a visible or palpable swelling. This is a frequent presenting sign of malignant disease.

## DIFFERENTIAL DIAGNOSIS OF A NECK LUMP

- *Skin lumps* (e.g. sebaceous cyst, lipoma).
- *Cystic* (e.g. branchial cyst, thyroglossal duct cyst).
- *Lymphadenopathy* or swelling of lymph nodes, which may be:
  - *Secondary to suppurative disease* in the head and neck (e.g. skin, tonsils, teeth, sinuses, etc.)
  - *Infective: viral* (e.g. EBV (infectious mononucleosis), HIV); *bacterial* (e.g. TB); *parasitic* (e.g. toxoplasmosis, cat scratch disease).
  - *Inflammatory* (e.g. rheumatoid arthritis, SLE).
  - *Primary malignancy* (e.g. lymphoma or leukaemia).
  - *Metastatic malignant disease: from head and neck* (usually a squamous cell carcinoma); *from distant sites* (e.g. Virchow's node from gastric malignancy, breast, etc.).
- *Salivary gland* (e.g. submandibular and parotid gland swellings).
- *Thyroid gland: goitre* – physiological, pathological; *cyst*; *tumour*, benign or malignant.
- *Vascular* (e.g. carotid body tumour).
- *Lymphangiomatous* (e.g. cystic hygroma).

## HISTORY IN PATIENTS WITH A NECK LUMP

### Symptoms suggestive of malignancy

Any patient who complains of a neck lump along with weight loss, night sweats, hoarseness or dysphagia has malignant disease until proven otherwise. Any neck lump in a smoker must similarly be regarded with suspicion.

### Is there infection elsewhere?

Next, it is important to ascertain if there is infection elsewhere that may be causing secondary lymph node swelling. Ask about dental problems, ear discharge, sore throat and sinus pain. Painful neck swellings are unusual and if pain is present it is usually secondary to suppuration which may progress to abscess formation.

### Duration

Lumps that have been present and static for years are often not worrying, for example calcified lymph nodes following TB. A short, painful history suggests infection. Progressive painless enlargement, however, suggests neoplastic disease, be it benign or malignant. Variation in size with mealtimes is seen in obstructive salivary gland disease.

## Thyroid-related symptoms

If you suspect the patient may have a thyroid lump then ask about heat intolerance, weight gain, weight loss, change in mood, lethargy, etc.

## EXAMINATION OF THE PATIENT WITH A NECK LUMP

### General examination

Observe the patient, looking for signs of anaemia including pallor, glossitis, cheilitis, koilonychia, etc. Look for cachexia and jaundice, which may indicate malignancy. Listen to the patient speak; hoarseness may be a sign of laryngeal cancer or recurrent laryngeal nerve palsy secondary to mediastinal lymphadenopathy. Facial weakness is sometimes associated with malignant parotid gland neoplasms.

### Examine the lump

Use a standard scheme for describing any lump. For head and neck lumps the following are important.

### Number of lumps

Multiple neck lumps usually represent lymph node enlargement (lymphadenopathy). There are, however, multiple causes (see above).

### Site

This frequently gives a clue to the nature of the lump. Anterior neck swellings include thyroglossal cysts, thyroid masses, ranulae and occasional submental lymph nodes. Lateral neck swellings include most lymph node swellings, salivary gland lesions, branchial cysts, carotid body tumours and cystic hygromas. If there is a suspicion that neck lumps may represent malignant lymphadenopathy then their position may indicate the likely primary sites (Fig. 49.1).

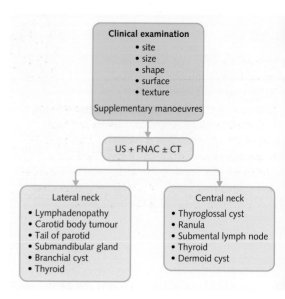

**Fig. 49.1** Algorithm for the investigation of a neck lump.

### Texture

A lot of information can be gained from the way the lump feels. Lymphoma is described as rubbery, carcinoma as rock hard; salivary neoplasms are often firm. Cystic lesions, lipomas and cystic hygromas may demonstrate fluctuance.

### Supplementary manoeuvres

Thyroid lesions will move on swallowing (offer the patient a glass of water) and thyroglossal cysts move upwards on tongue protrusion. Cystic hygromas will often trans-illuminate. Listen with a stethoscope; bruits may be heard overlying carotid body tumours and some thyroid masses.

### Full head and neck examination

It is necessary in all patients with a neck lump to examine the skin, ears, nose, oral cavity, pharynx and larynx looking for evidence of infection or malignancy. This would routinely include flexible naso-endoscopic examination (see Chapter 65). In all patients in whom you suspect lymphadenopathy, examine other lymph node areas and palpate for hepatosplenomegaly.

Lymphoma is an important cause of cervical lymphadenopathy. Hodgkin's lymphoma often presents initially as swollen cervical lymph nodes. It is important to ask in the history about weight loss, fevers and night sweats ('B' symptoms). In a patient in whom you suspect lymphoma examine all the other lymph node areas, especially axillae and groins, and palpate for hepatosplenomegaly. A lymph node biopsy will usually be required to confirm the diagnosis.

## FURTHER INVESTIGATION OF PATIENTS WITH A NECK LUMP

### Haematological investigations

In all patients in whom the cause is not immediately obvious haematological investigations may be useful, particularly when looking for infective causes. A full blood count and white cell count, liver function tests, and serological testing for cat scratch disease, toxoplasmosis and other infections may be performed. Erythrocyte sedimentation rate and lactic acid dehydrogenase are also performed if lymphoma is a possibilty.

### Fine needle aspiration cytology (FNAC)

This is the investigation of choice in all neck lumps (except vascular!). With the help of a good cytologist it is usually possible to diagnose the cause of the lump using FNAC.

### Open biopsy

This is generally to be avoided in the diagnosis of neck lumps owing to the risks of seeding malignancy and the potential damage to underlying structures (accessory nerve, etc.). Exceptions are where FNAC is unhelpful, principally in the diagnosis of lymphoma and occasionally in the diagnosis of tuberculosis.

### Imaging

The most widely used investigation is ultrasound which can delineate lumps, confirm if they are cystic or solid and locate them for subsequent FNAC. It is also readily used in even young children. CT and MRI scanning are also frequently used. These investigations are useful in the diagnosis and staging of a suspected malignant neck lump. Angiography can help in the diagnosis of carotid body tumours. If a lymph node is confirmed as malignant on FNAC it is sometimes the case that no obvious primary site is found (an unknown primary). In these cases it is increasingly common to use positron emission tomography (PET scan) to try and find the primary cancer.

Stridor is the audible, monophonic, musical airway noise produced by a narrowed upper respiratory tract. It is a worrying sign and in all cases warrants further thorough investigation. Stridor is usually inspiratory in nature but may be biphasic if there is narrowing of the intrathoracic trachea (Fig. 50.1). Wheeze is produced by narrowing of bronchiolar smooth muscle, and is usually widespread, polyphonic and expiratory.

## DIFFERENTIAL DIAGNOSIS OF STRIDOR BY AGE OF ONSET

### Birth/early infancy

- Subglottic stenosis (congenital and acquired).
- Congenital laryngeal abnormalities (cysts, haemangiomas, webs, etc.).
- Recurrent laryngeal nerve (RLN) palsy (possible spinal cord abnormality).
- Laryngomalacia.

### Childhood

- Inhaled foreign body.
- Croup.
- Epiglottitis.

### Adults

- Epiglottitis.
- RLN palsy – unilateral or especially bilateral.
- Laryngeal carcinoma.
- Acquired subglottic stenosis – secondary to intubation.
- External compression, e.g. lymphadenopathy, thyroid malignancy.

## HISTORY IN THE PATIENT WITH STRIDOR

The cause of stridor varies markedly with age. In the neonate a congenital cause is most likely. Infants tend to inhale things and get infections. Adults still get infections but malignancies (affecting the larynx or RLNs) become more common.

### Neonatal and early infancy

It is important to take a full pregnancy and birth history. A history of premature birth and endotracheal intubation increases the likelihood of acquired subglottic narrowing or stenosis. In the non-intubated infant, stridor from near birth with an abnormal cry, feeding difficulties and failure to thrive may indicate congenital laryngeal pathology. Severe stridor near to birth leading to ventilatory difficulties and requiring intubation is also seen in congenital vocal cord palsy. Laryngomalacia is the most common cause of mild stridor in this age group. The stridor is caused by a floppy larynx and often improves with growth.

### Childhood

In any child with sudden onset stridor, foreign body inhalation must be considered. The other two common causes in this age group are croup and, more rarely, epiglottitis. Croup is of gradual onset, the stridor is usually mild and associated with attacks of a seal-like cough.

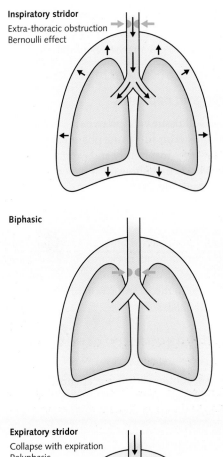

**Inspiratory stridor**
Extra-thoracic obstruction
Bernoulli effect

**Biphasic**

**Expiratory stridor**
Collapse with expiration
Polyphasic

**Fig. 50.1** Characteristics of abnormal airway noises.

Epiglottitis is of much more sudden onset with painful swallowing, pyrexia, malaise and often severe stridor.

## Adult

Ask about prolonged or difficult intubation or tracheostomy which may have caused a subglottic stenosis. If there is an associated hoarseness the level of the obstruction is either within the larynx or is due to a RLN palsy. Also ask about symptoms of

tracheobronchial malignancy, e.g. cough, haemoptysis or weight loss. Previous neck or chest surgery may produce a RLN palsy.

## EXAMINATION OF THE PATIENT WITH STRIDOR

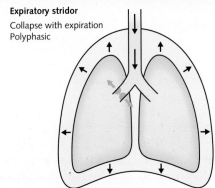

*Epiglottitis*. The essential difference between the management of a neonate or child versus an adult patient with stridor is the urgency of the situation. Any child with acute onset stridor which is present *at presentation* must be considered to have epiglottitis until this is ruled out. Your management should be calm but decisive. Call for senior help. Get the parent to hold high flow, humidified oxygen below (not over) the child's face. *Do not attempt to examine the child or get i.v. access* – a crying fit at this stage can occlude an already critically narrowed glottis. Arrange for the urgent transfer of the child on the parent's lap, with an anaesthetist present, to a suitable environment where the child can be intubated. The treatment is intubation and antibiotics. You will never regret over-reacting in this situation. Indecision, however, can prove fatal.

## The neonate or infant

- Assess stridor – phase, severity, positional changes, changes with feeding.
- Look for signs of respiratory distress – cyanosis, tachypnoea, recession, tracheal tug.
- Examination of the larynx – 2 mm flexible nasoendoscope, or microlaryngoscopy under general anaesthetic.

## The child

- *If epiglottis is suspected do not try to examine the mouth or pharynx. Call for help from an experienced anaesthetist, ENT surgeon and a paediatrician!*
- Assess respiratory distress (as above); listen to the chest.
- If croup, assess severity clinically.

## The adult

- Look for respiratory distress – hypoxia, confusion, tachypnoea, accessory muscles, inability to complete sentences.
- Examine the chest.
- Examine the larynx – using flexible naso-endoscopy look for laryngeal pathology, vocal cord movement (RLN palsy) and subglottic stenosis.
- Examine the neck – look for thyroid enlargement, cervical lymphadenopathy and tracheal displacement.

## INVESTIGATION OF THE PATIENT WITH STRIDOR

In any patient, child or adult, showing signs of respiratory distress do not waste time performing investigations. The definitive treatment is to secure the airway and for this you will need a friendly anaesthetist, with or without an ENT surgeon. Call them early! If they consider the patient is stable enough for further investigations they will tell you.

## Respiratory investigations

- Pulse oximetry
- Arterial blood gas analysis in adults

## Radiological investigations

### Children and neonates

- Lateral soft tissue view pharynx.
- Anteroposterior soft tissue pharynx.
- Chest X-ray – inspiratory and expiratory. Airway foreign body may show up as hyperinflation of the affected side.

### Adults

- Chest X-ray, posterior-anterior and lateral views
- CT fine cuts of head, neck and chest – if there is a suspicion of airway malignancy, adult subglottic stenosis or in the investigation of recurrent laryngeal palsies.

## Rigid laryngoscopy/bronchoscopy

Used for:
- Emergency intervention, e.g. epiglottitis, foreign body removal.
- Assessment of the adult airway.
- Assessment of non-infectious stridor in children, e.g. subglottic stenosis.

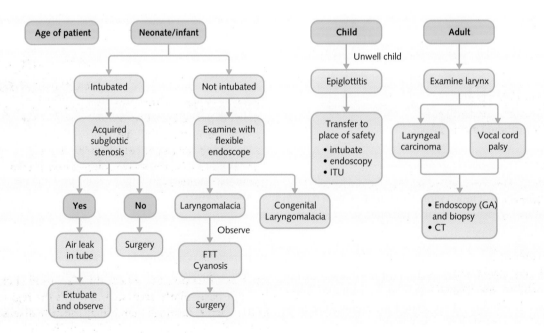

**Fig. 50.2.** Algorithm for the investigation of stridor.

## Objectives

You should be able to:

- Describe dysphagia.
- Tell the difference between dysphagia and odynophagia.
- Have an idea about the differential diagnosis of dysphagia.
- Recognize the warning signs associated with malignant causes of dysphagia.
- List the investigations to perform in dysphagia.

Dysphagia is the feeling of difficulty swallowing. It is surprisingly common and does not always equate with identifiable pathology. It is vital to distinguish it from odynophagia, which is painful swallowing.

## DIFFERENTIAL DIAGNOSIS OF DYSPHAGIA (Fig. 51.1)

### Central neurological causes of dysphagia

- Bulbar palsy.
- Pseudobulbar palsy.
- CVA.

### Peripheral neurological causes of dysphagia

- Multiple sclerosis.
- Motor neurone disease.
- Myasthenia gravis, etc.

### Oral

- Inflammatory lesions, e.g. herpes stomatitis.
- Tumour.

### Pharyngeal

- Tumour.
- Pharyngeal pouch.
- 'Globus pharyngeus'.

### Oesophageal

- Food bolus.

- Dysmotility disorders, e.g. achalasia, diffuse oesophageal spasm.
- Benign strictures.
- External compression, e.g. by thyroid mass or aberrant major blood vessel.
- Tumour.

### Gastric

- Tumour.

## HISTORY TO FOCUS ON IN DYSPHAGIA

*Warning symptoms*. These are suggestive of malignant disease and are vitally important. They are dysphagia that is progressive, weight loss and lymphadenopathy. Equally worrying is dysphagia in a patient who smokes.

### Site of dysphagia

Patients often point to where they feel food stick. It is not particularly accurate but if it is the region of the cricoid cartilage then it may indicate disease of the pharynx. 'Low' dysphagia usually indicates oesophageal disease.

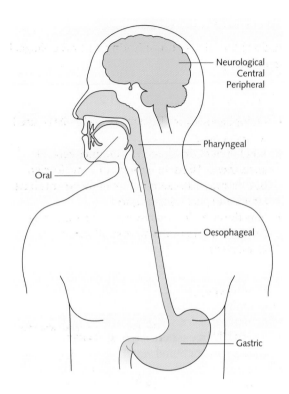

**Fig. 51.1** Differential diagnosis of dysphagia.

## Associated oropharyngeal symptoms

Disease of the oropharynx leading to dysphagia may also cause changes in the voice or dysarthria due to restricted tongue movement. This is a characteristic muffled voice sometimes resembling 'a mouthful of marbles' or the more common 'hot potato' voice heard in someone who has a large mass in their oropharynx.

## Laryngopharyngeal symptoms

Patients will commonly describe a feeling of food sticking at the level of the cricoid along with mild discomfort and fleeting hoarseness in globus pharyngeus. These problems are never sufficient to cause weight loss. In some patients so-called 'globus' symptoms may be due to reflux of stomach contents. Persistent or progressive hoarseness along with dysphagia may be caused by a carcinoma of the larynx. These are nearly always found in smokers.

A pharyngeal pouch is a pulsion diverticulum found in elderly patients. It nearly always presents with dysphagia as the pouch presses on the oesophagus.

Other classic symptoms include regurgitation of recently eaten food and gurgling in the neck on lying down.

## Gastro-oesophageal symptoms

Burning epigastric and retrosternal pain along with acid regurgitation are suggestive of gastro-oesophageal reflux disease (GORD) which can produce an oesophagitis with dysphagia and odynophagia. Regurgitation of food or saliva which is immediate or slightly delayed is secondary to either oesophageal dysmotility or tumour.

## EXAMINATION OF THE PATIENT WITH DYSPHAGIA

### General examination

Looking for signs of: anaemia, cachexia, jaundice or hepatosplenomegaly.

The patient with marked weight loss and dysphagia has malignancy of oesophagus or gastric antrum until proven otherwise.

### Examine the neck

Looking for:

- Lymphadenopathy, e.g. Virchow's node.
- Thyroid mass.

### Examine the upper gastrointestinal tract

Including:

- *Mouth*: using a headlight and dental mirror paying special attention to the tongue, tongue base and soft palate. Observe palatal elevation and tongue movement, abnormalities or asymmetry of which may indicate neurological disease.
- *Nasopharynx, oropharynx and larynx*: using a flexible naso-endoscope look for signs of laryngeal disease, for example tumour. It is also possible to observe the 'post-cricoid' region

which is the entrance to the oesophagus; there may be signs of inflammation, tumour or retained secretions visible here.

## INVESTIGATION OF THE PATIENT WITH DYSPHAGIA

### Haematological investigations

- Full blood count – anaemia may represent a dietary deficiency secondary to the dysphagia. However, it must be taken seriously as it may represent the anaemia commonly seen in cachectic patients. Plummer–Vinson syndrome is the combination of iron deficiency anaemia and post-cricoid webbing or even carcinoma and is more common in female patients.
- Liver function tests – if there is a suggestion of liver disease.
- Inflammatory markers, e.g. erythrocyte sedimentation rate, C-reactive protein – usually negative in globus pharyngeus and are therefore used by some to discriminate organic from non-organic disease. These markers are completely nonspecific, however, and may be normal even where malignancy is present.

Most patients with true dysphagia will require endoscopy to establish a diagnosis. Do not delay referral by requesting lots of extraneous investigations.

### Radiological investigations

- Plain radiographs – useful if you suspect a radio-opaque foreign body, such as a chicken bone (i.e. acute onset dysphagia).
- Ba swallow – can demonstrate oesophageal lesions in wall, intraluminal problems, extraluminal compression, dysmotility and gross reflux. It can also diagnose a pharyngeal pouch.
- CT – used for the diagnosis and staging of malignancy.
- Videofluoroscopy – dynamic assessment useful in dysmotility.

### Tests of GI function

Include 24 hour pH monitoring and oesophageal manometry.

### Endoscopic examination

- Oesophago-gastro-duodenoscopy (OGD) – used for most cases.
- Rigid upper GI endoscopy – requires general anaesthesia. Used for removal of some foreign bodies and a full examination of the tongue base, larynx and post-cricoid region.
- Functional endoscopic evaluation swallowing (FEES) – specialist dynamic swallowing assessment.

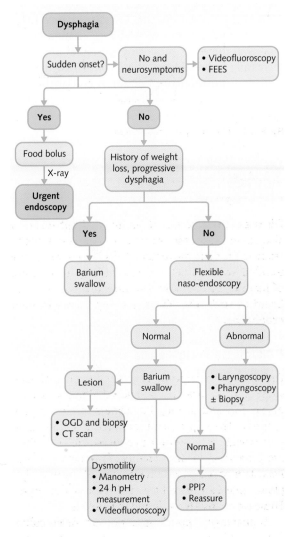

Fig. 51.2 Algorithm for the investigation of dysphagia.

## Objectives

You should be able to:

- Describe the causes of hoarseness.
- Describe the examination of a hoarse patient.
- Recognize the warning signs of malignant disease in hoarseness.
- Say which investigations to perform on the hoarse patient.

The vibratory mucosa of the vocal folds is only 0.3 mm thick; even the smallest disturbance in its structure or function can lead to a change in the quality of the voice, producing a rougher texture or increasing its breathiness. It is also the case that the voice is an instrument of emotion and at this site more than most emotional or psychological factors can have a large impact.

## DIFFERENTIAL DIAGNOSIS OF HOARSENESS

### Neurological

- Recurrent laryngeal nerve paralysis.
- Dystonia, either generalized or localized (spasmodic dysphonia).

### Laryngeal

- Functional/physiological.
- Muscle tension dysphonia – improper voice use.
- Reinke's oedema.
- Inflammatory – laryngitis, laryngopharyngeal acid reflux, sarcoidosis.
- Vocal cord nodules/cysts/polyps.
- Laryngeal papillomatosis.
- Laryngeal carcinoma.

## HISTORY IN THE PATIENT WITH HOARSENESS

Hoarseness in a smoker or persistent hoarseness for more than 3 weeks should make you suspect laryngeal cancer. Weight loss, neck swelling or associated dysphagia should also prompt referral and investigation.

### General

A history of cardiac, thoracic or neck surgery may indicate recurrent laryngeal nerve (RLN) damage. This is much more likely on the left side where the RLN wraps around the arch of the aorta before ascending to the larynx. Similarly a history suggestive of bronchial carcinoma such as cough, haemoptysis or weight loss may identify a further site of RLN compression.

It is important to ask all patients about acid reflux-related symptoms such as epigastric pain, regurgitation and indigestion. Laryngopharyngeal acid reflux may, however, produce hoarseness in the absence of these symptoms.

## Duration and character of hoarseness

Hoarseness lasting more than 3 weeks should prompt specialist referral. Constant hoarseness suggests laryngeal pathology whereas hoarseness that comes and goes may indicate a functional cause, i.e. stress or vocal misuse.

## Hobbies and habits

Vocal cord nodules are caused by voice overuse and misuse, and are more common in teachers and singers. Muscle tension dysphonia and other functional causes are also more common in professional voice users, especially if there is an element of stress.

## EXAMINATION OF THE HOARSE PATIENT

## General examination

Look first for general signs of malignancy, such as anaemia, cachexia, clubbing, etc. Look for signs of previous neck or chest surgery. Hypothyroidism also sometimes causes voice changes (Reinke's oedema) so look for signs associated with this. Some voice disorders (the spasmodic dysphonias) are associated with generalized dystonic reactions such as torticollis or writer's cramp.

## Examine the neck

It is important to feel specifically for a thyroid mass. Cervical lymphadenopathy may occur as a result of metastatic chest or laryngeal malignancy or may be due to a lymphoma.

## Examine the larynx

First listen to the voice. Does it sound abnormal to you? Next examine the larynx. This is most commonly now performed using a flexible naso-endoscope which also allows visualization of the larynx during normal speech. Look specifically for pathology of the vocal folds and at their movement, noting particularly any asymmetry.

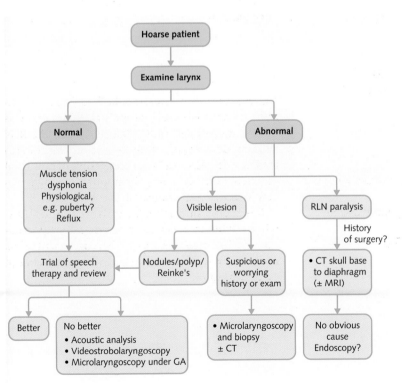

**Fig. 52.1** Algorithm for the investigation of hoarseness.

## INVESTIGATION OF THE HOARSE PATIENT

Any patient with audible hoarseness lasting more than 3 weeks needs visualization of the larynx. Do not delay this by requesting lots of extra investigations.

### Haematological

A full blood count and thyroid function test usually suffice.

### Radiological

CT scanning is the most useful radiological investigation. It is used in the diagnosis and staging of laryngeal and chest malignancy. If RLN palsy is seen clinically then it is necessary to image the whole length of the vagus/RLN from skull base to mediastinum.

## Microlaryngoscopy and biopsy

In cases where the diagnosis is not apparent or where malignancy is suspected, the laryngeal structures are examined under general anaesthesia. A rigid endoscope and a microscope are used to magnify the vocal folds. This may be supplemented with bronchoscopy.

## ALGORITHM FOR THE MANAGEMENT OF HOARSENESS

An algorithm for the management of hoarseness is shown in Fig. 52.1

# Disorders of the external ear

## 53

### Objectives

You should be able to:

- Describe the basic embryology and anatomy of the external ear and ear canal.
- List common congenital conditions affecting the external ear.
- Say what causes a cauliflower ear and how it is treated.
- Discuss the diagnosis and management of otitis externa.
- Discuss the worrying causes of otitis externa and how they are diagnosed and managed.
- Describe what malignant otitis externa is, what causes it and how it is managed.

## THE EXTERNAL EAR

### Anatomy and embryology

The pinna of the ear arises in utero from the growth and fusion of six swellings or 'auricular hillocks' derived from the first and second branchial arches. It is mainly composed of a cartilaginous skeleton and an overlying stratified squamous epithelium.

### Disorders of the external ear

#### Congenital disorders

Prominent ears ('bat ears') are most often caused by a lack of development of the normal antihelical fold (Fig. 53.1). As a result, one or both ears appear more prominent. This cosmetic defect can be corrected by the operation of otoplasty.

Of the various conditions which can result from inadequate growth or fusion of the auricular hillocks, pre-auricular pits and cysts are the most minor and most common. They are often asymptomatic but may present with pre-auricular swelling and pain if they become infected. If symptomatic they can be excised.

More severe developmental abnormalities may leave the pinna small and malformed (microtia). There may also be absence of the pinna, external ear canal (atresia) and deeper ear structures. These conditions may be isolated or associated with more widespread craniofacial anomalies such as Treacher Collins syndrome or hemifacial microsomia. Specialist reconstructive procedures may be used to fashion a new ear from costal cartilage; alternatively the deformed auricle is excised and replaced with a bone anchored prosthesis (Fig. 53.2). The associated conductive hearing loss is often treated with a bone anchored hearing aid (see later).

### Traumatic disorders

Given its prominent position it is not surprising that the external ear is prone to trauma. This can range from laceration to complete avulsion. An auricular haematoma may also result. This subperichondrial clot strips off the blood supply to the underlying

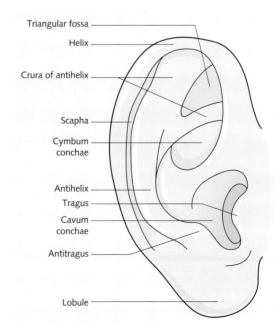

Fig. 53.1 Anatomy of the external ear.

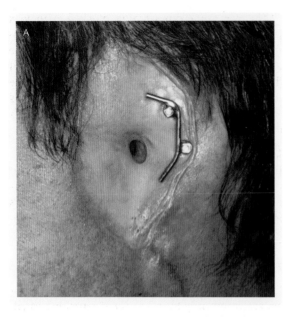
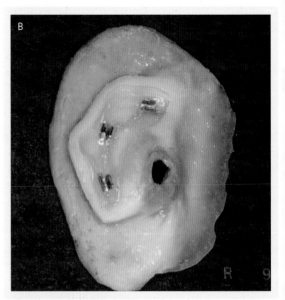
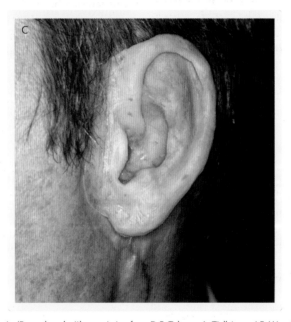

**Fig. 53.2** Bone anchored ear prosthesis. (Reproduced with permission from D.E. Tolman, A. Tjellstrom, J.E. Woods, Reconstructing the human face by using the tissue-integrated prosthesis, *Mayo Clin Proc*, 1998, 73:1171–1175.)

cartilage and can result in loss of cartilage, which is replaced by fibrous tissue. Unless drained promptly the result is the familiar 'cauliflower ear'.

## Inflammatory disorders

Relapsing perichondritis is an interesting but rare disease which is thought to be autoimmune in nature. It is characterized by recurrent inflammation of cartilaginous structures, particularly the external ear and the trachea. It results in brawny, tender swelling of the pinna and progressive deformity. If it affects the larynx and trachea it may produce hoarseness and airway compromise. Treatment is with high dose corticosteroids.

## Neoplastic disorders

The pinna is a common sight for sun-related cutaneous neoplasms. Basal and squamous carcinomas, along with malignant melanomas, are all seen at this site. Treatment is by excision.

## THE EXTERNAL AUDITORY CANAL

## Anatomy and embryology

The external auditory canal is formed by a tubular invagination of the first branchial cleft ectoderm. It meets up with the middle ear endoderm and, squashed between the two, the trilaminar structure of the tympanic membrane is formed (see Fig. 53.4).

In adult life the external auditory canal is around 2.5 cm in length and is lined throughout by stratified squamous epithelium; its lateral third is supported by cartilage and has frequent hair follicles, sebaceous and apocrine glands. The inner two-thirds of the canal are encased in bone and ends at the tympanic membrane. The tympanic membrane is a circular structure which lies obliquely at the end of the external canal. It comprises an outer layer of skin, a middle fibrous layer and an inner mucosal layer.

## Disorders of the external auditory canal

### Wax

Wax is a normal product of the external canal (though try telling some patients this). Keratinous debris forming deep in the ear canal has an ingenious way of finding its way to the outside. The desquamative process in the external ear produces an outward movement of skin products. As these 'squames' reach the cartilaginous canal they mix with glandular products to produce wax, which, encouraged by movements of the temporomandibular joint, is extruded from the ear canal.

> Wax is not dirt! It serves a useful bactericidal and mechanical cleansing role. 'Problems' caused by wax are usually the result of misguided attempts by the patient to remove it from the ear canal. Cotton ear buds should be discouraged and should never be inserted into the external canal. They serve only to compress wax into the deep portion of the ear canal making its removal more difficult.

The ear canal can become blocked with wax (impacted) and a minority of patients seem to produce wax in excess. Conditions which narrow the external ear canal or result in failure of the normal desquamative processes (keratitis obturans) may result in blockage of the external canal with wax and squamous debris. This may lead to recurrent otitis externa and a conductive hearing loss (see later).

#### Management

Impacted wax may be removed by the use of softening agents (ceruminolytics such as sodium bicarbonate and olive oil) followed by syringing of the ears (Fig. 53.3) or removed by suction under the microscope (microsuction).

### Foreign bodies

Foreign bodies such as paper, stones and pencil erasers are commonly found in the external ear canal. Children of school age are the usual perpetrators. In the cooperative child the object may be removed by syringing, microsuction, or the use of a small blunt hook. However, general anaesthesia is sometimes required.

Rarely, foreign bodies such as insects may wander in unassisted (a particularly irritating cause of tinnitus!). They may be killed by instilling alcohol solution into the ear and then removed as above.

## Infections of the external auditory canal (Fig. 53.4)

### Otitis externa

This extremely common condition results from infection of the external ear canal skin. Predisposing

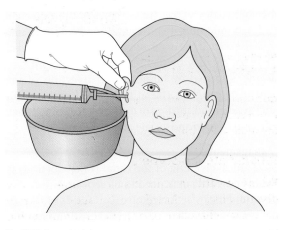

**Fig. 53.3** Ear syringing.

**Fig. 53.4** Structures of the ear.

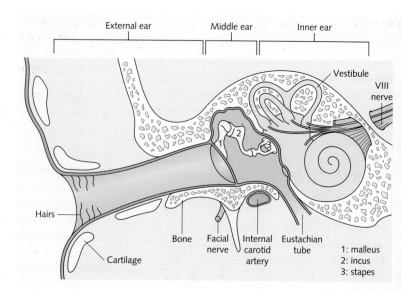

conditions include swimming, especially in non-hygienic conditions, and anything which interferes with the normal desquamative processes of the external ear canal, e.g. scratching with dirty fingernails, canal exostoses, etc. Common infecting organisms include *Pseudomonas* and *Staphylococcus aureus*. Fungi such as *Candida* and *Aspergillus* may also be responsible.

### Clinical presentation

Infection results in itching, blockage and a scanty discharge from the ear canal. More severe cases may cause pain and a spreading infection of the pinna (perichondritis). Examination typically reveals oedema of the canal with a scanty discharge and debris in the canal, in most cases the tympanic membrane is intact, although this may be difficult to determine. Fungal otitis externa presents largely in the same way. Examination characteristically reveals excessive amounts of debris with the consistency of wet tissue paper in the ear canal. Pathognomic fungal spores and hyphae can sometimes be seen. If the organism responsible is *Aspergillus* these spores may be pigmented. Ramsay Hunt syndrome is caused by herpes zoster infection of the geniculate ganglion (facial nerve) and may present with vesicles and crusting of the external ear and canal, followed by pain and facial palsy.

### Management

Mechanical cleaning of the canal (microsuction) is carried out. This may need to be repeated every few days until the infection resolves.

Topical antibiotic/corticosteroid ear-drops are prescribed (gentamicin/dexamethasone, etc.).

Its important to note that many ear drops, e.g. gentamicin, are potentially ototoxic, especially if used for prolonged periods and if there is a perforation of the tympanic membrane. It is now increasingly common in these cases to use topical ciprofloxacin or ofloxacin drops. These are, in theory, less ototoxic and are certainly the drugs of choice in children.

Choice of antibiotic can be guided by microbiological investigation of an ear swab. In fungal otitis externa topical antifungal drops are used. The patient is strongly advised to keep their ears scrupulously dry and to avoid scratching.

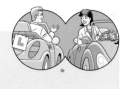

Following resolution of the acute stage, a chronic otitis externa commonly occurs.
This results in dry, flaky, intensely itchy ear canals. Scratching creates abrasions and re-introduces pathogens and a new acute episode occurs. In order to avoid this it is essential to inform the patient that it may happen and that it is very important to keep their ear canals dry and not to scratch or poke them. A topical corticosteroid ointment is often used temporarily to alleviate the itching.

## External canal furuncle

This results from blockage and infection of a hair follicle in the cartilaginous portion of the ear canal, leading to an acute localized infection or abscess. It is often seen as a complication of acute otitis externa. It leads to an exquisitely tender ear canal and even jaw movement may cause pain. Examination itself is painful and will often reveal relatively localized swelling in the canal. Treatment involves incision of the furuncle under local anaesthetic following which pain and oedema settle rapidly.

## Necrotizing otitis externa (malignant otitis externa)

This is a potentially life-threatening infection of the external ear and temporal bone. It is most often seen in the elderly and the immunocompromised, especially in poorly controlled diabetics. It is caused by a spreading infection of the skull base by *Pseudomonas aeruginosa*.

Beware the immunosuppressed, elderly or diabetic patient with otitis externa, especially if there is marked pain (otalgia) – they may have malignant otitis externa or a squamous carcinoma of the ear canal.

### Clinical presentation

The characteristic feature is a deep-seated otalgia in the presence of an apparent otitis externa which does not respond to the usual treatment regimes. Facial soft tissue swelling is not uncommon. Examination of the ear canal reveals suppuration, oedema and florid granulation tissue. Systemic signs such as pyrexia, malaise and loss of diabetic control are also common. The white blood cell count is raised as are other inflammatory markers. Spreading osteomyelitis of the temporal bone and skull base may produce cranial nerve palsies; the facial, vagus and hypoglossal nerves are the most commonly affected. Without aggressive treatment infection may spread intracranially and lead to death.

### Management

Diagnosis is mainly based on the clinical history and examination.

Other useful investigations include:

- Ear swabs for microbiology.
- High-resolution CT scanning.
- Technetium bone scanning.

Treatment involves admission to hospital and the following regimen:

- Careful control of diabetes is essential.
- Daily microsuction of the ear canal.
- Intravenous antibiotics for up to 6 weeks. Ciprofloxin is a popular choice.
- Analgesia.

Failure to respond to these measures as judged by continuing pain, progression of neuropathies, or continuing or progressive infection on CT or bone scanning necessitate surgical debridement.

## External canal exostoses

These lesions are really hyperostoses rather than neoplasms. They cause fusiform swelling of the deep bony canal and are often bilateral and multiple. Cold water swimmers are especially prone to exostoses. They are usually asymptomatic but if big enough or multiple may trap keratinous debris in the deep canal, predisposing to recurrent otitis externa. If symptomatic they can be removed surgically.

## Malignancy of the external ear canal

This is a fortunately rare condition seen in elderly patients. The cause is usually a squamous cell carcinoma. Deep-seated, intractable otalgia and serosanguinous discharge results; cranial neuropathies may be seen as the disease spreads. Diagnosis depends on a high degree of suspicion in cases where otitis externa fails to respond to therapy. Histopathology and high resolution CT scanning confirm the diagnosis.

Treatment is with surgery and/or radiotherapy. The prognosis is, however, poor.

## DISORDERS OF THE TYMPANIC MEMBRANE

Disorders of the tympanic membrane (TM) are seldom primary in nature but more often reflect disease and dysfunction of the underlying middle ear and Eustachian tube. However, it is important for the student to recognize the characteristic and common tympanic membrane abnormalities.

### Perforations (Fig. 54.1)

These are usually relatively easy to see and are located in the pars tensa. They may be incidental findings or may be associated with active middle ear infection. Trauma, middle ear infection and previous surgery may all leave perforations, many of which will heal spontaneously. The presence of a perforation makes ingress of potential pathogens into the middle ear easier and may result in frequent bouts of chronic suppurative otitis media (CSOM). Once the infection has been dealt with the tympanic membrane perforation can be repaired by the operation of myringoplasty.

### Retraction pockets

These are 'sucked in' areas of tympanic membrane caused by negative middle ear pressures and Eustachian tube dysfunction. They are most commonly seen in the pars flaccida or attic region. If they become deep enough they may begin to accumulate keratinous debris from the squamous epithelial cells of the TM and ear canal skin. It is thought that this is the first step in the pathogenesis of cholesteatoma (see below).

### Tympanosclerosis

This common finding is thought to be the result of inflammatory or post-traumatic changes within the tympanic membrane. An increased deposition of hyaline and calcified tissue within the TM produces a characteristic chalky white horseshoe inferiorly in the membrane. It is an innocuous finding.

### Disorders of the middle ear and mastoid

The middle ear cavity is lined by ciliated columnar respiratory epithelium. It contains the three ossicles – the malleus, incus and stapes – and their supporting ligaments. Connected to the ossicles are the two muscles of the middle ear, the tensor tympani and stapedius. The middle ear is connected to the nasopharynx by the mucosally lined Eustachian tube which acts as a pressure equalizer. Posterosuperiorly it is continuous with mastoid aditus and air cells.

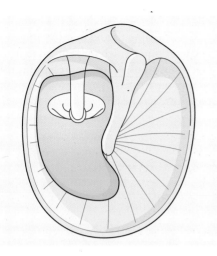

**Fig. 54.1** Perforation of the eardrum.

## Acute suppurative otitis media (ASOM)

Colonization of the middle ear cleft by pathogenic bacteria is a common childhood event that few of us escape. The bacteria may colonize the middle ear via the Eustachian tube, via a perforation or rarely by haematogenous spread. Bacterial infection may be a primary event or may follow initial viral infection. The common pathogens include *Streptococcus pneumoniae*, *Haemophilus influenzae* and *Moraxella* spp. The result is a suppurative process which is self-limiting in the vast majority of cases; for the unfortunate few ASOM can progress to major and life-threatening complications.

### Clinical presentation

The patient is most often a child. There is commonly a preceding viral upper respiratory tract illness. Infection of the middle ear results in severe otalgia, conductive deafness and a pyrexial illness. In the very young ASOM may present with more vague signs such as ear pulling and restlessness. Examination of the eardrum shows an initial hyperaemia which progresses to suppuration and a bulging drum. Untreated ASOM normally leads to ischaemia of part of the tympanic membrane and a perforation results. After this occurs there is a mucopurulent ear discharge and eventual resolution of symptoms. Rarely complications of ASOM may become apparent (see below).

### Investigation

#### Clinical examination
Reveals a hyperaemic or bulging drum. At a later stage there is obvious ear discharge and a TM perforation.

#### PTAs/tympanometry
These tests are seldom available in the acute setting. Prior to perforation the audiograms will show a conductive deafness. Tympanometry would be inappropriate because of the discomfort it would cause, but would be flattened, confirming the presence of fluid in the middle ear.

Imaging is rarely required in the uncomplicated case; however, CT scanning is invaluable in the diagnosis of complications.

### Management

- Analgesia – simple analgesics and non-steroidal preparations are useful symptomatic treatments.
- Antibiotics – recently there has been a great deal of debate about whether antibiotics are effective in this common and often self-limiting disease. If they are used, amoxicillin is as effective as more expensive drugs as first-line therapy. Failure to respond indicates possible drug resistance and the need for second-line agents such as co-amoxiclav or a cephalosporin; however, this is rarely necessary.
- Myringotomy – in some countries, notably the USA, the availability of access to specialist ENT surgeons means that interventions such as myringotomy to pre-empt perforation and drain the middle ear in its suppurative phase are possible, but, evidence suggests, of little benefit.
- Some children develop recurrent bouts of acute otitis media requiring frequent medical attention. For some of these children surgical insertion of grommets to ventilate the middle ear can alleviate the pain associated with frequent infection.

## Complications of suppurative otitis media

### Intratemporal complications

- *Otitis media with effusion* (OME). In 10% of patients middle ear effusion may persist for longer than 3 months leading to otitis media with effusion and conductive hearing loss.
- *Hearing loss*. As well as OME, acute suppurative OM may have direct toxic effects on the cochlea producing a sensorineural hearing loss. Pressure necrosis of the ossicles or their fixation from post-inflammatory tympanosclerosis may result in a conductive loss. The same conductive loss may be seen with a large perforation.
- *Dizziness*. Acute infection may involve the labyrinth resulting in dizziness.
- *Facial nerve palsy*. In around 4% of the population the facial nerve traverses the middle ear cavity without its normal casing of bone, i.e. it is dehiscent. These patients are at risk of facial nerve paralysis during a bout of ASOM. This is normally transient.
- *Mastoiditis/petrositis*. In every case of ASOM there is spread of infection into the air cells of the mastoid. Mastoiditis, however, refers to the clinical picture of persistent infection of the mastoid with or without ear discharge and swelling and or an abscess over the mastoid. This requires surgical drainage and a mastoidectomy operation. Petrositis is a progression of mastoiditis and clinically may present as Gradenigo's syndrome. This comprises otitis media, retro-orbital pain and an ipsilateral abducens nerve palsy.

### Extratemporal complications

These conditions are rarely seen following acute suppurative otitis media but are more common following chronic disease.

- *Neck abscess*. A Bezold's abscess forms when pus tracks from mastoiditis down the sternomastoid muscle to point at its anterior border. Similarly, a Citelli's abscess is formed by pus tracking into the digastric fossa to produce a submandibular swelling.
- *Intracranial complications*. These are the much feared complications of suppurative ear disease. The relative proximity of the cranial cavity to the ear and the often flimsy bony barrier of the tegmen tympani, or roof of the middle ear, mean that intracranial spread of infection is often easier than extracranial spread. Complications include brain abscess, subdural and extradural collections, meningitis and infective thrombosis of the lateral sinus which may spread to involve the cavernous sinus. All of these complications, unless they are treated by aggressive surgical intervention, may be fatal.

It is vitally important that all clinicians involved in treating children should have a high index of suspicion for complications following acute otitis media. All children with a recent history of ear discharge and the onset of nonspecific neurological complaints such as dizziness, headaches, lethargy, drowsiness, etc., are taken seriously and investigated thoroughly. Most often this will involve imaging (CT and MRI ) of the temporal bone and brain.

## Otitis media with effusion (OME)

Otitis media with effusion (OME) or glue ear is an extremely common disease of children. It is estimated that it will affect around 80% of children before their 4th birthday. The number of these children in whom OME is present over a prolonged period is, however, much lower. A middle ear effusion commonly follows an episode of acute otitis media; however, it is best thought of as a non-infective inflammatory sequel to this. OME is thought to be prevalent in young children as they have a relatively inefficient Eustachian tube. Certainly it is seen even more frequently in children in whom Eustachian function is compromised further, for example those with a cleft palate. Large adenoids are thought to act as a source of infection and therefore continued inflammation and may also contribute to OME.

### Clinical presentation

The presentation of OME is in most cases insidious. It causes nothing other than a conductive hearing loss. However, its effects may be profound. Due to the young age of the population it affects the presence of OME is often not noted until the child fails a school hearing test or has a delay in acquiring speech. Occasional episodes of mild, short lived otalgia are not uncommon but are not associated with the severe pain and systemic upset seen in AOM. Clinical examination reveals a dull grey-looking tympanic membrane (Fig. 54.2) which may look retracted. The nasal airway may be reduced or blocked if large adenoids are present.

## Investigation

A conductive hearing loss on pure tone audiogram along with a flattened trace on a tympanogram (Fig. 54.3) confirms the diagnosis.

## Management

Intervention is usually recommended for children with bilateral OME with hearing thresholds below 20 dBHL for more than 3 months. The usual intervention is a period of watchful waiting followed if necessary by surgical drainage of the effusion via a small anteroinferior incision in the ear drum (myringotomy) and the insertion of small ventilation tubes (grommets). This re-aerates the middle ear cavity and usually results in a speedy return of normal hearing and often a dramatic improvement in speech and overall behaviour. Grommets are expelled naturally by the normal desquamative processes of the ear drum after a few months. Some children require multiple sets of grommets while normal Eustachian function is awaited. This normally occurs in the early teens. Adenoidectomy has been shown to reduce rates of recurrent OME and need for subsequent grommets; it is normally reserved for children requiring a second set of grommets.

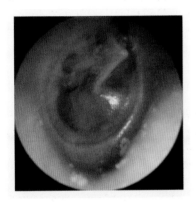

**Fig. 54.2** Otitis media with effusion. (Reproduced with permission from R.S. Dhillon, C.A. East, *Ear, Nose and Throat and Head and Neck Surgery: An Illustrated Colour Text*, 2nd edn, 1994, Churchill Livingstone, Edinburgh.)

Fluid can accumulate in the middle ear of adult patients producing a conductive hearing loss. This is usually described as a middle ear effusion. It is important to rule out disease affecting the opening of the Eustachian tube in the nasopharynx and causing this effusion. This can vary from a mild allergic rhinitis to the more sinister nasopharyngeal carcinoma.

## Chronic suppurative otitis media

Chronic suppurative middle ear disease is of two common types. These are known by many different names. The first, mucosal (alternatively 'safe' or tubotympanic) CSOM follows on from acute suppurative otitis media. A perforation is formed in the pars tensa which then allows ingress of pathogens from the ear canal and recurrent bouts of painless suppuration. These may be precipitated by swimming or syringing the ears. The second is called attico-antral or cholesteatomatous CSOM and is a much more serious disease (thus its previous epithet of 'unsafe').

Cholesteatoma is a disease where skin squames form in the middle ear. Rarely it is congenital and thought to be due to the inclusion of rests of epithelial cells within the TM. More commonly it is acquired. The most likely cause of cholesteatomatous CSOM is accumulation of keratin squames within a retraction pocket of the tympanic membrane (Fig. 54.4).

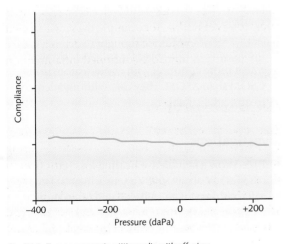

**Fig. 54.3** Tympanogram in otitis media with effusion.

231

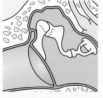

1 Attic retraction pocket forms

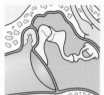

2 Continued formation of keratin in retraction pocket

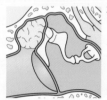

3 Repeated infection and enlargement of cholesteatoma

**Fig. 54.4** Stages in the formation of a cholesteatoma.

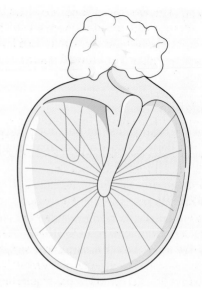

**Fig. 54.5** Attic cholesteatoma.

## Clinical presentation

Cholesteatoma can present from childhood onwards. It is more common in patients who have had previous suppurative ear disease or OME or who have risk factors for these diseases.

The most common presentation is of a chronic foul smelling ear discharge. However, progression to the complications of suppurative ear disease may occur and may be the presenting feature.

Careful clinical examination of the uncomplicated case will reveal debris in the attic region of the tympanic membrane. Removal of this debris with microsuction often reveals the 'cheesy' cholesteatoma matrix extending into the middle ear (see Fig. 54.5).

Always suspect cholesteatoma in any patient with recurrent or chronic ear discharge that does not settle readily with antibiotics. Carefully look for the site of a perforation; any abnormality in the attic region is likely to represent a cholesteatoma. If in doubt refer for further investigation.

## Complications of CSOM

These are essentially the same as seen in acute suppurative otitis media but they are more common.

- *Hearing loss.* Conductive due to ossicular erosion or sensorineural if cochlea is eroded.
- *Dizziness.* The vestibule may be eroded to produce a fistula and dizziness. Or infection may spread via this fistula to produce a bacterial labyrinthitis.
- *Facial nerve paralysis.* Cholesteatoma can involve the nerve directly, or acute infection may supervene and compress the nerve. May be permanent.
- *Mastoiditis/petrositis.* Cholesteatoma can block the normal mastoid drainage pathways and lead to spread of infection within and outside the mastoid air cells.
- *Neck abscesses* (see above).
- *Intracranial complications* (see above). These are much more common with cholesteatomatous CSOM than ASOM. They can, without adequate treatment, be fatal.

## Investigations

- PTAs show a conductive hearing loss (erosion of ossicles) or occasionally a sensorineural loss.
- Microbiology of an ear swab will often show *Pseudomonas* spp. or other anaerobes.
- Fine-cut CT scanning of the temporal bones will show soft tissue within the middle ear

cleft and often erosion of bone or ossicles by the cholesteatoma. It is also invaluable in the diagnosis of complications. MRI is used for the diagnosis of intracranial complications.

## Management

- *Conservative.* Early disease may sometimes be stabilized by the judicious use of topical antibiotics and microsuction of the keratinous debris from the retraction pocket.
- *Surgical.* This is frequently required for more established disease, especially if there are complications. This normally takes the form of a mastoidectomy procedure under general anaesthetic. Following this procedure these patients require regular follow-up and toileting of any mastoid cavity created. Intracranial complications require the intervention of a neurosurgeon and the drainage of any infected collections via a craniotomy.

Risks of mastoidectomy:
Hearing loss.
Tinnitus.
Vertigo.
Injury to seventh nerve.
CSF leak.

## Traumatic injuries of the tympanic membrane and temporal bones

The tympanic membrane is well protected by the external ear canal. However, traumatic injures are not that uncommon. They are usually caused by cotton buds or other implements being pushed into the canal. Blast injuries may also perforate the eardrum. No active treatment is required and most of these injuries will heal spontaneously.

Blunt trauma to the temporal bone is much less common. The bone here is extremely thick and considerable force is required to fracture it. In the past injuries were usually due to road traffic accidents. The routine use of seatbelts and airbags has made temporal bone trauma much less common. The fracture line may run longitudinally, often along the roof of the ear canal disrupting the tympanic membrane and middle ear, or it may run transversely across the temporal bone, in which case structures such as the

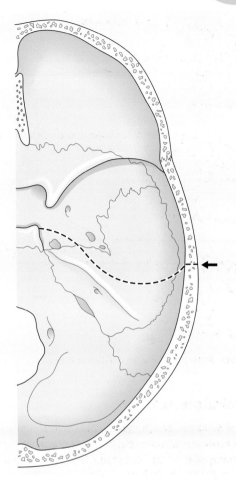

**Fig. 54.6** Longitudinal fracture of the temporal bone. (Adapted with permission from C. W. Cummings, *Otolaryngology: Head and Neck Surgery*, 4th edn, 2005, Mosby, Edinburgh.)

facial nerve and vestibulocochlear (seventh) nerve may be transected (Figs 54.6, 54.7).

## Clinical presentation

See Fig. 54.8.

## Otosclerosis

### Background

This is a relatively common disease which produces a progressive, conductive or mixed hearing loss secondary to abnormal bone metabolism in the remnants of the otic capsule in the inner ear. The initial pathology is most often bone resorption followed by abnormal bone deposition. Its site of attack in the ear is most often at the *fistula ante fenestra* at the anterior part of the stapes footplate (Fig. 54.9). Abnormal bone deposition

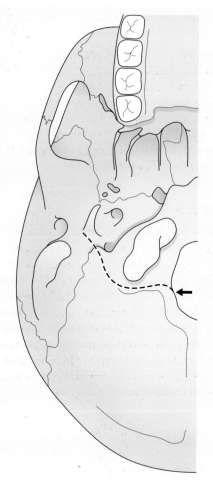

Fig. 54.7 Transverse fracture of the temporal bone. (Adapted with permission from C. W. Cummings, *Otolaryngology: Head and Neck Surgery*, 4th edn, 2005, Mosby, Edinburgh.)

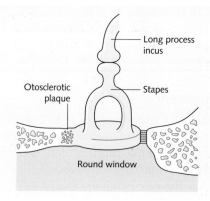

Fig. 54.9 Otosclerosis.

here 'anchors' the stapes in the round window preventing normal conduction of sound. It affects about 1% of the British Caucasian population but is less common in other ethnic groups. Females are affected twice as often as males. Its aetiology is unknown but it is familial and is most often transmitted as an autosomal dominant disease with incomplete penetrance.

## Clinical presentation

This disorder most often presents in the third decade with slowly progressive, bilateral, conductive deafness, tinnitus and occasional mild vertigo. Longstanding disease may also affect the cochlea, producing an added sensorineural hearing loss. Otoscopy reveals a normal ear drum in most cases. In the early bone resorptive stages the hypervascularity of the middle ear may be noted as a reddish 'blush' to the tympanic membrane this is known as Schwartze's sign.

| Fig. 54.8 Clinical presentation of fractures of the temporal bones | | |
|---|---|---|
| | **Longitudinal fractures 70–90%** | **Transverse fractures 10–30%** |
| Otoscopy | Bleeding from the external ear Tympanic membrane often perforated | Bleeding in the middle ear Tympanic membrane intact causing *haemotympanum* |
| CSF leak | CSF otorrheoa sometimes | CSF into nasopharynx – common |
| Hearing loss | Conductive hearing loss due to disruption of the ossicles SNHL relatively uncommon | Severe SNHL |
| Facial nerve paralysis | Rare, often delayed | In 50%, immediate |
| Vestibular symtoms | Mild | Severe |

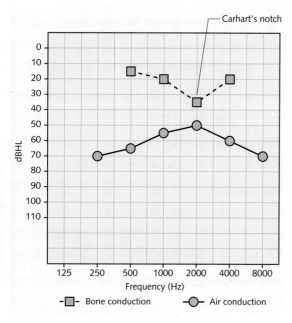

Fig. 54.10 Audiogram in otosclerosis.

If tuning fork tests or an audiogram suggest a conductive deafness and you can see a normal eardrum the diagnosis is either a middle ear effusion or otosclerosis. If tympanometry is then normal the diagnosis is otosclerosis (rarely other forms of ossicular discontinuity or fixation). If the tympanogram is flat then there is a middle ear effusion.

## Management

- *Conservative.* Hearing aids may be advised.
- *Surgical.* Stapedectomy can be carried out under local or general anaesthesia using the operating microscope. It involves the removal of the stapes superstructure and the creation of a 'fenestra' or hole in the fixed stapes footplate into which a piston-like prosthesis is inserted. The other end is connected to the long process of the incus (Fig. 54.11). Good closure of the air–bone gap is reliably achieved. There is a less than 1% risk of creating a 'dead' ear, i.e. complete sensorineural hearing loss.

## Investigations

- *Audiograms* show a typical conductive loss (Fig. 54.10). A 'Carhart's notch' may also be present; this is a 10–30 dB depression in bone conduction at 2 kHz. In late disease there may be a superimposed sensorineural hearing loss. Speech discrimination audiometry is typically much better than expected from the hearing loss. Stapedial reflexes are absent in established disease.
- *Tympanograms* are typically normal but may show decreased compliance.
- *CT scanning* may show abnormal bone deposition around the cochlea with areas of radiolucency. This is called otospongiosus.

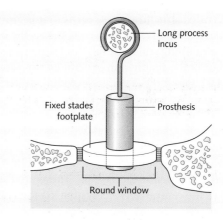

Fig. 54.11 Stapedectomy.

# Disorders of the inner ear and facial nerve

## Objectives

You should be able to:

- Describe the basic structure and physiology of the inner ear.
- Discuss the aetiology and presentation of presbyacusis.
- Give an account of cochlear implantation.
- Say what a vestibular schwannoma is.
- Appreciate the importance of unilateral hearing loss.
- List the three most common causes of vertigo.
- Give a differential diagnosis of facial palsy.
- Discuss Bell's palsy.

## THE INNER EAR

The structures of the inner ear are encased in the petrous temporal bone and include the cochlea and the membranous labyrinth (Fig. 55.1). The cochlea is a coiled structure of 2½ turns that is around 35 mm in length. In cross-section it reveals the perilymph containing scala vestibuli and scala tympani either side of the endolymph containing scala media (Fig. 55.2). Vibration of the stapes footplate is transmitted via the oval window to the scala vestibuli and thence to the scala tympani causing a distortion of the basilar membrane. Specialized hair cells in the organ of Corti are activated by this mechanical distortion and are responsible for the generation of cochlear nerve action potentials. These are transmitted to the central nervous system via the eighth cranial nerve.

The membranous labyrinth contains the anterior, posterior and lateral semicircular canals which detect angular accelerations, i.e. rotation. The otolith organs, the macula and saccule, detect acceleration or deceleration forces. Action potentials generated in these organs are transmitted via the vestibular nerves (part of the eighth nerve).

## DISORDERS OF THE VESTIBULOCOCHLEAR NERVE (EIGHTH NERVE)

### Sensorineural hearing loss

Congenital hearing loss affects around 1 in 1000 births. Acquired disease or degeneration of the eighth nerve or cochlear hair cells is more common and typically presents with the symptom of hearing loss. This may be accompanied by tinnitus and less commonly vertigo. For a discussion of the differential diagnosis and investigation of sensorineural hearing loss see Chapter 43, p. 196.

### Presbyacusis

This is irreversible sensorineural hearing loss due to age-related degeneration of hair cells. It is extremely common and frequently debilitating. The patient often reports a gradual onset of bilateral hearing loss which may be accompanied by tinnitus. Speech discrimination is affected first and it is often difficulty understanding speech when there is background noise that leads patients to seek attention.

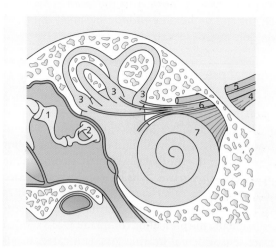

**Fig. 55.1** The inner ear: 1. incus; 2. stapes; 3. semicircular canals; 4. auditory nerve; 5. facial nerve; 6. vestibular nerve; 7. cochlea.

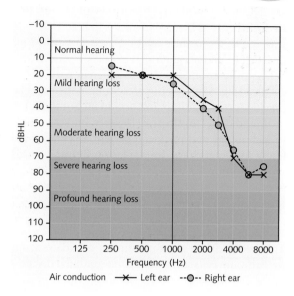

Air conduction    —✕— Left ear    --○-- Right ear

**Fig. 55.3** Audiogram in presbyacusis.

## Management

Provision of an appropriate hearing aid is the first step. Management also encompasses advice about the use of environmental aids such illuminated door bells and useable telephone equipment.

Occasionally hearing loss occurs not gradually but suddenly, so-called sudden onset sensorineural hearing loss. This is usually unilateral but may affect both ears. It is important to rule out a vestibular schwannoma as a cause (MRI scan). In the vast majority of cases the cause is unknown; autoimmune disorder, a herpes neuronitis and vascular compromise have all been postulated as causes. Most cases are treated with a course of corticosteroids. In bilateral cases it may be worth admitting the patient for investigation and more extensive support and intervention such as inhaled carbogen (a $CO_2/O_2$ mixture); there is, however, little evidence for the efficacy of more extensive treatment.

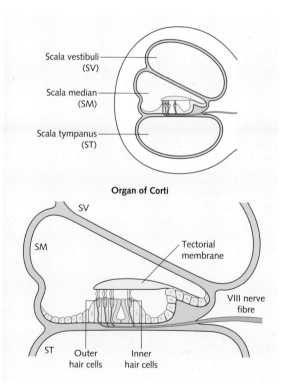

**Fig. 55.2** Cross-section of the cochlea and the organ of Corti.

## Diagnosis

This is based on audiological evidence of bilateral sensorineural hearing loss that is more marked in the higher frequencies (Fig. 55.3).

## Cochlear implantation

Increasingly this technology is being used in profoundly hearing impaired children and adults. It is possible because sound recognition in the spiral of the cochlea is organized 'tonotopically'. High frequencies are detected towards the tip of the spiral with low frequencies at its base. This means that an electrode with multiple channels can be placed surgically into the cochlea and programmed to encode sounds and deliver different frequencies to different parts of the cochlea (Fig. 55.4). At the present time the expense precludes cochlear implantation in all but the most profound of hearing losses. However, improvements in technology and price and patient acceptance are likely to see cochlear implantation become much more common.

## Vestibular schwannoma (acoustic neuroma)

This benign, slow growing tumour originates from the Schwann cells surrounding the vestibular division of the eighth cranial nerve. The most common sites

are just before the nerve exits the internal auditory meatus and in the cerebellopontine angle. Bilateral tumours may be seen in neurofibromatosis type 2.

## Clinical presentation

Interestingly, although this is a vestibular nerve lesion, most patients present with unilateral progressive sensorineural hearing loss and tinnitus. Careful history taking will reveal mild early imbalance but the ability of the vestibular system to accommodate means that this is usually transient. Increasing size may precipitate other cranial nerve neuropathies with loss of corneal reflexes occurring relatively early. Occasionally the presenting complaint is of a sudden onset sensorineural hearing loss. Untreated, headaches, photophobia, and death from intracranial expansion may occur but this is now rare.

**Fig. 55.4** Cochlear implant. 1. External speech processor captures sound and converts it to digital signals. 2. Processor sends digital signals to internal implant. 3. Internal implant turns signals into electrical energy, sending it to an array inside the cochlea. 4. Electrodes stimulate hearing nerve, bypassing damaged hair cells, and the brain perceives signals; you hear sound.© (Copyright Cochlear Ltd, 14 Mars Road, PO Box 629, Lane Cove, NSW 2066 Australia. Telephone: 61 2 9428 6555. Fax: 61 2 9428 6353.)

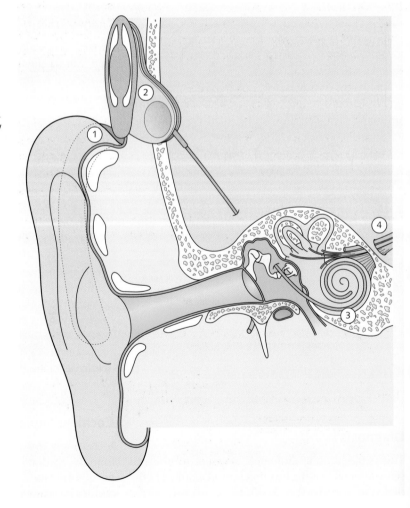

Never ignore the patient who complains of a unilateral hearing loss. Arrange a hearing test. If this shows asymmetric hearing loss imaging of the eighth nerve should be arranged.

## Diagnosis

Suspicion is often aroused incidentally when asymmetric sensorineural hearing loss is noted on pure tone audiometry. In these cases gadolinium-enhanced MRI scan of the internal auditory meatus will reveal an enhancing lesion if a vestibular schwannoma is present.

## Management

Observation with serial scanning may be appropriate for slowly growing lesions in elderly patients. Otherwise the choice is between surgical excision and targeted radiotherapy, the so-called 'gamma-knife'. Each has its vocal proponents.

The internal auditory meatus can be accessed surgically via the temporal bone, the trans-labyrinthine approach, or by more conventional neurosurgical routes such as the retrosigmoid approach.

## TINNITUS

Tinnitus is the perception of sound in the absence of external stimuli. It may be objective and caused by noise in structures surrounding the ear, e.g. heart murmurs and vascular abnormalities of the temporal bone. More commonly it is subjective and heard only by the sufferer. The most useful theory of the aetiology of tinnitus is the neurophysiological model proposed by Jastreboff (Fig. 55.5).

## Clinical presentation

Tinnitus may be associated with hearing loss. It may be unilateral or bilateral. Objective tinnitus may be pulsatile if associated with vascular anomalies. There is an association with depression, although a cause and effect relationship is not proven.

## Diagnosis

Diagnosis is based upon the clinical history. An audiogram is performed in all cases. In cases of unilateral tinnitus with unilateral sensorineural hearing loss it is important to exclude a vestibular schwannoma; a gadolinium enhanced MRI scan is the most useful investigation for this. If the tinnitus has a pulsatile element then a CT is ordered to look for vascular abnormalities of the temporal bone.

## Management

In the vast majority of patients with tinnitus there is no underlying pathology except perhaps a degree of hearing loss. Reassurance is extremely important. For many patients this is all that is required. There is, however, a small group of patients in whom tinnitus is intrusive and extremely troublesome. They often benefit from contact with a trained hearing therapist. Correction of any hearing loss using a hearing aid

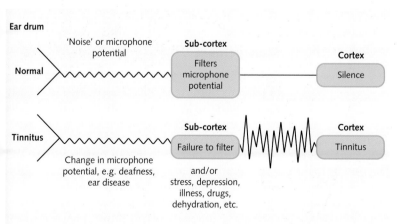

Fig. 55.5 Neurophysiological model of tinnitus.

should be attempted. Tinnitus masking devices either placed in the bedroom or worn in the ear may help to attenuate tinnitus for some.

## VERTIGO

See Chapter 44, Vertigo.

Vertigo is the erroneous impression of movement caused by disease of the vestibular system. It is typically rotatory in nature.

### Benign paroxysmal positional vertigo (BPPV)

This is the most common type of vertigo seen in ENT clinics. It may follow viral URTI or a full-blown labyrinthitis. It is thought that it is caused by the deposition of calcific debris in the posterior semicircular canal following inflammation, so-called canalithiasis. This debris causes momentary stimulation of balance centres with particular head movements.

### Clinical presentation

The patient experiences severe rotatory vertigo lasting seconds. This is typically precipitated by rolling over in bed. The patient will often volunteer that it is caused by turning in one direction but not the other.

### Diagnosis

This is usually obvious from the history. The Dix–Hallpike test is diagnostic. This attempts to induce torsional nystagmus by creating a sudden change in head position. The patient will experience dizziness. A positive test will, after a short latent period, produce an observable nystagmus which will then fatigue and disappear while at the same time the patient's dizziness subsides.

### Management

The Epley manoeuvre is designed to rotate the calcific material out of the posterior canal via a series of head and body movements performed usually in the clinic setting. It is said to be effective in 75% of cases of BPPV. It is especially useful as it is repeatable and the patient can be taught to perform it themselves at home.

## Ménière's disease

Ménière's disease has for years puzzled and excited the otology community. That is largely because it is relatively common, frequently troublesome, and there is no effective cure. It is thought to be due to recurrent increases in endolymph pressure within the vestibule leading to bouts of otological and vestibular hyperstimulation.

### Clinical presentation

Ménière's disease presents clinically as a triad of symptoms:

1. *Vertigo* – this comes in bouts lasting usually for a number of hours at a time. It is rotatory and may cause nausea and vomiting.
2. *Tinnitus* – this may precede the onset of a bout of vertigo and often acts as a warning to the patient that an attack is imminent. It may also become higher in pitch just before an attack.
3. *Sensorineural hearing loss* – unusually the sensorineural loss may fluctuate, worsening during an attack and then improving as the dizziness improves. There is, however, a tendency towards progressive hearing loss.

### Diagnosis

Despite the well known classical features of this disease it is often difficult to diagnose. There is no one test that is specific for the presence of Ménière's disease. A history of episodic vertigo lasting hours with tinnitus and hearing loss is extremely suggestive as is the finding of asymmetric sensorineural hearing loss on audiograms. Vestibular function testing (see p. 309) shows reduced vestibular function in most patients.

### Management

Although there is no cure it is said that around 80% of patients improve spontaneously. This obviously makes objective evaluation of therapy difficult. The progressive hearing loss is not amenable to treatment. Most therapy is symptomatic and aimed at reducing vertigo during attacks. To this end salt restriction and diuretics are used to counteract the increased endolymphatic pressure. Antihistamines which act as 'vestibular sedatives', such as betahistine are routinely prescribed, although there is little evidence for their effectiveness. Anti-emetics are also popular.

For the resistant 10% of patients with intractable vertigo, various surgical procedures have been suggested. The multitude of techniques indicates that none is ideal. They either aim to decompress the endolymphatic sac or to destroy and therefore 'quieten down' the affected labyrinth using drugs (intratympanic gentamicin) or surgery (labyrinthectomy). The unfortunate side effect of the surgical ablative procedures is a deaf ear.

## Vestibulitis/labyrinthitis

Probably a more accurate term is vestibular neuronitis, although the terms vestibulitis and labyrinthitis are more commonly used. This clinical entity is thought to be the result of infection of the vestibular apparatus, possibly with a herpes type virus.

### Clinical presentation

The patient complains of a sudden-onset debilitating vertigo, often with nausea. There may be a preceding upper respiratory tract infection. There are usually no other otological symptoms and the hearing is normally preserved. The key to the diagnosis is that the vertigo persists for days even though it gradually improves. After the acute vertigo has settled the patient may suffer from persistent imbalance. They may also develop BPPV.

### Diagnosis

This is based on the clinical history. Audiometry is normal. During the acute attack the patient will demonstrate nystagmus.

### Management

Management is supportive. The great feature of the vestibular system is its ability to adapt. Given time and encouragement vertigo will nearly always settle. In the acute period anti-emetics such as prochlorperazine are used. They also have a vestibular sedative effect and can be very helpful. However, it is important that they are used only in the first few days. Continuation beyond this period interferes with normal adaptive processes. The patient is encouraged to mobilize in order to encourage adaptation. Specific exercises called Cawthorne–Cooksey exercises can also speed this process. Following the acute attack, if imbalance persists specific balance orientated physiotherapy is helpful.

The facial nerve enters the temporal bone through the internal auditory meatus and then passes through the hiatus of the facial canal. It runs forward to its geniculate ganglion and then passes above the stapes footplate, turning inferiorly at its second genu to run vertically through the mastoid posterior to the tympanic membrane (Fig. 55.6). It emerges from the temporal bone at the stylomastoid foramen before passing forward into the substance of the parotid gland. Within the gland it splits into its five terminal branches, temporal, zygomatic, buccal, mandibular and cervical, which supply the muscles of facial expression.

## Facial paralysis

Causes of facial paralysis are listed in Fig. 55.7.

Middle ear disease is discussed elsewhere; here we concentrate on the most common form of facial nerve pathology, namely Bell's palsy.

## Bell's palsy

This is used to be thought of as idiopathic facial nerve palsy. It is likely that it is a mononeuritis caused by herpes simplex virus infection. It is thought that viral replication within the facial nerve leads to oedema and swelling. As the nerve is contained within the tight confines of the temporal bone this oedema results in axonal degeneration and failure to conduct impulses.

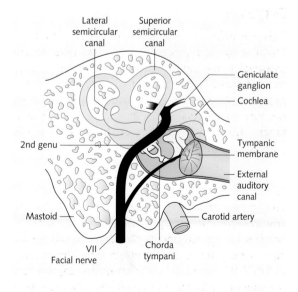

**Fig. 55.6** Intratemporal course of the facial nerve.

**Fig. 55.7** Causes of facial paralysis

**Upper motor neurone**
a.　CVA
b.　Cerebello-pontine angle tumour

**Lower motor neurone**
a.　Intratemporal
　i.　Bell's palsy
　ii.　Ramsay Hunt syndrome
　iii.　Acute or chronic suppurative otitis media
　iv.　Tumour
　v.　Trauma
　vi.　Nerve infiltration, e.g. sarcoidosis
b.　Extratemporal
　i.　Malignant parotid neoplasms
　ii.　Traumatic

## Clinical presentation

There is commonly an aching pain in the mastoid which precedes the onset of facial weakness. Progressive unilateral facial palsy then follows. It is complete in 70% and partial in the remainder. Paralysis of other intratemporal branches results in decreased taste sensation on the ipsilateral tongue (chorda tympani), hyperacusis (nerve to stapedius) and decreased tearing (secretomotor fibres to the lacrimal gland). Full recovery occurs in around 85%. This may take up to 3 months. Where the orbicularis oculi muscle is paralysed ocular complications such as corneal ulceration may occur if eye care is neglected.

## Diagnosis

This rests mainly on the clinical findings combined with the absence of other neurological findings. Otological examination should be normal. Audiograms are usually performed to rule out more extensive cranial nerve involvement and thus more serious pathology. In the UK MRI scanning is reserved for those with polyneuropathies, unusual presentations and those in whom the palsy shows no sign of resolution at 3 months.

## Management

1. *Steroids* – oral prednisolone is usually prescribed for a period of 2 weeks. It should be commenced as soon as possible.
2. *Aciclovir* – the viral aetiology of Bell's is increasingly accepted and the use of aciclovir is much more common. There is little evidence that it is effective.
3. *Eye care* – as most cases recover spontaneously this is perhaps the most crucial aspect of care. Lubricants such as hypromellose drops and Lacri-Lube ointment are usually required. The patient should be shown how to tape the eye closed at night. More serious cases (i.e. complete palsy) may need partial surgical closure of the eyelids (tarsorrhaphy) while recovery of function is awaited.
4. *Surgical decompression* of the facial nerve. There are some vocal proponents of surgery in cases of complete palsy with other poor prognostic signs. Electrophysiological studies such as EMG (electromyography) and ENOG (electroneuronography) can help decide which patients are likely to constitute the minority who are unlikely to recover spontaneously.

## RAMSAY HUNT SYNDROME

This, like Bell's palsy, is a viral neuropathy. It is caused by reactivation of herpes zoster infection in the geniculate ganglion. It is, however, a more serious condition than Bell's palsy.

Pain in the ear is a more marked feature. There is usually a vesicular eruption on the pinna, ear canal or ipsilateral soft palate. Involvement of other cranial nerves (V, VIII, IX, X, XI) may occur. Permanent paralysis is much more likely, especially if the paralysis is complete at presentation.

Treatment comprises eye care, steroids and antivirals, as for Bell's palsy.

# Disorders of the nose and paranasal sinuses

## Objectives

You should be able to:

- Describe the anatomy and physiology of the nose.
- List the common congenital malformations of the nose.
- Discuss nasal trauma and how it is managed.
- Understand the importance of a septal haematoma and know how it should be managed.
- Discuss epistaxis.
- Describe rhinosinusitis and its management.
- Give a brief account of nasal tumours.
- Understand anosmia and know how to investigate it.

The paired nasal cavities serve the dual purposes of olfaction and preparation of inspired air for delivery to the lower airway. The olfactory mucosa found in the roof of the nose contains specialized nerve endings which connect with the first cranial nerve via the cribriform plate.

In order to warm and humidify inspired air the nasal cavities have a large surface area and a rich blood supply. The mucosa is ciliated columnar epithelium. The cilia play a vital role in filtering out particulate foreign matter and transporting it to the nasopharynx where it is swallowed.

Similar ciliary pathways operate within the paranasal sinuses from where mucus and other debris is transported mostly into the middle meatus and thence to the nasopharynx.

## CONGENITAL NASAL DEFECTS

The nose develops in utero from the frontonasal process and the invagination of paired nasal placodes to form pits which deepen to produce blind-ending tubes. The primitive nasal cavities are separated from the nasopharynx by the bucconasal membrane which usually breaks down at between 5 and 6 weeks in utero to form the posterior choanae.

### Choanal atresia

This occurs when there is failure of the bucconasal membrane to rupture and the nasal cavities remain separate from the nasopharynx. It is usually a unilateral problem and may not present until later in life. If bilateral it causes severe respiratory difficulties in newborns, who are obligate nose breathers. It is twice as common in females. Particularly in bilateral cases it may also be associated with craniofacial and other congenital anomalies, for example the CHARGE association of coloboma, hearing deficit, choanal atresia, retardation of growth, genital defects (in males) and endocardial defects.

### Clinical presentation

There is breathing difficulty and cyanosis within hours of birth. The obstruction is relieved by crying and worsened by attempts at feeding. There may be other congenital anomalies.

### Diagnosis

Failure to pass a naso-endoscope or Foley catheter through the nose into the nasopharynx confirms the diagnosis. CT scanning is helpful in determining the extent of the anatomical abnormality.

### Management

*Airway control.* This is the priority in the early stages. Initially it can be accomplished by the placement of an appropriate oropharyngeal airway. However, this does not allow feeding unless a orogastric tube is placed. Devices such as the McGovern nipple allow feeding and airway maintenance. Rarely intubation or even tracheostomy may be required if early definitive repair of the defect cannot be attempted. This is usually due to coexisting anomalies.

*Surgical management.* The atretic plate may be removed as soon as is practicable, usually via the transnasal route. Fibreoptic endoscopy has made early intervention in the neonate much easier.

## Nasal dermoid cyst

These congenital lesions contain skin, hairs and sebaceous material. They usually form a midline mass on the dorsum of the nose which presents in childhood. They may also be noted as a midline sinus. Some of them connect intracranially.

MRI is performed to rule out cranial extension prior to surgical excision.

The differential diagnosis of nasal dermoids includes two other congenital abnormalities. These are nasal gliomas and encephalocoeles, both of which connect intracranially (Fig. 56.1). Diagnosis is confirmed by MRI.

## NASAL FRACTURES AND OTHER INJURIES

Given its prominent situation it is hardly surprising that fractures of the nose are the most common

maxillofacial bony injury. The injury is usually the result of interpersonal violence but may also occur as the result of falls, sports and motor vehicle accidents. Fractures of the cartilaginous septum are just as common but less well recognized.

## Clinical presentation

Significant injuries to the nasal skeleton usually result in obvious cosmetic deformity with lateral deviation. This may not be immediately evident owing to periorbital and soft tissue swelling. Immediate epistaxis usually occurs but is mostly self-limiting. Nasal obstruction may occur due to bony injury, septal displacement or septal haematoma.

## Diagnosis

History and examination are usually all that is required to make the diagnosis of a nasal bone fracture. It is important to look into the nose to exclude septal injuries and especially to exclude a septal haematoma.

Routine nasal bone radiographs are not useful as they do not alter management. The need for manipulation is based upon the presence of deformity. This is best assessed once soft tissue swelling has settled, at around 5–7 days.

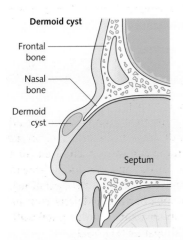

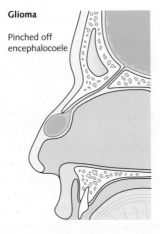

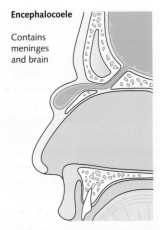

**Fig. 56.1** Congenital nasal abnormalities.

## Management

Displaced nasal bone fractures are best treated within 2 weeks of the injury. The usual strategy is to manipulate the bones back into place under anaesthetic (MUA). If presentation is delayed or if there is significant septal deformity then it is customary to let the acute injury heal and deal with any residual functional or cosmetic problems around 4–6 months later. This usually involves a septoplasty procedure to correct the septum, with or without rhinoplasty to correct bony deformity. Some advocate early septal surgery with MUA.

## SEPTAL HAEMATOMA

It is vital to examine for a septal haematoma in all cases of nasal injury. A missed diagnosis results in significant long-term cosmetic deformity and potential litigation.

The nasal septal cartilage depends for its blood supply on the overlying mucoperichondrium. In a septal haematoma an expanding blood clot in the subperichondrial plane 'strips off' the mucoperichondrium, leaving the cartilage denuded of its blood supply. Septal necrosis and abscess formation may then occur with collapse of support for the tip of the nose and an ugly saddle deformity.

## Clinical presentation

A high degree of suspicion is required. An additional feature that would alert you to the presence of a septal haematoma would be severe bilateral nasal blockage following a nasal fracture; this is rare following simple injuries. Also, pain that worsens in the days following the injury may suggest septal abscess formation.

## Diagnosis

A septal haematoma is seen as a cherry red fluctuant swelling of the anterior part of the septum. It is usually bilateral. It can be distinguished from the much more common deviated septum by gentle pressure with a cotton bud. A haematoma is soft, the septum is not.

## Management

This should be treated as an emergency if necrosis of the septum is to be avoided. The haematoma is drained via an intranasal incision under local anaesthetic and a gentle pack is inserted into the nose to prevent reaccumulation. Prophylactic antibiotics are given orally.

## NASAL FOREIGN BODIES

Although fly larvae and other exotic specimens have been known to make their own way into the nasal cavity, most cases involve a young child who has inserted a toy, a bead or a pencil eraser into their nose.

## Clinical presentation

If the foreign body goes unnoticed the child may present some time later. The classical findings are of a foul-smelling unilateral nasal discharge. There may also be excoriation of the skin of the upper lip. The offending object is usually visible just inside the nostril.

## Management

Inexpert attempts at removal are to be discouraged as they usually just produce an upset child with a foreign body even further back in the nose. Careful removal in clinic is usually possible utilizing a small curved hook, or a paediatric Foley catheter inserted past the object, the balloon inflated and then slowly withdrawn. If this is not possible general anaesthesia is required.

## EPISTAXIS

See also Chapter 48, Epistaxis.

Nosebleeds are extremely common; nearly all of us will have one during our lifetime. They occur at all ages but are more common in children (due to nose picking and URTIs) and the elderly (due to vascular fragility and coexistent anticoagulation). Predisposing factors include platelet defects, clotting abnormalities and abnormalities of the vessel wall. Most, however, are idiopathic (Fig. 56.2).

The nasal mucosa has a prolific vascular supply to aid in its role of rapid humidification and warming of inspired air. It has contributions from the external

**Fig. 56.2** Predisposing factors for epistaxis

**Systemic factors**

Coagulopathy, e.g. warfarin, liver disease, haemophilia

Platelet abnormality, e.g. aspirin, thrombocytopaenia, Von Willebrand's

Vessel wall abnormalities, e.g. hypertension, hereditary haemorrhagic telangiectasia (HHT, see text)

**Local factors**

Trauma

Drying and atrophy, e.g. septal perforation, septal deviation, steroid sprays

Idiopathic

Inflammation – rhinitis, sarcoidosis, drugs, e.g. cocaine

Neoplasms – juvenile angiofibroma (see text), SCC, adenocarcinoma, melanoma

carotid artery via the maxillary artery which supplies the antero-inferior part of the nose. There is also a supply from the ophthalmic branch of the internal carotid artery via the anterior and posterior ethmoidal arteries which supply the supero-posterior part of the nose. There is a rich anastomosis between these two supplies which is most marked on the anterior septum at Little's area. This is the most frequent site of epistaxis (Fig. 56.3).

## Clinical presentation

Many patients are referred routinely to out-patients with troublesome intermittent epistaxis which may be precipitated by nose blowing or exertion.

However, a significant number of patients present as an emergency with acute epistaxis.

In acute epistaxis the bleed can be anterior, and therefore visible, or posterior, in which case the major symptom may be expectorated or swallowed blood. Epistaxis is frequently severe enough to cause haemodynamic changes and shock, especially in the elderly.

## Diagnosis

In the non-acute setting it is important to look at the other mucous membranes such as the lips to rule out conditions such as hereditary haemorrhagic telangiectasia (see later). Look for bruising around belt lines, etc., which may suggest a coagulopathy

**Fig. 56.3** Vascular anatomy of the nasal septum.

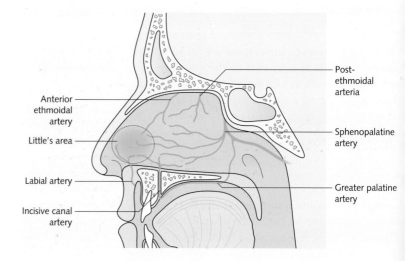

Anterior ethmoidal artery

Little's area

Labial artery

Incisive canal artery

Post-ethmoidal arteria

Sphenopalatine artery

Greater palatine artery

Finally examine the nose (see p. 309). Often there is evidence of a recent bleed in Little's area, or other anatomical abnormalities that may predispose to epistaxis (see above).

## Management

In the acute setting management commences as for any emergency, with attention paid to Airway, Breathing and Circulation (ABC) while the patient or an assistant applies pressure to the anterior septum.

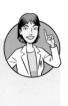

Before getting 'stuck in', it is vital that you don protective clothing including glasses, mask, gloves and a gown. It is also a good idea to protect the patient's clothing.

- ABC
- Assess for signs of shock and treat as appropriate.
- Insert i.v. access and full blood count, clotting and cross match.
- Pressure to bleeding point.
- Examine the nose.
- Obvious bleeding point – cautery using silver nitrate or diathermy.
- No obvious bleeding point – apply nasal packs (see below).

## Nasal packs

If it is not possible to stop a nose bleed using cautery, then a nasal pack has to be inserted (Fig. 56.4). These may be placed anteriorly in the nasal cavity and may need to be combined with a posterior pack in the nasopharynx. Anterior packs may be ribbon gauze soaked in iodoform paste, or specially made sponge tampons. Posterior packing may be made from gauze packs or utilize a Foley catheter inflated in the nasopharynx (Fig. 56.5). This is not a pleasant procedure for the patient but may be life-saving.

All patients with packs should be admitted to hospital and face mask oxygen should be given. It is customary to leave the packs in place for 24 hours prior to removal. If retained longer than this, antibiotics should be given to prevent staphylococcal toxic shock. Any haematological or clotting abnormalities should be corrected. Failure to arrest epistaxis with simple cautery and/or nasal packing necessitates intervention; this usually means endoscopic ligation of the sphenopalatine arteries within the nose plus sometimes clipping the ethmoidal arteries via a medial orbital incision. (See Fig. 48.1, Algorithm for management of epistaxis, p. 210.)

## Hereditary haemorrhagic telangiectasia (HHT)

HHT is transmitted in an autosomal dominant fashion. Multiple knots of abnormal fragile capillaries are found throughout the mucosa of the nose and

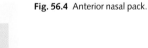
**Fig. 56.4** Anterior nasal pack.

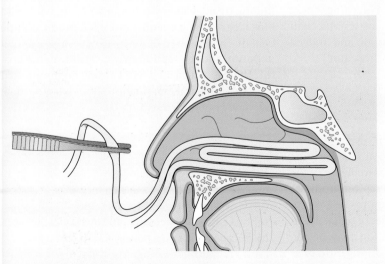

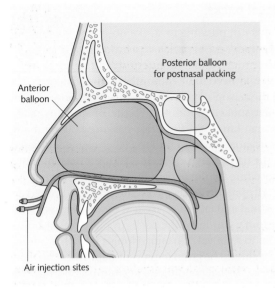

Fig. 56.5 Anterior and posterior nasal packing with balloons.

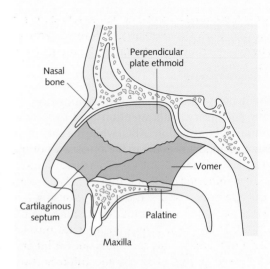

Fig. 56.6 Anatomy of the nasal septum.

gastrointestinal tract and viscera. There may also be pulmonary arteriovenous malformations. The lesions usually appear around puberty. Epistaxis is extremely common and may produce anaemia.

## Clinical presentation

Epistaxis may be the presenting complaint. Examination reveals characteristic telangiectases on the lips and on the nasal mucosa. Even minor trauma from examination may provoke bleeding.

## Management

Various management strategies have been tried in an attempt to limit the episodes of bleeding. These include argon laser cauterization of lesions, skin grafting of the entire nasal septum, and indeed closure of the nasal cavity (Young's procedure).

## SEPTAL DEVIATION

The nasal septum divides the nasal cavity, plays an important role in the humidification and warming of inspired air and provides support to the tip of the nose (Fig. 56.6). Deviation of the septum from the midline is extremely common – up to 50% of the population is affected. Minor degrees of septal deviation are therefore normal. Deviation may be the result of trauma acquired in utero, during birth or as a result of a blow to the nose. Alternatively it may be

a consequence of asymmetric growth of the septum and nasal structures.

## Clinical presentation

The main symptom of severe septal deviation is unilateral or sometimes bilateral nasal blockage. The obstruction is typically constant and not cyclical. However, it may be made worse with URTIs.

## Diagnosis

In the history it is important to rule out other common causes of nasal blockage before ascribing symptoms to septal deviation. All too often the normal finding of a deviated septum in a patient with mild blockage results in an operation that produces little benefit. Examination of the nose may show external deviation and the septum may be visible in the nostril. There is a decreased nasal airway on the affected side and intranasal examination should demonstrate a deviated or buckled septum.

A useful diagnostic procedure is to examine the nose before and after topical decongestion using oxymetazoline. This will make little difference to a mechanical septal obstruction but may temporarily relieve obstruction caused by mucosal swelling, i.e. rhinitis.

## Management

Obstruction caused by septal deviation is best treated by the operation of septoplasty. Deformed cartilage can be either removed or straightened and the nasal airway improved.

Almost all asthma patients have allergic rhinitis. Of patients diagnosed with allergic rhinitis, 15% have asthma. It is important to look for both diseases together.

## RHINOSINUSITIS

Inflammation affecting the mucosal surfaces of the nose is likely to similarly affect the paranasal sinuses, a so-called rhinosinusitis. Many different disease entities can affect the nose and cause rhinosinusitis. It is conventional to refer to rhinitis as a separate clinical entity, while the term rhinosinusitis encompasses acute sinusitis and chronic conditions such as inflammatory nasal polyps, and chronic rhinosinusitis, among many others.

## Allergic rhinitis

Around a quarter to a half of the British population suffer from allergic rhinitis. It may in fact be the most common chronic disease. There are numerous potential allergens but the most common are grass and tree pollens followed by allergy to house dust mite. Symptoms may be described as intermittent if present for less than 4 weeks or persistent if present on most days for more than 4 weeks. Allergic rhinitis is a cause of significant morbidity and workplace absenteeism.

It is mediated by a classical type 1 hypersensitivity reaction to inhaled allergen. Contact with allergen to which the host has been previously sensitized results in IgE linkage and mast cell degranulation, producing the immediate symptoms of sneezing, itching, rhinorrhoea (runny nose) and congestion. In common with asthma there is also an eosinophil mediated late phase response which results in a 'winding up' of the immune response, producing persistent background inflammation and hyper-reactivity even when the allergen has long gone.

## Clinical presentation

The classical symptoms are of nasal congestion, rhinorrhoea, hyposmia and sneezing. There may also be itching of the eyes, nose and throat. The rhinitis may also have secondary effects such as bacterial sinusitis, otitis media and difficulty sleeping. The patient may suffer from other atopic diseases such as eczema or asthma.

Examination of the nose reveals pale, oedematous nasal mucosa often with marked enlargement of the inferior turbinates, sometimes mistaken by the unwary for nasal polyps. The mucosa is usually wet.

## Diagnosis

The clinical history and characteristic appearances on nasal examination will usually suggest the diagnosis. However, it is often useful to supplement this with formal tests for allergy. Skin prick testing is simple, cheap and safe and provides the patient with a good demonstration of some of the changes that occur within the nose upon contact with allergen.

Ten common allergens, including pollens and house dust mite, along with a negative and positive control are introduced into the dermis. A wheal and flare reaction suggests allergy (Fig. 56.7). Serological testing for allergy is also sometimes used (e.g. RAST). Pulmonary peak flow measurements are a good way to screen for asthma in these patients.

## Management

The management of allergic rhinitis has two main components

### 1. Allergen avoidance

If at all possible the patient should minimize their exposure to allergen. In pollen allergy avoidance is difficult but involves staying indoors with the windows closed when the pollen count is highest. Hardly

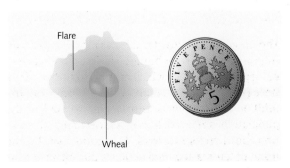

Fig. 56.7 Wheal and flare skin reaction.

an ideal way to spend a hot summer's day! For other allergens such as house dust mite avoidance is more feasible. It involves minimizing soft furnishings in the bedroom, regularly replacing pillows, weekly boil washing of bedding (including duvets), and regularly vacuuming the mattress. This requires a considerable input of both time and money by the patient and their family; it is, however, frequently successful in improving symptoms.

## 2. Medical treatment

This includes:

- Regular corticosteroid nasal sprays (relieves nasal blockage, rhinorrhoea, and sneezing to some extent)
- Regular oral antihistamine, e.g. fexofenadine or azelastine or other second-generation non-sedating drug (will relieve itching eyes and throat and sneezing but will not relieve nasal blockage).
- Allergen immunotherapy – delivers regular small systemic doses of an allergen with the aim of producing anti-IgE blocking antibodies and producing tolerance. At present its use is limited to patients who fail with standard avoidance measures and medical therapy.
- Surgery is rarely required for uncomplicated allergic rhinitis. Occasionally, surgery to the inferior turbinate (cautery or surgical reduction) is used to reduce its bulk and improve the airway but any gains are soon lost if the patient does not comply with their medical treatment.

## Other causes of rhinitis

There are many conditions that may produce similar symptoms. It is important that in taking a history from a patient with rhinitis other potential causes are considered. These are listed in Fig. 56.8.

| **Fig. 56.8** Causes of rhinitis |
| --- |
| Infectious – viral, bacterial |
| Allergic – persistent/intermittent |
| Occupational exposures – allergic or non-allergic |
| Drug induced – aspirin, ACE inhibitors, rhinitis medicamentosa (see text) |
| Hormonal – pregnancy induced |
| Idiopathic or vasomotor rhinitis |

Many patients, if they develop rhinitis, will use over-the-counter vasoconstrictor sprays such as xylometazoline. Unfortunately , although extremely effective at quickly relieving congestion, they produce a rebound increase in congestion after they wear off. Patients become 'addicted' to their sprays and may have blockage that becomes chronic. This is rhinitis medicamentosa. It is extremely common.

## Rhinosinusitis

Rhinosinusitis is inflammation of the nasal and paranasal sinus mucosa. Two of the following symptoms should be present alongside endoscopic or CT evidence of disease:

- Rhinorrhoea.
- Nasal blockage.
- Hyposmia/anosmia (reduction/loss of smell).
- Facial pain.

Classification is based on duration of symptoms:

- <10 days – acute viral rhinosinusitis.
- >10 days <12 weeks– acute bacterial rhinosinusitis.
- >12 weeks – chronic rhinosinusitis (CRS):
  - CRS with polyps
  - CRS without polyps
  - Others, e.g. Wegener's, sarcoidosis.

## Acute bacterial rhinosinusitis

Alteration or blockage of normal mucociliary drainage pathways from the paranasal sinuses results in stasis of secretions and secondary bacterial infection. The majority of the sinuses drain into the cramped ostiomeatal complex (OMC) under the middle turbinate (Fig. 56.9). Preceding conditions may include a viral rhinosinusitis or allergic rhinitis. Both may cause physical blockage within the OMC or may impair mucociliary clearance.

Causative organisms are common upper respiratory tract pathogens, including *Streptococcus pneumoniae*, *Haemophilus influenzae* and *Moraxella catarrhalis*.

### Presentation

Most patients presenting with sinusitis have a combination of facial pain (often worse on bending

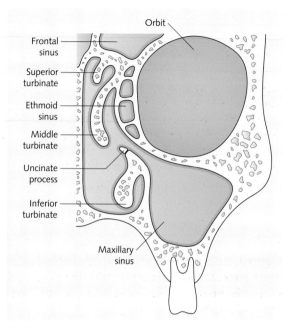

**Fig. 56.9** Anatomy of the ostiomeatal complex.

forward), nasal blockage, rhinorrhoea, and a bad smell (cacosmia); there are often systemic symptoms of malaise and pyrexia.

### Diagnosis

In the acute case the finding of the above symptoms along with tenderness on pressure over the affected sinuses and constitutional symptoms should alert you to the diagnosis. In most cases examination with an endoscope reveals pus in the ostiomeatal complex.

Pain from sinusitis should be anatomical, and should conform to an infective cause; the patient who has frontal sinus pain lasting for an hour at a time with no nasal blockage does not have sinusitis. Examination of the nose with an endoscope and CT scans of the sinuses can be very helpful to confirm or refute the diagnosis in these cases.

### Management

- *Antimicrobial* – amoxicillin, co-amoxiclav or cephalosporin.
- *Topical decongestant* – ephedrine drops or xylometazoline nasal spray.
- *Rarely surgery* – sinus washout or middle meatal antrostomy to drain the sinus, especially if there are complications. Recurrent bouts of acute rhinosinusitis may be treated with FESS (see below, Functional endoscopic sinus surgery) in an attempt to improve sinus drainage.

## Complications of rhinosinusitis

Prompt antibiotic treatment means that complications are relatively rare. However, they are still seen most often in paediatric patients where the diagnosis of sinusitis is often delayed and the bony barriers to spread of infection from the sinuses are thin and easily breached. They include:

- Orbital complications – ranging from periorbital cellulitis to cavernous sinus thrombosis. May result in vision loss or even death if not treated appropriately.
- Osteomyelitis of the frontal bone – 'Potts puffy tumour'.
- Intracranial complications – meningitis, subdural and extradural empyema, encephalitis, brain abscess. All may be fatal.

## Chronic rhinosinusitis

This is a common problem affecting 2–15% of the population. The symptoms are of nasal blockage, rhinorrhoea, anosmia and facial pain lasting more than 12 weeks. There are many underlying issues which may contribute. And all of these factors should be taken into account in the history and examination. They include:

- Local anatomical abnormalities within the paranasal sinuses.
- Ciliary impairment – secondary to viral infection or congenital, e.g. Kartagener's or cystic fibrosis.
- Immunocompromise.
- Genetic factors.
- Micro-organism factors – some bacteria and fungi seem able to excite a deleterious host reponse leading to chronic inflammation in predisposed individuals.

## Chronic rhinosinusitis with polyps

CRS with polyps is a chronic inflammatory condition of unknown aetiology. The polyps are multiple oedematous outgrowths of mucosa with a profuse eosinophilic reaction. There is an increased incidence of asthma in these patients and both conditions are likely to represent an alteration in immunological surveillance. The combination of asthma, nasal polyps and aspirin intolerance is well described and known as Samter's triad. Severe nasal polyposis may also be caused by hypersensitivity to fungal species (allergic fungal sinusitis). Despite being a difficult disease to eradicate, this entity is not to be confused with the invasive fungal sinus infection associated with immunosuppressed states. These cases run a much more virulent course and may be fatal.

### Clinical presentation

> Nasal polyps in children are rare and when they are seen a generalized mucociliary clearance disorder such as Kartagener's syndrome or cystic fibrosis must be excluded.
>
> Grape-like polyps are formed in the nose from early adulthood onwards resulting in progressive bilateral nasal blockage, rhinorrhoea and anosmia.

### Diagnosis

Careful examination with an endoscope reveals the characteristic glistening grey–white polyps, usually originating from the ethmoid sinuses and emerging under the middle turbinate. In severe cases the polyps may be seen emerging from the nostril and may fill the nasal cavities, even causing widening of the inter-canthal distance. Inflammatory polyps are usually bilateral; unilateral nasal polyps raise the possibility of a neoplastic disorder.

> If a patient has unilateral nasal polyps on examination, it is important to exclude a neoplastic process. The most common of these is an inverted papilloma. A CT scan is obtained. If this raises the possibility of a neoplastic process, i.e. unilateral bone destruction, a biopsy is performed.

CT scanning is the radiological investigation of choice and demonstrates polyposis extremely well; it is essential before operative intervention but is seldom required for diagnosis.

### Management

Inflammatory nasal polyposis is incurable but is generally steroid responsive. Treatment should be based on a stepped approach, often called a therapeutic pyramid, the patient going up each step until control is gained (Fig. 56.10).

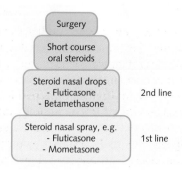

Fig. 56.10 The therapeutic pyramid for nasal polyposis.

Surgery for polyposis ranges from simple endoscopic polypectomy through to more extensive clearance of disease from the nose, frontal, ethmoid, maxillary and sphenoid sinuses as part of a functional endoscopic sinus surgery (FESS) procedure. It is important that the patient is counselled about the importance of regular long-term preventative medication in order to avoid frequent surgical intervention.

## Functional endoscopic sinus surgery (FESS)

There has been an increasing tendency to treat refractory chronic rhinosinusitis with minimally invasive endoscopic surgery. The principle behind this FESS is to leave as much mucosa behind as possible and to remove only grossly diseased tissue within the ethmoid sinuses and the OMC. This is thought to retain the integrity of mucociliary drainage pathways and allow a speedier return of normal nasal and sinus function. These endoscopic procedures have largely supplanted external approaches to the sinuses such as the Caldwell–Luc procedure.

## Wegener's granulomatosis

This is a multisystem granulomatous disorder of unknown aetiology. It can affect the whole of the respiratory tract as well as causing a focal necrotizing glomerulonephritis. Nasal symptoms include blockage with marked rhinosinusitis and crusting. Granulomatous necrosis within the nose may occur, leading to necrosis of the septum with perforation and a saddle deformity of the nose. Diagnosis may be suggested by the finding of non-caseating granulomas on biopsy and is confirmed by a raised cANCA level. Treatment is with immunosuppressive chemotherapy.

## Sarcoidosis

This is another idiopathic multisystem disorder which may have prominent nasal symptoms. Granulomatous inflammation is found throughout the respiratory tract and at multiple other sites. The nasal skin may be infiltrated 'lupus pernio' or there may be nasal blockage due to granuloma formation. Diagnosis is by finding a raised serum angiotensin converting enzyme (ACE) level, or by biopsy of an active lesion. Chest X-ray may also show characteristic hilar lymphadenopathy.

## NASAL AND SINUS TUMOURS

The nose is a relatively uncommon site for neoplasms. However, they do occur. Suspect neoplasia in any patient with a unilateral nasal blockage and bloody discharge, especially if there is facial pain, numbness in the infraorbital region or loosening of teeth. Tumours, especially inverted papilloma, may present as asymptomatic unilateral nasal polyposis.

Common sinonasal tumours include:

- *Benign tumours* – inverted papilloma is analogous to a basal cell carcinoma of the nose. They tend to occur under the middle turbinate and present as a friable unilateral polyposis which is locally invasive and recurs after surgery but does not metastasize. There is a small rate of malignant change. Diagnosis is by CT scan and histology. Other common benign tumours include viral papillomata or warts which occur in the vestibule of the nose and osteomata which tend to occur in or around the frontal sinuses.
- *Malignant tumours* – both adenocarcinoma and squamous cell carcinoma can occur within the sinuses. They both tend to present late with nasal blockage, bleeding, sinus and facial pain, loosening of teeth, infraorbital nerve anaesthesia and eventual cheek swelling. Examination often reveals a fungating mass arising from the sinuses and destroying bone. Treatment is by radical excision, i.e. extended maxillectomy with or without orbital exenteration, followed by primary reconstruction or a prosthesis. Survival rates are poor.

Other malignant sinonasal tumours include melanomas, olfactory neuroblastomas, and lymphomas.

## Juvenile angiofibroma

This is a rare benign vascular tumour of the nasopharynx found in young boys.

### Presentation

Common clinical complaints are unilateral epistaxis and nasal blockage. Other symptoms may occur if there is local invasion, e.g. of the skull base.

### Diagnosis

Clinically a vascular mass may be observed in the nasopharynx. Due to the risk of major bleeding, biopsy should be avoided. MRI scanning is extremely useful and may show characteristic features, including widening of the sphenopalatine foramen and erosion of the pterygoid plates.

Any young male with recurrent epistaxis should be suspected of having a juvenile nasal angiofibroma. Examination of the nasopharynx with an endoscope is mandatory.

### Management

Surgical excision is the treatment of choice. Large tumours may be shrunk preoperatively using angiography and embolization.

## ANOSMIA

Lack of or decrease in the sense of smell is a relatively common symptom. The olfactory nerve fibres leave the olfactory bulb and cross the cribriform plate to enter the olfactory mucosa in the roof of the nose. They are easily torn in even minor head injuries. Anosmia may also be caused by tumours of the olfactory groove, e.g. meningiomas, and by tumours, polyps and inflammation within the nose, especially if the roof of the nose is involved. Often no cause is identified even after MRI scanning. It is likely that some of these patients have post-viral damage to the olfactory apparatus. Smoking also seems to have a long-term deleterious effect on the sense of smell.

In the short space available it is impossible to cover all disorders of the oral cavity. However, it is important that all doctors and especially ENT surgeons have some knowledge about these common problems.

## DISORDERS OF THE TEETH AND JAWS

The calcified structures of the teeth comprise the living, sensate dentine and its external covering of crystalline enamel. The teeth are anchored in the bone of the jaws by the fibrous periodontal ligament which inserts into the cementum of the tooth root. Each tooth has a nerve supply from the trigeminal nerve and an arteriolar and venous supply, all of which enter the dental pulp at the root apex. There are 20 deciduous and 32 permanent teeth (Figs 57.1, 57.2).

### Dental caries and dental sepsis

Dental caries is caused by demineralization of enamel and invasion of dentine by acid-forming oral bacteria especially of the *Streptococcus mutans* species. These bacteria colonize the surface of teeth, forming dental plaque. They then utilize dietary sugar in order to create an acid milieu. Once demineralization spreads beyond the enamel, bacteria can gain entry to the porous dentinal tubules and thence to the dental pulp, leading to death of the tooth and periapical inflammation, in lay terms toothache. Further suppurative inflammation may occur at the root apex leading to abscess formation. Spread may occur to the deep tissue planes of the neck.

'Ludwig's angina' is the name given to cellulitis affecting the sublingual, submandibular and deep neck spaces. It is usually caused by dental sepsis of the lower jaw. Cellulitis may be severe enough to cause airway compromise and necessitate emergency tracheostomy.

Dental caries may be prevented by avoiding dietary sugars. Fluoride strengthens enamel resistance to attack by acid. Geographical areas with high natural fluoride levels in drinking water, e.g. Newcastle upon Tyne, have very low rates of dental caries. Fluoride supplements (in toothpaste or added to drinking water) have the same effect.

### Periodontal disease

Periodontal disease is inflammation of the supporting structures of the teeth and is also caused by plaque bacteria. Nearly all adults have some inflammation of the gums or gingivitis. More serious disease of the periodontal ligament, periodontitis, is also regularly seen and is a frequent cause of tooth loss in adults.

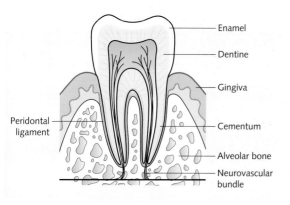

**Fig. 57.1** Anatomy of the teeth.

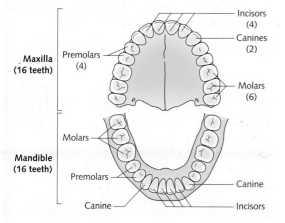

**Fig. 57.2** Adult dental arch.

## Cysts of the jaws

Cysts of the jaws are relatively common. They are often seen as incidental findings on dental radiographs. Some, however, may be large enough to cause thinning of the bone and pathological fractures. Types of jaw cyst are listed in Fig. 57.3.

### Radicular cysts

These inflammatory lesions are by far the most common of the jaw cysts (around 60%). They are formed at the root apex of non-vital teeth. Inflammation spreads from pulpal necrosis and causes apical inflammation and proliferation of epithelial rest cells. They may disappear if root canal therapy is used to remove the dead pulp.

### Dentigerous or follicular cysts

These are also common and form around the crown of unerupted teeth. They are therefore more common around teeth which are frequently impacted (unable to erupt), i.e. lower wisdom teeth and upper canines. The cystic elements sometimes must be removed surgically to allow the tooth to erupt.

### Odontogenic keratocyst

This is an important lesion due to its frequently large size and its tendency to recur after treatment. It is thought to be derived from rest cells of the dental lamina (the primitive organ which gives rise to the tooth 'buds'). It is most often seen as a unilocular lesion in the posterior ramus of the mandible and on exploration is seen to contain cheesy keratinous debris. It may be large enough to compress the alveolar nerve causing anaesthesia of the chin. It may also lead to pathological fractures. Treatment is by careful surgical removal; however, recurrence rates are high.

### Fissural cysts

These developmental cystic lesions are thought to arise from 'rests' of epithelial cells left behind after fusion of the primitive facial processes in utero. They tend to occur in children. The nasopalatine duct cyst is usually an incidental finding on X-ray and is seen as a heart-shaped radiolucency visible between the roots of the upper central incisor teeth. The nasolabial cyst is soft tissue lesion seen near the alar rim of the nose. It most often presents as an infected cystic lesion in a child.

## Ameloblastoma

This rare but infamous lesion is not really a cyst but a benign tumour arising from the primitive odontogenic tissues. However, it often presents in the same way as the jaw cysts and is part of the differential diagnosis of any radiolucency in the jaws. It is usually a multilocular radiolucent lesion at the angle of the mandible; it may also occur in the maxilla. Bony erosion and expansion of the cortex occurs and may lead to pathological fracture. Resorption of adjacent tooth roots may leave many teeth mobile. Alveolar nerve involvement may cause numbness of the chin or cheek.

Diagnosis is usually by the finding of the above features on radiographs or especially the finding of a 'soap bubble' radiolucency. Diagnosis can only be made with certainty by histological analysis following a biopsy.

Management is by careful removal of the tumour along with involved teeth. Some authors advocate block resection of involved bone with a margin of healthy tissue. Recurrence may occur and deaths due to intracranial spread (usually from maxillary lesions) have been described.

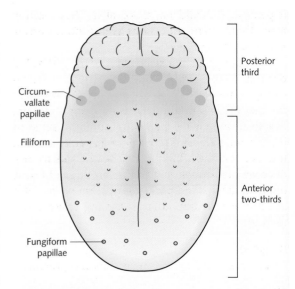

**Fig. 57.4** Surface anatomy of the tongue.

## DISORDERS OF MUCOSA

The oral cavity is lined by pseudostratified squamous epithelium in areas subject to masticatory forces, e.g. the gums and palate, there is keratinization. The dorsum of the tongue is covered with specialised keratinizing mucosa containing taste buds and numerous papillae (Fig. 57.4).

### Oral ulceration

An ulcer is a loss in continuity of an epithelial surface. They are extremely common within the oral cavity. The worry for the clinician is whether an ulcer may represent malignancy. The main risk factor for malignancy is smoking. Causes of oral ulceration are listed in Fig. 57.5.

### Herpes simplex

Around 80% of the population carry antibodies to the herpes simplex virus. Herpes simplex type 1 is the organism traditionally associated with oral disease.

#### Clinical presentation

There are two main forms of oral disease associated with this virus. The first, herpetic gingivostomatitis,

---

**Fig. 57.5** Causes of oral ulceration

Infection
– Viral, e.g. coxsackie virus, herpes simplex
– Bacterial, e.g. TB
– Treponemal, e.g. syphilis (chancre, snail track ulcers and gumma)
– Fungal, e.g. candida

Trauma
– Physical, e.g. burns, radiotherapy
– Chemical, e.g. aspirin burns, pizza burns to hard palate

Inflammatory
– Recurrent aphthous ulceration
– Behçet's syndrome
– Lichen planus (see white patches)
– Crohn's disease – linear ulcers and anaemia
– Coeliac disease and dermatitis herpetiformis

Vesiculobullous disorders
– Pemphigus
– Pemphigoid

Neoplastic
– Neutropenia
– Squamous cell carcinoma

---

represents the primary infection. It is commonly seen as a febrile illness in young children. Oral manifestations may be severe with marked ulceration affecting the whole of the mouth and particularly the gums (gingivostomatitis). Swallowing may be difficult due to pain and the child may drool saliva. The condition is self-limiting and the lesions heal without scarring in around 10 days.

A proportion of those infected go on to develop recurrent herpes simplex infection. The virus is neurotropic and epitheliotropic and may lie dormant for many years in the trigeminal root ganglion. Reactivation may be sparked by sunlight, stress or intercurrent illness. The virus then replicates and travels back down the sensory nerve roots to produce vesicle formation and the familiar cold sore, often on the lips (herpes labialis). Lesions may also affect oral mucosal surfaces causing vesicles and ulceration.

### Diagnosis
Diagnosis is usually made on the clinical appearances.

### Management
Recurrent herpes labialis may be treated with topical aciclovir which may abort attacks if applied early enough.

## Recurrent aphthous oral ulceration

These are the most common oral ulcers. They can affect all age groups from childhood onwards. Their cause is unknown but they are likely to be an expression of immune overactivity. They may be associated with anaemias of various types.

### Clinical presentation
Minor aphthae typically appear as small (<1 cm) shallow but painful ulcers of the buccal, labial and lingual mucosa; they often have a yellow fibrinous base surrounded by a small area of erythema. The ulcers tend to appear in groups which last for a week or so and then heal without scarring. Herpetiform (multiple tiny ulcers) and major aphthae (>1 cm, heal slowly with scarring) also occur but are more uncommon.

### Diagnosis
This is usually made on the clinical history. It is important to ask about ocular and genital ulceration (Behçet's) and also bowel disorders (Crohn's, coeliac and ulcerative colitis). It is also important to ask if the patient is anaemic as iron metabolism particularly seems to affect mucosal turnover. It is usual to perform a full blood count along with serum iron, $B_{12}$ and folate levels. Major aphthae may require biopsy to exclude oral carcinoma.

### Management
There is little effective treatment:

- Good oral hygiene and prescription of chlorhexidine mouthwash to prevent secondary bacterial infection.
- Steroid lozenges/Adcortyl in Orabase. Can be tried to alleviate an attack. There is little evidence for their effectiveness.

## Vesiculo-bullous disorders

In these rare conditions there is a loss of normal cell to cell adhesion as a result of autoimmune destruction. This results in bulla (blister) formation and loss of epithelium leaving ulceration of mucosal surfaces.

## Pemphigus vulgaris

This is an autoimmune disorder usually seen in the elderly. Autoantibodies are directed at desmogleins, the proteins that stick epidermal cells together. Inflammation causes loss of cell to cell adhesion and bulla formation within the epidermis and mucosa.

### Clinical presentation
Bullae are formed initially in the mouth, pharynx and larynx and then on the skin. These are fragile and the surface is readily lost to leave large patches of coalescent and painful ulceration.

### Diagnosis
- *Clinical signs.* Lateral forces (rubbing) on mucosa or skin may produce shearing of the epidermal layer. This is Nikolsky's sign.
- *Immunofluorescence.* A biopsy of oral mucosa is typically taken. Direct immunofluoresence labels the anti-desmoglein autoantibodies and allows them to be seen attacking intracellular attachments in the epidermis. This is diagnostic.

### Management
This is with steroids or other immunosuppressants.

## Pemphigoid

The type of pemphigoid seen in the mouth is cicatricial pemphigoid. It is also an autoimmune disease though in this case the autoantibodies are directed at the mucosal basement membrane.

### Clinical presentation

Patients are typically elderly. Bullae or ulcerations are seen within the oral cavity. The larynx, pharynx, eyes and nose are also affected; 20% have skin lesions. The lesions heal slowly with scarring.

### Diagnosis

*Immunofluoresence.* Autoantibodies are seen attacking the basement membrane of epidermis or mucosa.

### Management

Eye, laryngeal and oesophageal involvement all necessitate aggressive immunosuppressive treatment.

## Oral squamous cell carcinoma

More people die in the UK every year from oral cancer than from cervical cancer. However, it is not a disease that attracts much publicity. Of these 1700 deaths most are associated with tobacco smoking and alcohol consumption, both often acting together in a synergistic relationship. In other parts of the world, and especially South Asia, oral cancer is one of the most common cancers. This is attributed to high rates of smoking and consumption of *paan* or betel nuts.

### Clinical presentation

The peak age of presentation is the 6th decade and males have previously been affected more commonly than females. Worrying recent trends have seen an increase in the number of female patients, young patients and patients with no recognized risk factors.

Oral cancer is initially painless. It may present as a crater-like ulcer, a white patch (leukoplakia) or a red area (erythroplakia). Due to the lack of pain many oral cancers go undiagnosed until they have caused considerable local destruction and invaded local nerves (causing a neuralgia) or they have metastasized to the cervical lymph nodes. The most common sites for oral cancers are the floor of the mouth, tongue, retromolar and tonsillar areas.

### Diagnosis

*Biopsy.* Histopathology shows squamous cell carcinoma with varying degrees of differentiation.

All oral ulcers present for more than 2 weeks should undergo biopsy to exclude squamous carcinoma.

*Radiology.* Orthopantomogram (OPG) may reveal bony erosion or invasion. Increasingly CT scanning is used instead as it also allows concomitant assessment of the neck for metastases. All patients with proven oral cancer should also have a chest X-ray (or CT) to exclude lung metastasis (quite rare) or second primary lung tumours (more common). MRI may be used to assess depth of invasion especially in tongue lesions.

### Management

Most oral cancers are unfortunately advanced at the time of diagnosis. The main curative options are surgery or radiotherapy, with surgery being favoured by most clinicians owing to the disabling side effects of radiotherapy within the mouth. 5-year survival rates of 80–90% are possible with early tumours. However, in the presence of lymph node metastasis this rate drops to around 40%.

## White patches

White patches in the mouth are extremely common but are of concern as some of them may represent pre-malignant disorders. True leukoplakia is a diagnosis of exclusion and represents an increase in the keratin layers of the mucosa, hyperkeratosis. It is thought to carry an increased risk of oral malignancy.

The differential diagnosis of white patches is shown in Fig. 57.6.

## Candidal infection

Candida albicans is saprophytic yeast that is a common commensal in the oral cavity. In the very young, the unwell or the immunosuppressed it may become pathogenic.

**Fig. 57.6** Differential diagnosis of white patches

Congenital
– Sponge naevus

Infective
– Candidiasis
– Hairy leukoplakia

Immune mediated
– Lichen planus
– Discoid lupus erythematosus

Idiopathic
– Leukoplakia (erythro-leukoplakia)

Neoplastic
– Squamous cell carcinoma

## Pseudomembranous candidiasis

The commonest oral manifestation is 'thrush' or pseudomembranous candidiasis. This superficial mucosal infection is seen in neonates, the immuno-suppressed and sometimes following broad spectrum antibiotic therapy. The typical appearances are of cream coloured plaques of fungi which can be wiped off the mucosa to leave an erythematous, sometimes bleeding base. Diagnosis is usually made on clinical grounds and treatment commenced with topical antifungal medication such as nystatin or miconazole.

## Chronic hyperplastic candidiasis

This is a more unusual manifestation of infection and is seen as white patches, often on the tongue or the commissure, which are thickened and hyperkeratotic. Unlike thrush they cannot be wiped off. Diagnosis usually requires biopsy. Treatment is with topical and occasionally systemic antifungals.

## Other candidal infections

Chronic atrophic candidiasis is more often called denture stomatitis. It causes sore erythematous areas beneath dentures. It is associated with poor denture hygiene in patients who wear their dentures at night. It is due to candidal overgrowth in the porous acrylic of the denture surface. Treatment is with denture hygiene measures and topical antifungals applied to both the mucosa and the denture. Often seen with this is angular cheilitis. This is soreness and macera-tion of the skin at the corners of the mouth it is asso-ciated with fungal infection, loss of facial height due to ill-fitting dentures and anaemias. It may be treated with topical antifungals in most cases.

Median rhomboid glossitis is a minor fungal infec-tion which is usually asymptomatic. It causes a dia-mond shaped area of depapillation on the dorsum of the tongue.

# Hairy leukoplakia

This is an important but asymptomatic condition. Leukoplakic areas are seen on the lateral tongue borders. Its importance lies in its association with HIV infection and co-infection with Epstein–Barr virus. It may be the first manifestation of immuno-suppression.

# Lichen planus

Many disorders which affect the skin have oral mani-festations examples are discoid lúpus erythematosus and erythema multiforme. The most commonly seen skin disease in the oral cavity is lichen planus. This is thought to be an immune-mediated chronic inflam-matory disorder; the cause is, however, unknown. It is thought to affect around 1–2% of the population, women more commonly than men.

## Clinical presentation

The classical oral lesion is of reticulate or striate leu-koplakia most often affecting the buccal mucosa; this is often asymptomatic. However, erosive and atrophic forms exist and may lead to large areas of ulceration. These areas may be painful, especially when exposed to spicy foods. Oesophageal and laryngeal involve-ment is seen occasionally. Skin lesions in the form of itchy violaceous plaques are seen in around 15%. They most often affect the flexor surface of the fore-arms and the shins. Genital leukoplakic lesions or erosions may also occur. It is thought that the oral erosive and atrophic forms of the disease may be pre-malignant in a small proportion of patients.

## Diagnosis

In classical striate disease, especially if skin lesions are present, the diagnosis may be made on the basis of the clinical history and appearance. In erosive dis-ease biopsy it is important to rule out other causes of ulceration, e.g. SCC, vesiculo-bullous disease, and also to assess the presence of dysplasia which may predict pre-malignant potential.

## Management

For the vast majority of patients no treatment is required. Symptomatic disease, especially erosive varieties, may be treated with topical steroid prepara-tions, e.g. Corlan pellets, Adcortyl in Orabase.

# Disorders of the salivary glands

## Objectives

You should be able to:

- Describe the basic anatomy and physiology of the salivary glands.
- Understand the functions of saliva.
- Recognize acute bacterial sialadenitis and know about its management.
- Describe Sjögren's syndrome and other causes of dry mouth.
- Describe the 'cystic' disorders of the salivary glands, mucocoeles and ranula.
- Understand sialolithiasis (salivary stones).
- List salivary gland tumours.
- Discuss operations on the parotid glands (parotidectomy).

The salivary glands comprise the paired structures of the parotid, submandibular and sublingual glands along with the many thousands of minor salivary glands scattered throughout the mucosa of the oropharynx.

These glandular structures develop from epithelial ingrowth and are under the control of the autonomic nervous systems. They secrete saliva at a rate of 1.5 litres per day, 70% of this coming from the submandibular glands. The functions of saliva are lubrication of the food bolus and the digestion of starch by amylase. Saliva also serves a protective role by mechanically washing the oral cavity and teeth, by buffering changes in pH and by the secretion of lysozyme, peroxidase and IgA.

## ANATOMY

The parotid glands occupy a roughly pyramidal space between the angle of the mandible in front, the mastoid process and sternomastoid muscle behind and the overlying connective tissue (Fig. 58.1). The parotid duct runs forward and pierces the buccinator muscle to empty opposite the upper second molar tooth. Emerging from the stylomastoid foramen and entering the posteromedial part of the gland is the facial nerve. Within the gland the nerve splits into its five terminal branches. The facial nerve somewhat artificially divides the gland into deep and superficial lobes.

The submandibular glands lie between the lower border of the mandible and the floor of the mouth (Fig. 58.2). They comprise a superficial lobe, and a deep lobe that wraps around the posterior free edge of the mylohyoid muscle and ends in Wharton's duct. This duct runs forward, closely involved with the lingual nerve, in the floor of the mouth to end at the submandibular papillae on either side of the lingual fraenulum.

The sublingual glands lie in the floor of the mouth and are closely involved with both the submandibular duct and the lingual nerve. Numerous small ducts empty directly from the sublingual glands into the floor of the mouth.

## DISORDERS OF THE SALIVARY GLANDS

- *Infectious:*
  - *Viral* – mumps, CMV
  - *Bacterial* – sialadenitis, TB.
- *Inflammatory.* Sjögren's, post radiotherapy.
- *Obstructive.* Mucocoele, ranula, sialolithiasis.
- *Idiopathic.* Sialosis, necrotizing sialometaplasia.
- *Granulomatous.* Sarcoid.
- *Neoplastic.* Benign, intermediate and malignant.

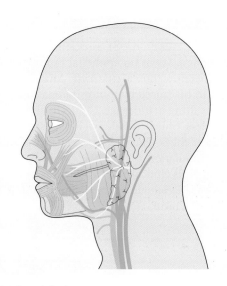

**Fig. 58.1** Parotid gland.

The key to establishing a diagnosis of bacterial sialadenitis is to express pus from the parotid ducts. Massage the gland while looking inside the mouth opposite the second upper molar.

The infecting organism is usually a *streptococcus* or *Staphylococcus aureus*. Adequate rehydration, oral hygiene measures (including denture hygiene and chlorhexidine mouthwashes), gland massage and appropriate antibiotics usually result in improvement.

Chronic parotitis is not uncommon and is associated with a damaged ductal system or 'sialectasis'. This results in repeated bouts of gland swelling and infection with further damage. The cause is unknown.

Bacterial sialadenitis of the submandibular gland is by contrast more commonly secondary to blockage of the duct by a calculus (see Sialolithiasis, below).

## Infectious disorders

Viral parotitis due to mumps infection was previously common. It is now rarely seen owing to the effectiveness of the MMR vaccination programme. Acute bacterial parotitis is unfortunately not rare. It is generally seen in elderly, dehydrated, post-surgical patients where debilitation and poor oral care allow an ascending bacterial infection of the parotid glands. The patient is systemically unwell and there is tender enlargement of the parotids.

## Sjögren's syndrome

This autoimmune disease is caused by lymphocytic infiltration and destruction of salivary and lacrimal gland tissue by activation of autoantibodies. It is commonly associated with other autoimmune disorders such as rheumatoid arthritis, systemic lupus erythematosus and primary biliary sclerosis; as such it almost exclusively a disease of women. Where there is no associated autoimmune disease the term primary Sjögren's is used.

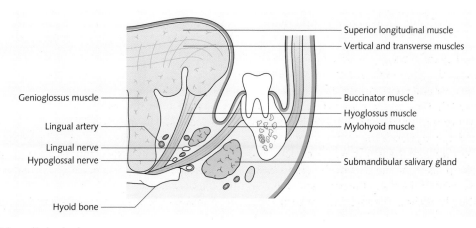

Genioglossus muscle

Lingual artery

Lingual nerve
Hypoglossal nerve

Hyoid bone

Superior longitudinal muscle
Vertical and transverse muscles

Buccinator muscle
Hyoglossus muscle
Mylohyoid muscle

Submandibular salivary gland

**Fig. 58.2** Submandibular gland.

## Clinical presentation

The patient who is usually a female in their 4th to 5th decade presents with a dry mouth and dry eyes and sometimes a dry vagina. There may be candidal infection of the mouth. The oral mucosa is often sore and atrophic and there may be rampant dental caries due to the loss of salivary protection. Diffuse enlargement of the parotid glands may be seen.

After a prolonged period with the disease there appears to be an increased risk of developing lymphoma within the salivary glands.

## Diagnosis

Sjögren's syndrome is suspected in all patients presenting with a dry mouth.

One of the most common causes of a dry mouth is prescribed medication. The most common culprits are antihypertensives, diuretics and antidepressants.

Salivary and lacrimal flow rates may be measured and are usually reduced. Positive autoantibody titres, especially antinuclear antibodies, rheumatoid factor, anti-double stranded DNA, anti-Ro and anti-La (salivary duct proteins), are suggestive but not diagnostic. Clinical suspicions can be confirmed by biopsy of minor labial gland under local anaesthetic. Periductal lymphocyte infiltration is diagnostic of Sjögren's.

## Management

Sjögren's is not curable. Treatment is symptomatic.

**Eyes**
- Ophthalmology opinion.
- Tear substitutes.

**Oral cavity**
- Dental opinion and regular fluoride treatments to prevent dental caries.
- Salivary substitutes occasionally helpful, e.g. Glandosane or Saliva Orthana.
- Antifungals if required.
- Sialogogues stimulate salivary secretion, e.g. pilocarpine; rarely helpful owing to significant incidence of unwanted effects.

## Mucocoele

This is an extravasation 'cyst' associated with a minor salivary gland. It has no epithelial lining, however, and is therefore not a true cyst. Mucocoeles are thought to be caused by minor trauma to the duct orifice resulting in blockage. Clinically they present as a painless, bluish, sessile swelling, usually of the lower lip or cheek. There may be a history of rupture and reaccumulation.

Diagnosis is clinical and treatment is by excision under local anaesthetic if they are troublesome. They can, however, recur.

Mucocoeles are more common on the lower lip because of trauma from teeth. They are rare on the upper lip. Salivary gland tumours, however, are more common on the upper lip.

## Ranula

This painless, translucent swelling in the floor of the mouth is caused by a sublingual gland retention cyst. Its name comes from the Latin for a small frog, owing to its resemblance to a frog's belly. It is most often seen in children and young adults.

In a 'plunging' ranula the cyst extends from the floor of the mouth through the mylohyoid muscle to produce a dumb-bell shaped lesion with a sublingual and submandibular component (Fig. 58.3).

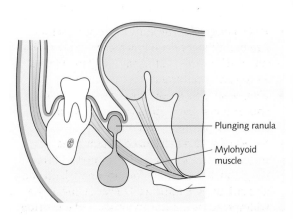

Fig. 58.3 A plunging ranula.

Treatment is by excision of the lesion along with the sublingual gland. Inexpert removal carries a risk of recurrence along with lingual nerve damage and ipsilateral tongue anaesthesia.

## Sialolithiasis

This condition is common. It particularly affects the submandibular glands, although it is also seen in the parotids (80% vs 20%). It is caused by the precipitation of calcium salts found in saliva to form stones. Submandibular saliva is more alkaline and contains increased concentrations of calcium and phosphate, making it more prone to stone formation. These occur within the gland substance or within the duct and lead to a ball valve effect with intermittent stasis and swelling of the gland. The stagnant saliva may then become secondarily infected leading to a bacterial sialadenitis.

### Clinical presentation

Most cases occur in middle age. There is usually painful gland swelling precipitated by mealtimes. The swelling settles spontaneously over a period of hours to days. Acute sialadenitis may supervene with an increase in pain, redness and pyrexia.

Examination is rarely coincident with gland swelling, although it may be precipitated in some patients by stimulating salivary flow with citrus sweets. A calculus may be palpated within the duct. Turbid saliva or pus may be observed emanating from the duct orifice.

### Diagnosis

This is usually suspected from the clinical history. The following investigations may also be useful:

- *Plain radiographs*. These are especially useful in submandibular calculi of which 90% are radio-opaque. However, in the parotid gland 90% of stones are radiolucent.
- *Ultrasound*. This is now the investigation of choice. It can reveal all calculi and also any associated pathology of the gland.
- *Sialography*. This specialized test involves injection of a contrast medium into the duct of the gland. It is excellent for showing calculi and also strictures of the duct. However, due to the widespread availability of ultrasound it is being used less and less.

### Management

The management usually involves surgical removal of the calculus or the gland. In recent years there has been much interest in endoscopic methods of stone removal but these are as yet not widely practised:

- *Intra-oral calculus excision*. For calculi in the submandibular duct which are more in front of the lower first molar tooth it is usually possible to excise them intra-orally via the floor of the mouth. The first molar marks the point where the duct is crossed by the lingual nerve. Many parotid calculi may be removed intra-orally.
- *Extra-oral gland excision*. Calculi which are behind the first molar or which are within the submandibular gland itself are best removed via a submandibular incision along with the gland. This lessens the possibility of ipsilateral tongue numbness due to lingual nerve damage.

## Sialosis

This is the name given to non-inflammatory non-neoplastic enlargement of the salivary glands, mainly the parotid. It is progressive and pain free, and as such is mainly a cosmetic embarrassment to the patient. The main association is with alcoholic cirrhosis, but it is also seen in anorexia nervosa, bulimia and malnutrition states. Perhaps the most common cause is fatty infiltration of the parotid often associated with generalized obesity. It is a diagnosis of exclusion.

## Necrotizing sialometaplasia

This is a rare, unusual but important disease of minor salivary tissue. It usually occurs on the hard palate of male smokers. It causes a crater-like lesion of the mucosa which resembles a squamous carcinoma both clinically and histologically. However, it is self-healing and will resolve spontaneously within a period of weeks. Diagnosis can be made by biopsy and careful histology.

## Neoplastic disorders of the salivary glands

Tumours of salivary gland tissue vary from benign, slow-growing lesions to invasive, metastatic malignancy with all variations in between. 80% of all salivary tumours are found within the parotid gland, 15% in the submandibular and the remainder in the sublingual and minor salivary glands. However, the smaller the gland the more likely it is that the tumour is malignant (60% in sublingual and minor glands, 50% submandibular and 20% parotid).

*Rule of 80s* – 80% (ish) of salivary tumours are benign; 80% occur in the parotid; 80% are pleomorphic adenomas.

## Clinical presentation

Most tumours (95%) occur in adults; however, they are seen in all age groups. Benign salivary gland tumours produce slow, gradual, painless enlargement of the gland; local nerves are not involved. In contrast malignant tumours produce rapid, painful swelling which in the parotid gland may involve the facial nerve leading to a palsy.

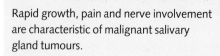

Rapid growth, pain and nerve involvement are characteristic of malignant salivary gland tumours.

## Diagnosis

- Examination reveals a firm swelling within the gland. There may be associated facial palsy in malignant disease.
- Fine needle aspiration is usually performed on all parotid masses. It may allow preoperative differentiation between malignant and benign tumours, thus allowing the appropriate intervention.

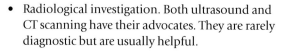

Open biopsy of the parotid gland is to be avoided at all costs. It risks unnecessary damage to the facial nerve and seeding of tumour.

- Radiological investigation. Both ultrasound and CT scanning have their advocates. They are rarely diagnostic but are usually helpful.

## Types of salivary tumour

Below is a list of salivary tumours. Some of the more important varieties are discussed in further detail below:

- Benign:
- Pleomorphic salivary adenoma
- Monomorphic adenomas
- Adenolymphoma (Warthin's tumour).
- Intermediate:
- Acinic cell carcinoma
- Muco-epidermoid carcinoma.
- Malignant:
- Adenoid cystic carcinoma
- Squamous cell carcinoma
- Carcinoma ex-pleomorphic adenoma
- Metastatic malignancy
- Lymphoma.

### Pleomorphic adenoma

This is the most common of all the salivary gland tumours. It is benign and metastasis is extremely rare. It is most commonly found in the parotid gland where it causes slow, gradual, symptom-free swelling. These tumours are often present for many years before the patient seeks advice. The facial nerve is not affected.

After 15–20 years a small proportion may undergo malignant change to a 'carcinoma ex-pleomorphic adenoma'. This is heralded by an increased growth rate with the onset of pain with or without facial palsy.

Histologically they are composed of many different cell types, hence their name 'pleomorphic'. Their expansile growth leads to a pseudo-capsule. However, they must be resected with a margin if recurrence is to be avoided as the capsule is penetrated by numerous microscopic pseudopodia.

Luckily most of these tumours occur in the superficial part of the parotid gland (above the facial nerve). They are thus best removed by the operation of superficial parotidectomy with only a small risk of facial nerve damage. Occasionally they may be in the deep portion of the gland and may even present as a 'dumb-bell' tumour with the deep portion causing swelling of the pharynx. These tumours must be resected by a total parotidectomy which carries a much greater risk to the facial nerve.

### Adenolymphoma or Warthin's tumour

These are relatively common benign tumours. They are usually completely asymptomatic and are found in older patients where they present as soft swellings of the lower part of the parotid glands. They are bilateral in around 10%. Surgical removal if required is most often via a superficial parotidectomy.

### Adenoid cystic carcinoma

This tumour represents the most common malignancy in the submandibular and minor salivary glands. It can invade local structures including nerves.

It is this perineural invasion which accounts for its malignant potential and, although 5-year survival rates are acceptable, following surgical resection many patients succumb to metastatic disease 10–15 years later. Management is with resection and post-operative radiotherapy.

## Parotidectomy operations

Total parotidectomy is the surgical removal of the whole of the parotid gland. It is rarely carried out in this form because of the loss of facial nerve function and particularly eye protection that ensues. It may be necessary in the treatment of malignant parotid tumours. If the nerve is sacrificed an attempt at primary re-anastomosis is usually made at the initial operation using another nerve (auriculotemporal or sural) as a graft.

Superficial parotidectomy is the most common operation on the parotid gland and involves removal of the part of the gland above the facial nerve leaving the nerve intact. It is possible because most parotid masses are pleomorphic adenomas and most of them are found superficial to the nerve.

It is important for the student to know some of the complications of superficial parotidectomy as this operation is commonly performed.

## Important complications

- Facial nerve damage – rarely permanent.
- Numbness of the ear – common and due to damage to the greater auricular nerve.
- Frey's syndrome – this complication is quite common but rarely disabling. It is caused by re-routing of the parasympathetic secretomotor supply to the gland innervating the overlying skin. It results in the curious complication of gustatory sweating, i.e. sweating of the cheek skin provoked by food. It can be treated by local application of antiperspirants or by injection of botulinum toxin.
- General complications, e.g. bleeding, haematoma, scarring.

# Disorders of the pharynx and larynx

You should know about:

- The anatomy of the pharynx and larynx.
- The adenoids and adenoidal enlargement.
- Why adenoids are removed surgically.
- Nasopharyngeal carcinoma.
- The tonsils, tonsillitis and tonsillectomy.
- Globus pharyngeus and laryngopharyngeal carcinomas.
- Pharyngeal pouches, how they are diagnosed and managed.
- The difference between vocal cord polyps and nodules.
- Recurrent laryngeal nerve palsy and its causes.
- Laryngeal papillomatosis.
- Cancer of the larynx, its diagnosis and management.

The pharynx and larynx serve as conduits transporting inspired air and ingested materials from the mouth and nose to the larynx and oesophagus, dividing these two streams and preventing contamination of the lower airway. In this chapter we will consider some of the more common conditions affecting these areas. See also Chapters 50, 51, 52.

## THE PHARYNX

The pharynx is a muscular tube running from the skull base to the oesophagus. It is open anteriorly to the oral cavity, nose and larynx. It comprises two muscular layers:

- The innermost longititudinal muscles, which elevate the larynx and pharynx during swallowing.
- The outer, circular layer of the paired superior, middle and inferior constrictors, which overlap each other from top to bottom and contract sequentially during swallowing.

The pharynx has three parts: the nasopharynx, the oropharynx and the laryngopharynx (Fig. 59.1).

### The nasopharynx

The nasopharynx (or postnasal space) connects the back of the nose (via the posterior choanae) with the rest of the pharynx; it lies above the level of the soft palate. Laterally it contains the paired openings of the Eustachian tubes and in between these, in the middle of its posterior wall, lies the adenoidal tonsil (adenoids).

## Disorders of the nasopharynx

The most important disorders of the nasopharynx are adenoidal hypertrophy, juvenile angiofibroma (see tumours of the nose, Chapter 56, p. 253) and nasopharyngeal carcinoma.

### Adenoidal hypertrophy

The adenoids are composed of lymphoid tissue and are involved in the immune response to antigens. As such they have a tendency to increase in size during childhood and in response to trivial upper respiratory tract infections. After childhood they involute and decrease in size.

*Clinical presentation.* Children between the ages of 2 and 6 years are most commonly affected. The increasing size of the adenoids blocks the child's nasopharynx leading to nasal blockage, discharge, snoring and sometimes obstructive sleep apnoea (OSA, see later). Adenoidal enlargement and infection may also be a factor in the development of glue ear. Long-term adenoidal hypertrophy and consequent mouth breathing may lead to skeletal changes in the developing child producing the so-called 'adenoidal facies'.

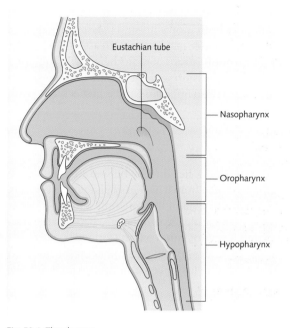

Eustachian tube

— Nasopharynx

— Oropharynx

— Hypopharynx

**Fig. 59.1** The pharynx.

Adults may also suffer from adenoidal enlargement, although it is much less common. It causes the same symptoms as in children. It can occur as a result of mycobacterial infection and immunosuppression. In adults it is important to rule out neoplasia as a cause and this usually requires a biopsy.

*Diagnosis.* Clinically one can confirm nasal blockage in the child by spatula test (see p. 310). Clinical suspicions can be confirmed even in the small child by examining the nasopharynx with a small flexible naso-endoscope. If this is not possible soft tissue radiographs of the postnasal space may show adenoidal enlargement and are occasionally useful:

*Management.* Adenoidal enlargement in childhood is normal and for most children with minimal symptoms no treatment is required other than reassurance that they are likely to grow out of the problem:

- *Medical.* In most children a trial of topical nasal steroids is appropriate before proceeding with surgery. This is especially the case if the child has known allergies to pollens or house dust mites.
- *Surgery.*

The following are some of the more common indications for adenoidectomy:

- Severe nasal symptoms that do not respond to medical therapy.

- Child with obstructive sleep apnoea (usually with tonsillectomy).
- As a therapy in otitis media with effusion (OME) (with grommet insertion).
- To exclude malignancy (mainly adults).

*Adenoidectomy.* This is a common procedure in children. It is performed under general anaesthetic. A bolster is placed beneath the shoulders and the neck extended. A catheter is placed through the nose to retract the soft palate and the nasopharynx visualized with a mirror. Enlarged adenoids may then be removed using a sharp curette, or a suction-diathermy may be used to ablate the adenoid. Complications include bleeding (rare) and nasopharyngeal scarring. The procedure is contraindicated in patients with cleft palate, even in quite mild forms such as a bifid uvula, as it may provoke disastrous leakage of fluids and air through the nose postoperatively.

### Nasopharyngeal carcinoma (NPC)

At birth the nasopharynx is lined with respiratory epithelium. Shortly after birth 60% of this tissue is transformed by the process of metaplasia into a squamous epithelium. It is within these cells that nasopharyngeal carcinoma can arise. Although rare in Europeans, it is seen with alarming frequency in areas of South China, Hong Kong and Shanghai where there are up to 50 cases per 100 000 of the population. The risk is also higher in anyone of Chinese ancestry including Eskimos. Other risk factors are high levels of consumption of salted fish and Epstein–Barr virus (EBV) infection.

*Clinical presentation.* NPC is two to three times as common in men as in women. It is seen from adolescence onwards. The tumour most often starts in the fossa of Rosenmüller behind the Eustachian tube orifice. Even very small tumours here may interfere with Eustachian tube function causing blockage and a middle ear effusion. Up to 30% of patients with NPC initially have a unilateral conductive hearing loss. Enlarging painless cervical lymphadenopathy is seen in 60%. Further growth of the tumour causes nasal blockage, epistaxis and eventually skull base invasion with cranial neuropathies (facial numbness, diplopia, ophthalmoplegia, vocal cord palsy, facial palsy, etc.). These are, however, late signs. Metastasis to distant sites may occur with even microscopic tumours. A frequent complication is bony metastasis. Without treatment the disease is fatal.

*Diagnosis*. In any patient with unilateral conductive hearing loss it is essential to thoroughly inspect the nasopharynx for carcinoma. In anyone of Chinese descent the fossa of Rosenmüller should be biopsied.

*Clinical examination*. Examination with a flexible naso-endoscope may reveal obvious friable tumour within the nasopharynx. However, around 10% of patients may have submucosal disease which, although it retains the ability to metastasize and kill the patient, may not be visible in the nasopharynx. It is essential to retain a high index of suspicion.

*Radiology*. In patients where there is high clinical suspicion of NPC but examination of the nasopharynx is normal, MRI may be useful in delineating any disease present and guiding sites for biopsy. CT is more commonly used for the staging of proven NPC and especially for assessing local bony and soft tissue invasion prior to treatment.

*Biopsy*. This is most often carried out under general anaesthetic either via the nose or in the same manner as adenoidectomy. Increasingly it is possible to use flexible naso-endoscopic biopsy in the awake patient for this purpose. Histopathology is diagnostic but may be difficult as the tumour is often poorly differentiated.

*Serological markers of HBV infection*. These are often used in high risk areas to monitor for disease recurrence.

*Management*. This is an aggressive disease and even with multimodal therapy overall 5-year survival remains at the 40–50% level:

- *Radiotherapy*. This is the primary treatment modality for NPC. External beam radiotherapy is directed at the nasopharynx and neck. Unfortunately this causes frequent side effects including chronic middle ear effusions, xerostomia, osteoradionecrosis and skin damage.
- *Surgery* plays little role in the management of NPC except in the setting of recurrent disease and residual neck disease after radiotherapy.
- *Chemotherapy* is used for patients with distant metastases and for palliation. It has little effect on overall survival.

Other supportive therapies are extremely important in order to limit morbidity and maximize quality of life. These include regular dental treatment to prevent further complications of radiotherapy. Treatment of middle ear effusion and the ensuing deafness that may result is also important and is best achieved with a hearing aid.

## Oropharynx

The oropharynx lies directly behind the oral cavity, being separated from it by the oropharyngeal isthmus. It ends at the level of the epiglottis and links below with the larynx and laryngopharynx. Between the anterior and posterior faucal pillars (formed by the ridges of the palatoglossus and palatopharyngeus muscles) are the tonsillar fossae containing the paired palatine tonsils.

### Pharyngitis

Infection of the pharynx is common and is often seen as part of a generalized upper respiratory tract infection. It is probably the cause of most episodes of sore throat. The responsible organism is most commonly viral but exotic bacterial and fungal disease may also occur. Examination will often reveal generalized erythema of the entire pharynx. Raised lymphoid aggregates may be visible especially on the posterior pharyngeal wall. Symptomatic treatment is usually all that is required.

### The tonsils

These small lymphoid aggregations on the lateral pharyngeal walls attract medical attention out of all proportion to their size. Their principal importance would seem to be the problems they cause. Like the adenoids they are composed of lymphoid tissue and are components of Waldeyer's ring. Childhood infection is common but unlike adenoidal infection is frequently painful.

#### Acute tonsillitis

In childhood recurrent acute tonsillitis is extremely common presumably as immunity to common pathogens is still developing. These pathogens include common upper respiratory tract viruses and bacteria including *Streptococcus pneumoniae* and *Haemophilus influenzae*. It is unclear whether bacterial infection follows initial viral infection. In adolescents it is necessary to consider infectious mononucleosis (EBV) as a cause of sore throat.

*Clinical features.* There is usually a systemic illness with pyrexia and malaise. Bilateral sore throat with difficult and painful swallowing is usually seen. Tender cervical lymphadenopathy is common. Examination of the tonsils may show generalized erythema or areas of suppuration arising from the tonsillar crypts. The illness is generally self-limiting and subsides within a week.

*Glandular fever* is a variable illness. Systemic malaise, headache and muscular pain are usually more marked. Cervical lymphadenopathy is a prominent feature and hepatosplenomegaly may also occur. Jaundice is seen in up to 10%. Intraoral findings may include tonsillitis, pharyngitis and petechiae on the soft palate.

*Diagnosis.* The diagnosis is usually made on the basis of careful history. It is worth bearing in mind that recurrent tonsillitis in adults is less common and other causes of throat pain such as anaemia, laryngopharyngeal acid reflux and carcinoma should be vigorously excluded. During the acute episode and especially in adolescent patients a leucocytosis, abnormal liver function tests and positive EBV serology helps to distinguish infectious mononucleosis.

*Management.* Management of the severe, acute attack (i.e. a patient who cannot swallow fluids and hence medication) is with antipyrexials, intravenous fluids and antibiotics. Penicillin will be effective in most cases but increasing resistance means that co-amoxiclav is a more common choice. It is important to avoid amoxicillin in glandular fever as it commonly produces a rash which may be mistaken for allergy.

*Surgery.* Tonsillectomy is reserved for those children with significant recurrent tonsillitis. The usual criteria for considering tonsillectomy in the UK are more than five episodes of significant tonsillitis (requiring time off school) per year or three episodes per year for 2 years.

### Complications of acute tonsillitis

These may be divided into local and systemic complications. Systemic complications are rare but include such post-streptococcal phenomena as scarlet fever, rheumatic fever and glomerulonephritis. Local complications are more common. In smaller children, especially if there is a background of obstructive sleep apnoea, the swelling associated with tonsillitis may precipitate stertor and upper airway compromise.

*Peritonsillar abscess (quinsy).* This results from spread of infection outside the tonsillar capsule where it forms an abscess. It is predominately seen as a complication of acute tonsillitis in young adults. The responsible organisms are usually a mixed bag of aerobic and anaerobic bacteria.

*Clinical presentation.* The patient usually gives a history of bilateral tonsillitis which has become unilateral. They usually feel extremely unwell and have severe unilateral throat pain which is commonly felt in the ear (referred otalgia). Examination reveals a sick-looking patient who is pyrexial and toxic. They may be dehydrated. The voice has a 'hot potato' quality due to oropharyngeal obstruction. The patient is often drooling and unable to swallow their saliva; foetor oris is usually marked. Examination of the oropharynx is difficult as trismus is nearly always present. However, careful inspection using a tongue spatula and a bright light reveals a unilateral swelling of the entire tonsil and soft palate. The uvula is usually displaced to the opposite side (Fig. 59.2). Tender cervical lymphadenopathy is often present.

> It is the general condition of the patient that gives away the diagnosis of quinsy. They feel, look, sound and smell unwell! Examination of the oropharynx usually confirms the presence of a quinsy.

*Diagnosis* is based on the characteristic clinical symptoms and signs.

*Management.* Resolution of the infection is only achieved following drainage of pus. This is achieved with either needle drainage or incision under local or topical anaesthesia. Pus should be sent to microbiology to assess microbial antibiotic sensitivities.

The patient is generally admitted to hospital for intravenous fluids and analgesia. An appropriate antibiotic with anaerobic coverage (e.g. co-amoxiclav) is

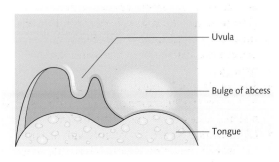

Fig. 59.2 Peri-tonsillar abscess.

given. The risk of a second subsequent quinsy is in the region of 20%. Most surgeons would offer prophylactic tonsillectomy following a second quinsy.

### Unilateral tonsillar enlargement
It is entirely normal for there to be a degree of asymmetry between the tonsils. However, painless unilateral tonsillar enlargement that is more marked cannot be ignored as it may represent serious pathology. Apparent tonsillar asymmetry may also be caused by masses in the parapharyngeal space pushing the tonsil medially.

Causes of unilateral tonsillar enlargement include:

- Normal variant.
- Recurrent tonsillitis.
- Quinsy (painful).
- Lymphoma.
- Squamous cell carcinoma (SCC).

*Clinical presentation.* Unilateral tonsil swelling is usually pain free and may be noticed by chance. One should ask about smoking habits, weight loss, night sweats and other lymphadenopathy. Except in the case of a quinsy, which is obviously quite different, it may be difficult to exclude serious disease without tonsillectomy and biopsy.

*Diagnosis.* CT scanning may help delineate parapharyngeal masses and SCCs of the tonsil; it may also show associated cervical lymphadenopathy. Tonsillectomy and biopsy is, however, often required.

### Tonsillectomy
The surgical removal of the tonsils is one of the most commonly performed surgical procedures. In the past the most common reason for performing tonsillectomy was recurrent acute tonsillitis; it is now increasingly common to remove the tonsils as treatment for obstructive sleep apnoea in a child. The main indications for tonsillectomy are:

- Recurrent acute tonsillitis – >5 significant episodes in a year.
- Recurrent peritonsillar abscess – usually after second episode.
- Treatment of OSA/snoring:
  - Children – adenotonsillectomy
  - Adults – usually with soft palate surgery (see sleep disorders).
- Exclusion of malignancy:
  - Obvious tumour of tonsil.
  - Unilateral tonsillar enlargement – cause?
  - Cervical metastasis with occult primary.

*The operation.* Tonsillectomy is performed under general anaesthetic. The patient is prepared as for adenoidectomy with the shoulders supported the neck extended and a mouth gag inserted. The tonsil is grasped by forceps and pulled medially. The anterior faucal pillar is incised and the tonsil dissected from the loose areolar tissue over the superior constrictor muscle. Bleeding is controlled with surgical ties or diathermy. Troublesome bleeding is most common at the base of the tonsil and it is usual to ligate this area prior to removal of the tonsil.

### Complications of tonsillectomy
*Pain.* Pain is usual, may be severe and lasts around 1 week. A combination of non-steroidal anti-inflammatory drugs and paracetomol is usually prescribed.

*Haemorrhage.* Bleeding is the most feared complication following tonsillectomy. It may occur immediately after the operation as a result of inadequate haemostasis (primary or reactionary haemorrhage). The patient most often requires a return to the operating theatre where the bleeding point may be identified and ligated. This may be a challenging situation and experienced anaesthetic help is essential.

*Secondary haemorrhage* is more common. It occurs at around 6–8 days after tonsillectomy and is often preceded by an increase in pain and pyrexia. It is speculated that secondary haemorrhage is the result of postoperative infection of the tonsillar bed. An intravenous cannula is inserted and blood sent for crossmatch and haemoglobin estimation. The patient is admitted to hospital and given intravenous antibiotics, analgesics and peroxide mouth washes. Rarely, if these measures are not successful, a return to the operating theatre is required.

## Laryngopharynx (hypopharynx)
The laryngopharynx is the part of the pharynx which lies below the hyoid and is behind the larynx (Fig. 59.3). Below it ends at the level of the cricoid cartilage where it joins the cervical oesophagus.

The laryngopharynx comprises the pyriform fossae, the post-cricoid area and the posterior pharyngeal wall.

The most important clinical disorders of the laryngopharynx are pharyngeal pouches and tumours. Globus pharyngeus, although not an isolated disorder of this area, shares many symptoms and is therefore considered here.

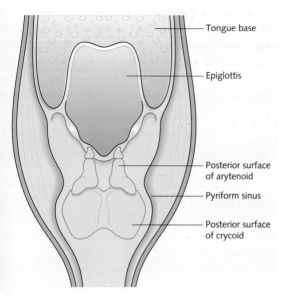

**Fig. 59.3** Hypopharynx – posterior view.

Labels: Tongue base; Epiglottis; Posterior surface of arytenoid; Pyriform sinus; Posterior surface of crycoid

## Pharyngeal pouch

In the posterior wall of the laryngopharynx there is a potential weak area between the cricopharyngeal and thyro-pharyngeal components of the inferior constrictor muscle. This is known as Killian's dehiscence (Fig. 59.4).

A pharyngeal pouch is a pulsion diverticulum that occurs in the elderly resulting from a combination of anatomical weakness combined with spasm in the cricopharyngeus.

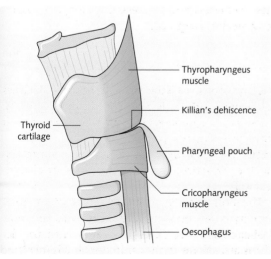

**Fig. 59.4** Pharyngeal pouch.

Labels: Thyropharyngeus muscle; Killian's dehiscence; Thyroid cartilage; Pharyngeal pouch; Cricopharyngeus muscle; Oesophagus

### Clinical presentation

The patient is most often elderly and reports progressive difficulty in swallowing. Classically, food is swallowed initially and then regurgitated some time later, often when lying down. The patient may report gurgling noises in the neck. The reflux of pouch contents into the airway may produce hoarseness and recurrent chest infections. With larger pouches there is frank dysphagia and weight loss.

### Diagnosis

The history is usually suggestive of a pouch. Occasionally a soft mass may be felt in the lower neck, more commonly on the left side. Diagnosis is based on the characteristic finding of a pouch on a lateral barium swallow film. This examination can also be used to exclude malignancy as a cause for the symptoms.

### Management

Previously the treatment was open diverticulectomy and nasogastric feeding for a week or so. This ran the risk of postoperative leakage and sepsis and was a risky procedure in patients who are often elderly and frail. This has been superseded by the operation of endoscopic diverticulotomy.

Under general anaesthesia a specially designed diverticuloscope is placed into the orifices of the pouch and the oesophagus. This demonstrates extremely well the 'bar' of mucosa and muscle between the two which may then be divided and at the same time sealed by a row of clips using an endoscopic stapling device. The patient can eat and drink normally a few hours after the procedure and is usually discharged home the next day.

## Globus pharyngeus

This is one of the most common reasons for attendance at an ENT department. Its importance, however, lies most often in the difficulty in distinguishing it from malignant disease of the pharynx or even oesophagus. It is a disease of exclusion. In the past it was considered to be primarily psychosomatic, 'globus hystericus', and, although in a proportion of patients it probably is, increasing emphasis has been placed upon laryngopharyngeal acid reflux (LPR) as a cause or precipitant.

### Clinical presentation

Patients most often complain of vague feelings of discomfort, or a 'lump' in the throat, usually at the level of the cricoid cartilage. There are usually feelings of intermittent hoarseness. Dysphagia is rare and weight loss does not occur.

Some patients may have symptoms of gastro-oesophageal reflux with epigastric burning and regurgitation. The patient may alternatively admit to stress and anxiety.

Examination of the neck is normal. Flexible naso-endoscopy is usually normal. Occasionally there may be subtle signs of reflux disease in the larynx such as interarytenoid swelling and supraglottic erythema.

### Diagnosis and management

- *History and examination.* Diagnosis is normally based upon the history and the lack of sinister findings on flexible naso-endoscopy, i.e. obvious tumour, cord palsy, pooling of secretions around larynx.
- *Full blood count* is generally normal; anaemia warrants further investigation.
- *Barium swallow.* If the patient has any suggestion of true dysphagia or weight loss then a barium swallow is traditionally ordered; however, it is not particularly helpful in diagnosing postcricoid tumours or showing reflux.
- *Diagnosis of LPR.* Although symptoms and signs may be suggestive they are frequently incorrect. The gold standard for diagnosing LPR is 24-hour pH monitoring. However, this is uncomfortable for the patient and not readily available in most ENT departments. An alternative is a trial of acid suppression using a proton pump inhibitor (PPI) for 8 weeks.
- *Endoscopy.* Persistent symptoms following PPI or anyone with sinister signs or symptoms (see Box below) should undergo rigid laryngoscopy, pharyngoscopy and oesophagoscopy (pan-endoscopy) under anaesthetic. This carries a risk of dental damage and perforation (<1%).

Ultimately some patients remain symptomatic after full investigation and treatment of reversible causes such as LPR and allergy. Stress and anxiety are certainly factors. In these patients the 'globus phenomenon' is likely to represent a disorder of interoception as is seen in other disorders such as irritable bowel syndrome and tinnitus.

## Laryngopharyngeal cancers

Cancers of the laryngopharynx (hypopharynx) are nearly all moderate to poorly differentiated squamous carcinomas. They spread early to surrounding structures, are frequently large at presentation, and often metastasize to cervical lymph nodes; they have a poor prognosis with only around 30% of patients surviving to 5 years.

Post-cricoid carcinoma is unusual among upper aero-digestive tract tumours in being more common in women than men. This is likely to be due to its association with Plummer–Vinson syndrome. This comprises iron deficiency anaemia and post-cricoid webbing which may progress to post-cricoid carcinoma.

### Clinical presentation

Tumours of the laryngopharynx most often present with dysphagia which is progressive. Pain is not unusual and may be felt in the ear (referred otalgia). There may be hoarseness or stridor as the larynx is invaded. Lymph node metastasis is common and the patient may be seen initially with a neck lump before major dysphagia occurs.

### Diagnosis

Many patients are seen in ENT clinics with minor difficulties in swallowing, throat discomfort and occasional voice difficulties. Most of these do not represent serious disease but more often may be ascribed to globus pharyngeus (see above). It is vitally important that patients with malignant disease are not missed.

Sinister symptoms and signs in patients with disordered swallowing:

- Smoking
- Anaemia
- True dysphagia
- Weight loss
- Pain (especially otalgia)
- Persistent hoarseness (vocal cord palsy)
- Cervical lymphadenopathy

The only way to exclude laryngopharyngeal malignancy in high-risk patients is with rigid endoscopy and biopsy under general anaesthesia. These lesions may not be visible on flexible endoscopic examination, CT or barium swallow.

### Management

The management of these tumours is complex and controversial and is either with chemo-radiotherapy or surgery. Surgery often necessitates removal of the larynx (laryngectomy) as well as the involved part of the pharynx (pharyngectomy). Morbidity after surgery or chemo-radiotherapy is often marked and most patients have ongoing difficulty with swallowing.

## THE LARYNX

The larynx is a beautiful example of tissue engineering and it is certainly worth considering its anatomy in more detail. It is present in all mammals but only in man is its evolution as a provider of speech so developed. Its primary function as an airway sphincter has largely been forgotten when placed next to its ability as an instrument of emotion. However, while one can easily survive without an operatic vocal range one cannot survive without adequate airway protection.

## Functions of the larynx

1. *Airway protection.* The larynx elevates, the epiglottis is pulled down and the cords adduct (close) during swallowing.
2. *Phonation.* Air from the lungs is propelled up to the larynx. Adduction of the vocal cords to within 95% of closure results in a 'mucosal wave' in the epithelium of the vocal fold. The gel-like nature of the lamina propria (Reinke's space) facilitates this movement. Laryngeal sounds are then modulated and articulated by the pharynx, oral cavity, lips, teeth and tongue to produce speech.
3. *Airway reflexes.* Abduction (opening) on inspiration, cough and control of intra-abdominal pressure (during heavy lifting, defaecation and childbirth) are all mediated by laryngeal reflexes.

## Anatomy

The framework of the larynx consists of three single rings of cartilage; the epiglottis, the thyroid and the cricoid cartilages. Perched on top of the cricoid cartilage are the three paired cartilages: arytenoid, cuneiform and corniculate (Fig. 59.5).

Attached to the vocal process of the arytenoid cartilage and the inner aspect of the thyroid cartilage is the thyro-arytenoid muscle. This muscle, the vocalis, and its overlying epithelium and lamina propria form

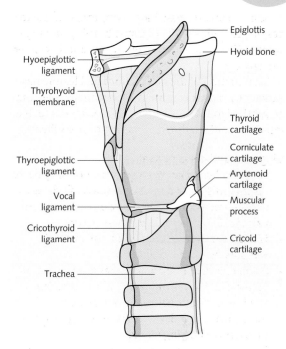

**Fig. 59.5** The laryngeal cartilages.

the vocal cord. The cover of the vocal fold is extremely delicate (only 0.3 mm thick) and is extremely susceptible to even small changes, producing hoarseness. The position of the vocal cords and thus airway patency is controlled by a series of muscles that insert into the muscular process of the arytenoid; the posterior crico-arytenoid is uniquely important as the only abductor of the vocal folds. Pitch is controlled by the tilting action of the cricoid on the thyroid cartilage (by the action of cricothyroid) and by the tension of the thyro-arytenoid muscle.

The nerve supply to all the intrinsic muscles of the larynx (abductors and adductors) is via the recurrent laryngeal nerve (a branch of the tenth nerve), except for cricothyroid muscle which is supplied by the superior branch of the external laryngeal nerve (again a branch of the vagus).

The lymphatic supply to the vocal folds is relatively poor. This has two effects, one bad and one good. It means that even relatively minor insults lead to oedema in the superficial lamina propria (Reinke's oedema) which may be slow to disperse and cause prolonged hoarseness. However, for the same reason vocal fold tumours have difficulty in metastasizing to lymph nodes, which accounts in some part for their good prognosis.

## Disorders of the larynx

The following list is not exhaustive:

### 1. Congenital (see Chapter 63)

- Laryngomalacia.
- Laryngeal clefts.
- Webs.
- Subglottic stenosis.
- Neonatal vocal cord paralysis.

### 2. Acquired

- Inflammatory:
  - Reflux laryngitis (see globus pharyngeus and LPR above)
  - Reinke's oedema.
- Infectious viral, bacterial, TB.
- Idiopathic:
  - Nodules
  - Polyps.
- Neurological:
  - Vocal cord paralysis
  - Dystonias – spasmodic dysphonia.
- Neoplastic:
  - Papillomatosis
  - SCC larynx.

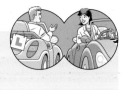

All patients with hoarseness persisting more than 2 weeks should have their vocal cords examined.

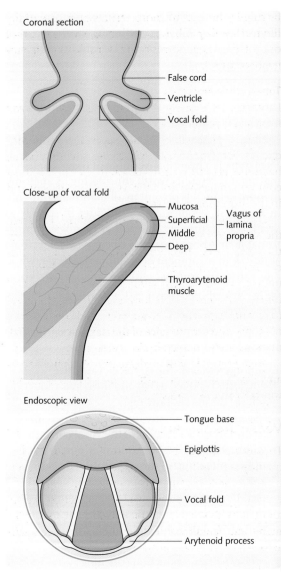

**Fig. 59.6** Laryngeal anatomy.

## Reinke's oedema

This is accumulation of fluid in the superficial lamina propria of the vocal fold, Reinke's space (Fig. 59.6). Predisposing factors include smoking, laryngeal reflux, vocal abuse (market traders, teachers, etc.) and hypothyroidism.

### Clinical presentation

The swelling and distortion of vocal fold anatomy leads to hoarseness, which is usually persistent.

### Diagnosis

Diagnosis is usually possible on flexible naso-endoscopic examination. The cords are swollen and oedematous, sometimes with a glassy appearance. Severe disease produces a 'saddle bag' appearance of the folds which may flop backwards and forwards with speech and breathing. It is usual to perform a thyroid function test.

### Management

It is necessary to stop any irritating factors. Speech therapy is also helpful. Severe unresponsive disease may be helped by reduction of oedematous areas under microscopic guidance; this requires general anaesthetic.

## Infectious laryngitis

A variety of organisms may produce an infective laryngitis. These vary from the relatively trivial viral aryngitis through to more serious and potentially ife-threatening tuberculous laryngitis (in the past one of the most common reasons for emergency tracheostomy).

## Tuberculous laryngitis

Laryngeal TB is nearly always associated with spread from active pulmonary TB.

*Clinical presentation.* Tuberculous laryngitis produces severe hoarseness with throat pain, dysphagia, haemoptysis, stridor and cough. In the UK it is most common in people from the Asian subcontinent and in the immunosuppressed.

*Diagnosis* is based on endoscopic findings. However, the signs may vary from mucosal oedema and erythema to frank ulceration mimicking laryngeal cancer. There are many cases in the literature of patients undergoing emergency laryngectomy for an 'obvious' cancer of the larynx only for histopathology to reveal tuberculous infection. Diagnosis is made on the basis of biopsy and the presence of the classical signs of TB, or more rarely on microbiological culture.

*Management* is with medical antituberculous therapy. Tracheostomy may still be needed if there is airway compromise and stridor.

## Vocal cord polyps and nodules

These are extremely common conditions and are frequently seen in the hoarse patient. Vocal cord nodules are most common in young female patients, especially in professional voice users such as singers and teachers. Vocal cord polyps are seen equally in males and females of any age group and are again associated with vocal misuse.

### Clinical presentation

Both conditions present with hoarseness that is usually persistent. There are no sinister features.

### Diagnosis

The diagnosis is easily made on fibreoptic endoscopic examination (Fig. 59.7). Nodules are typically bilateral and occur at the junction of the anterior and middle thirds of the vocal fold. Polyps are larger, unilateral and occur in the mid-third or posterior part of the vocal fold.

### Management

- *Nodules.* Patients' vocal problems are often cured with a course of speech therapy. Surgery is only necessary for persistent or large nodules which do not respond.

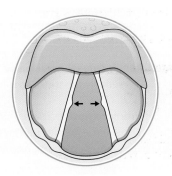

**Fig. 59.7** Vocal nodules.

- *Polyps.* Are usually larger and have a more profound effect on the voice. Surgical removal usually returns the voice to normal.

## Vocal cord paralysis

The nerve supply to the intrinsic laryngeal muscles is from the vagus via the superior laryngeal nerves (cricothyroid) and the recurrent laryngeal nerves (all other intrinsic muscles) (Fig. 59.8). Damage to the superior laryngeal nerve may occur following thyroid and parathyroid surgery resulting in subtle difficulty changing voice pitch. The recurrent laryngeal nerves take a more circuitous route to reach the larynx. On the left side the nerve loops around the arch of the aorta before travelling upwards in the tracheo-oesophageal groove to enter the larynx at the crico-arytenoid joint. On the right it wraps around the subclavian artery before ascending to the larynx. Especially on the left side the

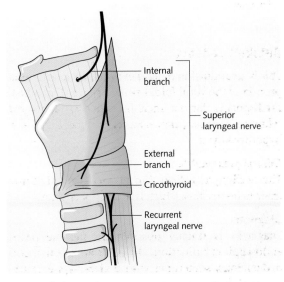

**Fig. 59.8** The laryngeal nerves.

nerve is at risk of damage anywhere from the skull base to the mediastinum. Consequently left vocal cord palsy is more common than right.

### Causes of recurrent laryngeal nerve palsy

- *Congenital* – presents with stridor in infancy (see paediatric ENT).
- *Neurological* – motor neurone disease, bulbar palsy.
- *Compression by tumour* – jugular foramen, neck, thyroid, laryngeal, mediastinum, bronchus, oesophagus.
- *Iatrogenic nerve injury* – especially cardiac operations and thyroid surgery.

### Clinical presentation

Unilateral vocal cord palsy results in a voice that is hoarse and breathy. There is often also mild difficulty with swallowing usually short-lived. Bilateral vocal cord palsy, especially if the cords are adducted, results in stridor and may present a surgical emergency.

### Diagnosis

- *Flexible naso-endoscopy* is diagnostic. The affected cord is seen to sit in the paramedian position (Fig. 59.9); there is no movement either with cough or phonation.
- *CT.* Except where the cause is obvious (post-thyroidectomy) the entire course of the recurrent laryngeal nerve should be imaged. This usually is done with CT scanning from brain to thorax.
- *Electrophysiology.* Occasionally where no cause for a palsy is demonstrated, laryngeal electromyography (EMG) is performed to confirm paralysis and exclude mechanical fixation of the arytenoids.

### Management

*Conservative.* Speech therapy may encourage the none paralysed cord to over-adduct and therefore improve the voice. This should be tried in all patients.

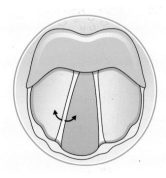

**Fig. 59.9** Right vocal cord palsy.

*Surgical.* In patients in whom conservative measures are not successful medialization of the paralysed cord may be performed surgically. There are two main methods:

1. *Injection medialization.* Under general or local anaesthetic a bulking material (e.g. silicone) is injected between the vocal cord and the laryngeal cartilage. This plumps out the cord and may return voice to near normal. This may be performed even in patients with limited life expectancy.
2. *Medialization thyroplasty.* A window is cut into the thyroid cartilage and the vocal cord medialized and held in place, usually with a silicone block or other prosthesis.

## Tumours of the larynx

Although there are numerous neoplastic conditions which can affect the larynx the most common are benign laryngeal papillomatosis and squamous cell carcinoma.

### Laryngeal papillomatosis

This is a condition that usually becomes apparent in childhood or early adulthood. It is a result of infection by human papilloma virus (HPV types 6 and 11) which is probably transmitted from the maternal vagina during delivery. There are multiple and recurrent raspberry like papillomas that affect the larynx and in severe cases the trachea and bronchi.

*Clinical presentation.* Hoarseness usually begins in childhood and in severe cases may be accompanied by stridor.

> All children with persistent hoarseness should be examined by an ENT surgeon. Laryngeal papillomatosis is an important and occasionally life-threatening cause.

*Diagnosis.* Diagnosis is usually confirmed by the flexible laryngoscopic appearance of typical papillomas (warts) which may affect the epiglottis, supraglottis or vocal folds.

Biopsy confirms the diagnosis.

*Management* can be surgical or medical.

*Surgery.* This condition is recurrent and at present incurable. The mainstay of therapy is microsurgical removal of papillomas using the $CO_2$ laser, mechanical shavers or conventional instruments. The voice seldom returns to normal and relapse is unpredictable.

*Medical treatment.* Various medical therapies have been tried including alpha-interferon and various antiviral drugs. At the present time intralesional cidofovir (an anti viral) seems to hold the most promise.

### Laryngeal cancer

Laryngeal cancer is the most common cancer of the head and neck region. It represents around 1–2% of all cancers in the UK. In some parts of Asia it is the most common cancer of all. Like most cancers of the upper aero-digestive tract there is a proven relationship between cigarette smoking and development of cancer. Heavy smoking and alcohol consumption have a synergistic effect, increasing the risk of cancer by a factor of 15–30 times. Laryngeal cancer is five times more common in males than females and tends to present in the 7th decade. It is most often a squamous cell carcinoma which may spread to local lymph nodes but rarely metastasizes to the lungs and liver.

*Clinical presentation.* There are three different sites which may be affected by cancer in the larynx and which, clinically behave differently. This is summarized in Fig. 59.10.

*Glottic cancer* is fortunately the most common as it has the best overall prognosis. It tends to produce hoarseness and due to the poor lymphatic supply of the vocal cord only spreads to lymph nodes when it is relatively advanced. Unfortunately in the UK it is still more common to see it in its advanced stages at presentation.

*Diagnosis* can usually be made on flexible nasoendoscopy. This is followed by pan-endoscopy for biopsy and also to exclude a second carcinoma in the upper aero-digestive tract (metachronous tumours are seen in 10% of patients).

*CT scan.* This is useful to stage the laryngeal cancer and also to assess the neck and chest for metastatic disease and synchronous tumours. It is necessary to have some idea of the staging system before we consider treatment. The system shown in Fig. 59.11 is based on the standard TNM classification (UICC).

*Management.* This is controversial and varies from country to country. The aim of therapy is cure with the best speech and swallowing outcomes possible. 'Organ sparing' using chemo-radiotherapy is increasingly common. We will consider the most common glottic tumours:

- Early tumours T1 N0. Spread to lymph nodes is rare and cure may be obtained with local therapy. Surgical excision or radiotherapy both give extremely good cure rates in excess of 90%.
- Moderate tumours T2–T3. Moderate-sized tumours offer an opportunity for organ preservation using either partial laryngectomy techniques, laser excision or radiotherapy. 5-year survival rates of 50–80% may be achieved.
- Advanced tumours T4. These are probably best treated by organ sparing combined chemo-radiotherapy, with laryngectomy reserved for failure following this.

### Surgical laryngectomy

Total laryngectomy is the surgical excision of the entire larynx. It is still a common treatment for laryngeal carcinoma. It is performed under general anaesthesia. Total

**Fig. 59.10** Cancers of the larynx

| Subsite | Glottis | Supraglottis | Subglottis |
|---|---|---|---|
| % of laryngeal cancers | 75% | 25% | 5% |
| Area affected | Vocal cords | Epiglottis, false cords | Area below cords |
| Hoarseness | Almost immediate | Late | Late |
| Stridor | Late | Late | Marked |
| Dysphagia | Late | Late | Medium |
| Pain | Rare | Common | Common |
| Lymph nodes | Rare (<10%) | Common and bilateral | Common and bilateral |
| Prognosis | Good if early | Poor | Very poor |
| 5 year survival | 40–90% (stage) | 60% | <40% |

**Fig. 59.11** Staging of laryngeal cancer (glottis)

| T stage (primary tumour) | N stage (cervical lymph nodes) | M stage (metastases) |
|---|---|---|
| T1 – tumour confined to vocal cords | N0 – no lymph nodes | M0 – no mets |
| T2 – spreads to supra- or subglottis, no cord fixation | N1 – single ipsilateral node <3 cm | M1 – mets present |
| T3 – limited to larynx with vocal cord fixation | N2 – nodes 3–6 cm a) 1 on same side b) >1 same side c) opposite or both sides | |
| T4 – spread outside larynx | N3 – any nodes >6 cm | |

laryngectomy involves the excision of all the laryngeal structures up to and including the hyoid and the proximal trachea. The trachea is brought out to the skin of the neck as a tracheostoma and the pharynx closed off entirely from the airway (Fig. 59.12). After the initial period the tracheostoma requires no tube to maintain its patency as the cartilage rings of the trachea hold it open; it is analogous to a 'nostril on the neck'.

*Partial laryngectomy* is possible maintaining some voice and swallowing function by retaining normal laryngeal structures. Transoral laser resection offers the chance to remove diseased tissue only, leaving other structures intact. In some centres it offers cure rates as good as or better than traditional surgery or radiotherapy with arguably better swallowing and speech results.

### Voice restoration after laryngectomy

Surgical voice restoration utilizes the laxity of the closed pharynx (the neo-pharynx) to generate vibration which is then articulated in the normal way to produce voice. Air is directed from the trachea via small one-way valve (tracheo-oesophageal valve) in its posterior wall (Fig. 59.13). Most patients have this procedure at the same time as their laryngectomy. A majority of them will achieve voice that is good enough to enable them to speak on the phone and hold down a job. This is a great improvement on the previously available methods. Oesophageal speech where air is swallowed and then belched back, and the 'electro-larynx' both produced non-fluent and difficult to understand speech and were not popular with patients.

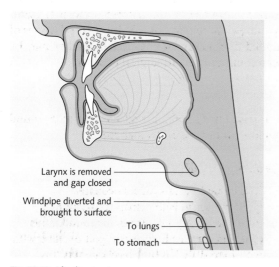

Larynx is removed and gap closed

Windpipe diverted and brought to surface

To lungs

To stomach

**Fig. 59.12** After laryngectomy.

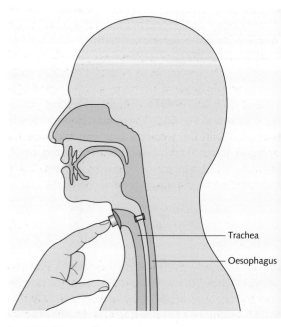

Trachea

Oesophagus

**Fig. 59.13** Voice prosthesis.

# Disorders of the thyroid and parathyroids

## Objectives

You should:

- Be familiar with the embryology and anatomy of the thyroid and parathyroid glands.
- Know a little about hyper- and hypothyroidism.
- Be aware of the main disorders of migration of the thyroid gland.
- Know about goitres and nodules.
- Know about thyroid cancer and its treatment.
- Know how hyperparathyroidism is managed surgically.

See also Chapter 65, p. 314, Examination of the thyroid gland.

## EMBRYOLOGY AND ANATOMY

The thyroid gland begins its development at around the 17th day of gestation as an out-pouching from the primitive stomatodeum. It leaves the foramen caecum at the junction of the anterior and posterior tongue and descends through the neck as the thyroglossal duct (Fig. 60.1). It eventually comes to lie anterior to the trachea at around 3 weeks. It is joined there by cells from the ultimobranchial bodies which form the calcitonin secreting C cells.

In adult life the thyroid gland is a butterfly-shaped organ. The isthmus overlies the second to fourth tracheal rings to which the gland is densely attached by the ligament of Berry. The blood supply and lymphatic drainage is shown in Fig. 60.2. The thyroid gland is closely associated with the recurrent laryngeal and superior laryngeal nerves. Lymphatic drainage is to paratracheal, pretracheal and mediastinal lymph nodes. Also closely associated are the parathyroid glands (see later).

## PHYSIOLOGY

The thyroid is organized into functional subunits called follicles. These take up iodine from the circulation and use it to produce the thyroid hormones T3 and T4. Hormone production is under the influence of thyroid stimulating hormone (TSH) produced by the pituitary (Fig. 60.3). T3 and T4 are stored in combination with thyroglobulin as colloid. They are released by pinocytosis when required before being separated from thyroglobulin and transported into the circulation. Most circulating thyroid hormone is in the form of T4 bound to protein. However, it is the unbound hormone that is active. Thyroid hormones act on many target cells, especially those involved in growth and metabolism.

## DISORDERS OF THE THYROID GLAND

Before moving on to consider some more typically 'surgical' diseases of the thyroid gland it is worth spending a little time considering medical causes of altered thyroid function, especially as they may be seen commonly in our surgical patients.

### Hypothyroidism

This is extremely common and affects women around ten times more frequently than men.

#### Causes

- Congenital aplasia – causes neonatal hypothyroidism with mental retardation.
- Iodine deficiency – common in mountainous areas; may cause enlargement (goitre) along with hypothyroidism if iodine levels are very low.

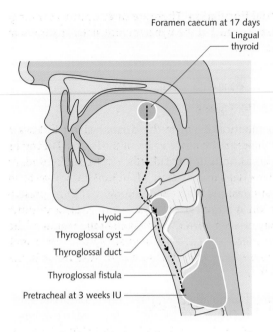

Foramen caecum at 17 days
Lingual thyroid

Hyoid
Thyroglossal cyst
Thyroglossal duct
Thyroglossal fistula
Pretracheal at 3 weeks IU

**Fig. 60.1** Embryology of the thyroid gland.

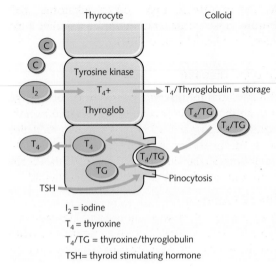

Thyrocyte
Colloid

Tyrosine kinase

$I_2$
$T_4+$
$T_4$/Thyroglobulin = storage

Thyroglob

$T_4$/TG
$T_4$/TG

$T_4$
$T_4$
$T_4$/TG

TG
$T_4$/TG
Pinocytosis

TSH

$I_2$ = iodine
$T_4$ = thyroxine
$T_4$/TG = thyroxine/thyroglobulin
TSH= thyroid stimulating hormone

**Fig. 60.3** Physiology of the thyroid gland.

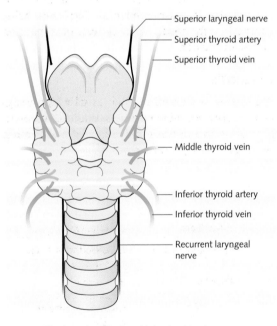

Superior laryngeal nerve
Superior thyroid artery
Superior thyroid vein

Middle thyroid vein

Inferior thyroid artery
Inferior thyroid vein

Recurrent laryngeal nerve

**Fig. 60.2** Blood supply of the thyroid gland and local nerves.

- Dyshormonogenesis:
  - Inherited abnormalities in the tyrosine kinase pathways make production of T3 and T4 impossible leading to hypothyroidism with a goitre.
  - Antithyroid drugs and others, e.g. amiodarone.

- Autoimmune:
  - Atrophic hypothyroidism – most common caused by microsomal auto-antibodies
  - Hashimoto's thyroiditis – high levels of thyroid microsomal antibodies causing atrophy and hypothyroidism with a goitre.
- Post-surgical and post-radioiodine.

## Clinical features

See examination of the thyroid gland.

## Investigations

- Elevated TSH – diagnosis depends on this finding along with decreased T4 level.
- Auto-antibodies – elevated levels of thyroid auto-antibodies may be demonstrable in the plasma.

## Management

Thyroxine is given by mouth and the TSH monitored until it returns to normal levels. Occasionally in the hypothyroid post-surgical patient T3 is given instead as this does not interfere with subsequent radioiodine scans (see later).

## Hyperthyroidism

This is less common than hypofunction of the thyroid gland. It again affects women more commonly than men at a ratio of around 5:1; most of those affected being relatively young. The common causes are Graves' disease, toxic solitary adenoma, toxic multinodular goitre and thyroiditis (either post-infective or Reidel's thyroiditis).

## Graves' disease

This autoimmune disease is caused by circulating IgG auto-antibodies. These bind to TSH receptors on the thyrocyte causing activation and excessive production of T4. The disease is commonly seen in young females and follows a relapsing course. Eventually the disease 'burns out' and the patient becomes hypothyroid.

### Clinical features

The patient presents with a goitre and the features of hyperthyroidism (see Chapter 65, examination of the thyroid gland). Eye signs are usually present and are often pronounced.

### Diagnosis

- *Thyroid function tests* show a depressed TSH and a high T3 or T4.
- *Auto-antibodies* – most often there is a raised level TSH receptor antibodies (LATS or long acting thyroid stimulating); other thyroid antibodies such as thyroid microsomal and anti-thyroglobulin may also be raised.

### Management

General medical management usually commences in the full-blown Graves' patient with symptom control. This is often done by administering a β-blocker such as propranolol. This controls the cardiovascular side effects such as tachycardia and

atrial fibrillation. There are three options for long-term control of the hyperthyroid state, as shown in Fig. 60.4.

## Disorders of migration

(e.g. thyroglossal cyst)

As mentioned above the thyroid gland follows a somewhat circuitous route in the foetus. During its descent, rests of thyroid cells may be left behind. At a later date, usually early adulthood, these may form cystic lesions. The most common clinical presentation is a thyroglossal cyst. More rarely a swelling may be seen within the tongue in the region of the foramen caecum. This lingual thyroid tissue may represent the only functioning thyroid tissue in the patient.

## Clinical presentation

The thyroglossal cyst usually presents in the second decade as a midline neck swelling. It may be completely asymptomatic but not uncommonly it is noticed after it becomes infected. The lesion being attached to the tongue base is seen to elevate on tongue protrusion.

## Diagnosis

The history and examination is usually highly suggestive. Ultrasound scanning is usually diagnostic. If there is still doubt then fine needle aspiration cytology (FNAC) is carried out.

**Fig. 60.4** Treatment of hyperthyroidism

| Treatment | Mode of action | Relapse rate | Advantages | Disadvantages |
| --- | --- | --- | --- | --- |
| Carbimazole (or propylthiouracil) | Block production T3/T4 | 50% relapse in 2 years | Safe, non-invasive | Agranulocytosis (0.1%) High relapse |
| Radioactive $^{131}$I | Destroys thyroid tissue | 15% | Effective | In-patient Hypothyroidism Not in pregnancy or breastfeeding |
| Surgery (total or subtotal thyroidectomy*) | Removes thyroid tissue | Subtotal thyroidectomy = 3% (in first year) then 1%/year | Extremely effective, esp. if other ways fail | Hypothyroidism Hypoparathyroidism (<1%) Recurrent laryngeal nerve palsy (1–10%) |

\* *Many specialist centres now perform total thyroidectomy which requires postoperative T4 but removes the possibility of recurrent hyperthyroidism.*
*Surgery is much more likely in toxic adenomas and multinodular goitres which are less likely to respond to other modalities.*

## Management

If thyroglossal cysts are symptomatic they are usually excised surgically. The body of the hyoid is removed as part of the operation (Sistrunk's procedure) as this has been demonstrated to produce lower (though still high) rates of recurrence when compared with standard enucleation. A more thorough central neck dissection with extension into the tongue base gives the lowest recurrence rates of all.

## Enlargement of the thyroid gland

This is the most common reason for referral to a surgeon. Causes are shown in Fig. 60.5. The term goitre is probably the only old Norse word you will be expected to remember in your medical career; it means 'neck' and is the term applied to diffuse enlargement of the thyroid gland. Discrete masses within the thyroid are commonly referred to as nodules; they may be solitary or 'dominant' (i.e. biggest) within a multinodular gland.

## Nodular thyroid disease

Nodules within the thyroid gland are extremely common, especially in females, and increase in frequency with age. Palpable nodules (usually greater than 1 cm) are present in around 7% of the population. However, ultrasound and post-mortem studies reveal nodules in up to 70%. Only one in 20 of these nodules represents malignancy. Common causes include multinodular goitre, thyroid cysts and benign colloid nodules.

## Clinical presentation

Most nodules are asymptomatic and the reason for consultation is concern about malignancy. Multinodular goitres and some very large nodules may cause compression of surrounding structures, e.g. trachea and oesophagus, leading to dyspnoea or dysphagia. This is especially true if they extend retrosternally. Hoarseness may be caused by tumours invading the recurrent laryngeal nerve; rarely, however, a large goitre may stretch the nerve leading to voice changes. Large lesions may also cause cosmetic concerns.

## Diagnosis

Fig. 60.6 lists factors which make malignancy more likely. As well as these risk stratification factors most patients will undergo additional tests, the most useful of which are:

- *FNAC (fine needle aspiration cytology)*. This is an extremely useful investigation in the hands of expert cytologists and can help greatly in the differentiation of cancer from benign nodular disease. A negative FNAC, however, does not exclude the presence of malignancy, especially in a larger nodule (>3 cm).
- *Ultrasound scanning* allows the differentiation of solitary nodules versus dominant nodules within a multinodular goitre (10% vs 6% risk of malignancy). It may also detect features suggestive of malignancy such as calcification, cervical lymphadenopathy or invasion of the thyroid capsule. If used to direct fine needle aspiration it increases the accuracy of cytological diagnosis.

---

**Fig. 60.5** Causes of thyroid enlargement

**Goitre**
Physiological – i.e. pregnancy/puberty
Dietary – $I^2$ deficiency, goitrogens, e.g. kale, cauliflower (block $I^2$ absorption)
Dyshormonogenesis – familial, drugs, e.g. amiodarone
Multinodular goitre
Autoimmune – Graves' disease, Hashimoto's
Thyroiditis – infective, Reidel's thyroiditis

**Nodular thyroid disease**
Cysts
Multinodular goitre and benign thyroid nodules (colloid nodules)

**Thyroid cancer**
Follicular neoplasms
Papillary thyroid cancer
Medullary thyroid cancer
Anaplastic thyroid cancer

**Fig. 60.6** Factors making malignancy more likely

**Patient factors**
Age (<20 or >65 years)
Male sex
Exposure to ionizing radiation
Family history thyroid cancer

**History**
Rapid growth
Hoarseness

**Examination**
Hard, fixed texture
Cervical lymphadenopathy
Vocal cord paralysis

- *Thyroid function tests and antibody screen.*
- *CT scan* (non-contrast enhanced); especially useful if there is suspicion of retrosternal extension.

## Management of nodular thyroid disease

There are a number of indications for surgery in nodular thyroid disease:

1. *Exclusion of malignancy.* Even with the above tests it is sometimes not possible to exclude malignancy without excision of the nodule. This is especially true for patients who have any of the risk factors listed in Fig. 60.6.
2. *Compressive symptoms.*
3. *Cosmetic concerns.* This is a common factor in younger patients; however, it is extremely important that these patients are counselled about the possibility of complications following surgery.

## Thyroid cancer

Thyroid nodules are extremely common. Thyroid cancer, however, is not; it represents around 2% of all cancers. The difficulty is finding the needle in the haystack. Factors that make a nodule more likely to be malignant are shown above.

Thyroid cancer is more common in women and may affect all age groups, even children. Differentiated thyroid cancer is more common in areas of iodine deficiency and in those exposed to ionizing radiation.

### Clinical presentation

Most patients with thyroid cancer present with an enlarging lump in the neck. This may have the worrying features mentioned above or may be asymptomatic. There may be features of local compression. Most patients with thyroid cancer are euthyroid. In

medullary carcinoma there may be a known family history of thyroid or other endocrine tumours.

### Diagnosis

The diagnostic process for suspected thyroid cancer is the same as detailed for thyroid nodules above. Cancer may present as a solitary nodule, a dominant nodule in a multinodular goitre, rarely in the wall of a thyroid cyst, or as multifocal lymphadenopathy (papillary cancer). The steps in the diagnosis, however, remain the same. They are:

- *FNAC* – often performed with ultrasound guidance. It is possible to differentiate between benign thyroid enlargement, follicular, papillary and other neoplasms.
- *Ultrasound scan* – looking for the features of thyroid malignancy, i.e. microcalcification, irregularity and haphazard vascularity. Also assesses the presence of lymphadenopathy.
- *Specific markers* – a raised calcitonin level may indicate medullary thyroid cancer. In patients with a known family history of medullary thyroid cancer screening for the RET proto-oncogene mutation may be carried out.

### Histological types of thyroid cancer

*Differentiated thyroid cancers:*

- Papillary – 80%.
- Follicular – 10%.
- Hurthle cell – 1%.
- Medullary – 7%.

*Undifferentiated cancer:*

- Anaplastic – 2%.

*Others:*

- Lymphoma.
- SCC.

### Papillary thyroid cancer

80% of all thyroid neoplasms are papillary thyroid cancer. All age groups are affected including children. Predisposing factors include iodine deficiency and exposure to radiation. The disease at presentation is commonly multicentric and has often spread to the cervical lymph nodes. Treatment is with surgery (usually total thyroidectomy and neck dissection if involved lymph nodes present) followed in most cases by a course of radioactive iodine and lifelong suppression of thyroid function with thyroxine. Surveillance may be carried out by repeat measurement of serum thyroglobulin. It has the most favourable prognosis of all thyroid cancers with more than 90% of patients alive after 5 years.

### Follicular neoplasms

Follicular neoplasms are of two types: the benign encapsulated follicular adenoma and invasive follicular carcinoma. Unfortunately they can only be differentiated on histology following excision and not by preoperative FNAC. Follicular cancer spreads haematogenously to distant sites in around 30% of patients. Treatment is the same as for papillary thyroid cancer. Survival, however, is worse for follicular cancers.

### Medullary thyroid cancer (MTC)

This tumour arises from the parafollicular or C cells which secrete calcitonin. It is seen more commonly as a sporadic form but it may be familial. Many familial cases are in combination with other endocrine neoplasms as part of the multiple endocrine neoplasia 1 or 2 syndromes. Most affected family members carry the RET proto-oncogene mutation and this is increasingly used for screening asymptomatic family members (often children). MTCs secrete calcitonin and this is a useful tumour marker, especially for disease recurrence following treatment. Treatment is with total thyroidectomy and meticulous neck dissection.

### Anaplastic thyroid cancer

This is an aggressive and invariably fatal neoplasm. It is seen in elderly patients who often present with a rapidly enlarging thyroid mass which may invade local structures causing dyspnoea, hoarseness and dysphagia. It is often difficult to diagnose as the clinical and FNAC appearances may be very similar to lymphoma. Occasionally core or open biopsy is necessary to secure the diagnosis. Treatment is palliative and most patients die from their disease within months of diagnosis.

## Thyroid surgery

There is a confusing array of terms for different thyroid operations. Most benign lesions may be treated by the removal of half of the thyroid gland, a hemi-thyroidectomy. Most malignant diseases (except for very small tumours) are best treated by total thyroidectomy, leaving behind the parathyroid glands. Occasionally

Grave's disease is treated by removal of $^4/_5$ of the thyroid gland – the so-called sub-total thyroidectomy.

### Thyroidectomy

The operation is generally carried out under general anaesthesia. A horizontal incision is made through the skin and platysma muscle down to the strap muscles. The dissection continues deep to these muscles to free up the thyroid lobe, dividing the middle thyroid vein as it is reached. The superior pedicle is divided, carefully preserving the superior laryngeal nerve. The inferior thyroid artery is identified and the relationship of the recurrent laryngeal nerve identified before this pedicle is cut. The parathyroid glands are identified and preserved.

### Specific complications of thyroidectomy

*Recurrent laryngeal nerve palsy*. Damage to one recurrent laryngeal nerve produces a hoarse voice due to paralysis of all the intrinsic laryngeal muscles except cricothyroid. The vocal cord palsy rate is mostly claimed to be less than 1%; however, there are few good objective studies. Bilateral paralysis results in stridor and airway compromise. Tracheostomy or other procedures to open the airway (laser arytenoidectomy) may be required. All patients should have a vocal cord examination before and after surgery.

*Superior laryngeal nerve palsy*. This results in paralysis of the cricothyroid muscle and subtle difficulties changing the pitch of the voice. This is only likely to cause problems in the professional voice user.

*Hypothyroidism*. This is not necessarily a complication except after partial surgery. It is readily treated with once daily thyroxine administration. Tri-iodothyronine is used in cancer patients awaiting radioiodine therapy as it does not interfere with iodine uptake.

*Hypoparathyroidism*. Transient hypocalcaemia is relatively common and normally stabilizes without treatment. More acute falls in calcium level may be seen following thyroidectomy. Clinically they initially present as tingling in the extremities and perioral region along with carpopedal spasm. Untreated this may progress to full blown tetany. Acute hypocalcaemia is treated with intravenous calcium. Chronic problems are treated with oral administration of calcium salts and vitamin D.

*Haematoma and airway compromise*. Causes of airway compromise following thyroidectomy are bilateral vocal cord paralysis and wound haematoma.

All patients with airway compromise following thyroid surgery should be re-intubated without delay and transferred back to theatre where wound exploration and evacuation of any haematoma, with or without tracheostomy, may be performed safely. This is a better policy than opening wounds on the ward. However, if the patient is in extremis then this may still be required.

# DISORDERS OF THE PARATHYROIDS

The four parathyroid glands are located on the posterior surface of the thyroid. They secrete a polypeptide parathyroid hormone (PTH). PTH increases serum calcium levels by encouraging osteoclastic bone resorption, increasing renal tubular reabsorption and facilitating calcium absorption in the small intestine.

## Hyperparathyroidism

Overactivity of the parathyroids results in an increased serum calcium level.

## Clinical presentation

The classic clinical picture is of:

- *Bones* – bone pain, pathological fractures, Brown's tumours, osteitis fibrosa cystica.
- *Stones* – renal stones, nephrocalcinosis, polyuria.
- Abdo *moans* – constipation, peptic ulcers, pancreatitis.
- Psychic *groans* – anorexia, malaise, confusion, depression, psychosis.

## Classification of hyperparathyroidism

- *Primary hyperparathyroidism* is caused most often by a parathyroid adenoma. More rarely gland hyperplasia or a carcinoma may be responsible.
- *Secondary hyperparathyroidism.* Chronic renal disease may cause excess loss of calcium in the urine and decreased vitamin D synthesis, precipitating glandular hyperplasia.
- *Tertiary hyperparathyroidism.* Correction of the renal defect (mostly by transplantation) usually results in resolution of parathyroid hyperplasia in some patients; however, the parathyroids continue to secrete PTH even in the face of a normal or high serum calcium.

## Diagnosis

- *Biochemical investigations.* Diagnosis is made by demonstrating an elevated serum calcium, alkaline phosphatase and PTH. Other conditions which may cause hypercalcaemia include metastatic bone disease, myeloma, sarcoidosis and ectopic PTH secretion by tumours.
- *Imaging.* Localization of the gland or glands responsible may be achieved with ultrasound scanning and thallium/technetium scanning.

## Management

Adenomas or carcinomas may be removed surgically. Cases with four gland hyperplasia are best treated with removal of three glands; alternatively four glands may be removed and calcium supplementation given.

# Sleep disorders and ENT

**Objectives**

You should know about:

- Obstructive sleep apnoea in adults.
- Snoring and its management.
- The presentation and treatment of obstructive sleep apnoea in children.

This is an increasingly important branch of ENT practice and the diagnosis of sleep disorders is becoming more common. The main conditions dealt with by ENT surgeons are:

1. Snoring.
2. Obstructive sleep apnoea (OSA).

These conditions are not discrete entities but represent a spectrum of airway collapse during sleep. OSA in children is quite different to that seen in adults and is considered separately.

## SNORING

30–50% of the population snore, the rate increasing with age. Snoring is more common in men. Snoring is noise produced by vibration and partial collapse of a lax upper airway during sleep. It is most commonly produced by vibration of the soft palate against the posterior pharyngeal wall, but it may also be caused by nasal, nasopharyngeal or tongue base obstruction. This is the least serious of the sleep disorders in that it has no serious ill effects on the snorer. The main effect of snoring is on the patient's family and sleeping partners, who bear the brunt of the disturbance.

### Clinical presentation

The history is from the patient's family or sleeping partner and they are the ones who usually persuade the patient to seek help.

### Diagnosis

The primary aim in history and examination of a patient who snores is to rule out obstructive sleep apnoea as this has serious medical consequences. The history and examination is therefore the same for both groups.

Obviously not all patients who snore require further investigation, but if they have any symptoms of obstructive sleep apnoea it is important that this is investigated further by polysomnography or a sleep study. Management of snoring is considered later with the management of sleep apnoea.

## OBSTRUCTIVE SLEEP APNOEA (OSA)

Apnoea is defined as cessation in air flow during sleep lasting more than 10 seconds. Sleep apnoea may be a) central b) obstructive or c) a combination of both. Central sleep apnoea is a problem with the centres that control respiratory drive; it is mainly a neurological problem. OSA is by far the most common form of sleep apnoea. This is a serious but treatable condition; OSA patients have an increased mortality from cardiovascular causes (up to 23 times the risk of a cardiac event) and also from road traffic accidents caused by falling asleep while driving.

The major factor in OSA in adults is obesity; a major predictor for the development of OSA is a collar size greater than 17 inches. OSA is more common in men, who tend to have fat distribution patterns that favour the neck and chest. As with other sleep disorders, sedatives such as alcohol or antidepressants exacerbate the problem.

### Pathophysiology

Obstructive apnoeas occur during the deep stages of sleep; muscle relaxation in the upper airway causes

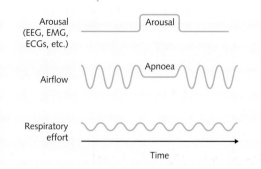

Arousal
(EEG, EMG,
ECGs, etc.)

Arousal

Airflow

Apnoea

Respiratory
effort

Time

**Fig. 61.1** Schematic diagram of apnoea.

complete airway collapse. The apnoea results in a drop in oxyhaemoglobin and a rise in $CO_2$. These changes are quickly detected by chemoreceptors, which increase central stimulation causing arousal and 'lightening' the stage of sleep. This leads to restoration of muscle tone and opens the airway thus restoring oxyhaemoglobin levels. This process may occur many times during the night leading to disturbed sleeping patterns (Fig. 61.1). A second effect is a chronic increase in negative intrathoracic pressure leading to increased pulmonary and systemic resistance and an increase in cardiac workload.

## Clinical presentation

Most patients are male and many are obese. The majority of patients with OSA are heavy snorers during the lighter stages of sleep. This is usually the presenting complaint. Sleeping partners may also volunteer that they appear to 'stop breathing' during sleep. The most obvious effect of OSA is to cause daytime somnolence; the patient reports that they never feel rested. They may also report headaches and falling asleep at inappropriate times, e.g. while driving, stopped at traffic lights or during meetings at work.

Chronic OSA may also produce serious cardiovascular complications such as hypertension, cor pulmonale and right heart failure and it is important to ask about these.

## Diagnosis

In the work-up of any patient with a history suggesting sleep apnoea the following are important:

## Physical factors

- General: weight, collar size, BMI, BP.

- ENT:
  - Dental malocclusion – retrognathia or mid-face hypoplasia
  - Nasal obstruction – septal deviation, polyps, rhinitis, etc.
  - Oropharyngeal obstruction – tonsillar enlargement, lax soft palate
  - Pharynx – excessive fat deposition in walls, collapse on inspiration
  - Larynx – any obstruction, e.g. cysts, papillomas.

## Medical investigations

FBC, TFTs, CXR, ECG.

## Polysomnography

This is the gold standard for the diagnosis of OSA. It is both expensive and time consuming. The patient is admitted to a sleep laboratory and during sleep the following parameters are generally measured:

- EEG – detects stage of sleep.
- EMG – detects limb movements.
- ECG.
- Airflow – at nose and lips.
- Abdominal and chest movements.
- $O_2$ saturation.
- Body position monitor – detects prone, supine, etc.
- Audio recording of snoring.

An obstructive apnoea is defined as cessation of breathing for 10 seconds or more with attempted respiratory effort. A hypopnoea is a decrease in airflow >50%. These are combined to give a score of events/hour known as the apnoea/hypopnoea index (AHI).

### Grading of OSA

AHI 5–20 = Mild OSA.
AHI 20–40= Moderate OSA.
AHI >40 = Severe OSA.

Less expensive and more convenient is a home sleep study which is essentially pulse oximetry. It is not as sensitive as polysomnography but may be useful for screening.

## Sleep nasoendoscopy (SNE)

This is generally performed on patients with snoring or mild OSA prior to surgical intervention. The patient is lightly sedated and allowed to drift off to sleep.

Observation with a flexible naso-endoscope during snoring helps to pinpoint the site of collapse. This may be at the soft palate, pharynx or tongue base or a combination of the three. It is also worthwhile attempting a jaw thrust manoeuvre – if snoring is relieved by this the patient may be helped by a simple mandibular repositioning splint.

## Management of sleep disordered breathing

### General

- It is vitally important that all patients are encouraged to lose weight and take regular exercise. In the obese patient other interventions will fail if they continue to put on weight. If necessary they should be referred to a dietician. In the morbidly obese consider referral to a bariatric (weight loss) surgery team.
- Obvious ENT abnormalities such as nasal blockage from a grossly deviated septum or obstructing tonsillar enlargement should be corrected, especially in the non-obese patient.
- Continuous positive airway pressure (CPAP) – moderate to severe OSA is best treated with CPAP delivered overnight via a nasal mask (Fig. 61.2). This keeps the airway inflated and prevents collapse. It reverses daytime somnolence and cardiovascular side effects. Compliance is, however, around 50%.
- Mandibular advancement appliances. These are custom-made dental splints that are worn over

the teeth at night. They advance the mandible, performing a 'jaw thrust' and pulling the tongue base and soft palate away from the pharyngeal wall. They may be helpful in snoring/mild OSA whether it occurs at the tongue base or soft palate.

### Surgery

- Snoring and mild OSA. Surgery is possible for snoring and mild OSA. It is guided by the findings of sleep naso-endoscopy. Most procedures are directed at the soft palate and oropharynx. These include laser-assisted uvulo-palatoplasty (LAUP) and uvulo-velo-pharyngo-palatoplasty (UVPPP) (Fig. 61.3). Both of these procedures produce scarring of the soft palate and increase its stiffness, making it less likely to vibrate. It is also conventional to remove the tonsils at the same time. Successful abolition of snoring occurs in around 90% immediately postoperatively; however, this drops to 50% at 3 years. It is notoriously painful and there is a risk of postoperative haemorrhage and nasopharyngeal incompetence. If the problem is at the tongue base, procedures that advance or reduce the tongue base may also be considered.
- Severe OSA. In these patients there is significant morbidity without treatment. In patients who cannot tolerate CPAP, tracheostomy may be curative. More extensive maxillo-mandibular advancement procedures are also becoming more popular, but this is major surgery. Bariatric surgical opinion should be considered.

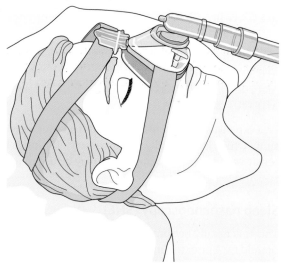

**Fig. 61.2** Nasal CPAP.

## OSA IN CHILDREN

Paediatric OSA is considered separately to adult OSA as the aetiology, symptomatology and treatment of this condition in childhood are completely different.

Unlike in adults there is usually an identifiable cause of airway obstruction and for the vast majority of children the cause is adeno-tonsillar hypertrophy. More rarely maxillary or mandibular disproportion may contribute, e.g. Down's syndrome or cranio-synostoses. Children with neuromuscular disorders may have severe sleep apnoea. The peak age for OSA in children is between the ages of 2 and 7 when the small size of the upper airway and lymphoid hyperplasia combine to cause airway obstruction.

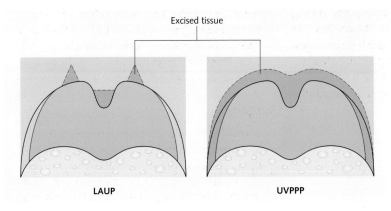

Excised tissue

LAUP                    UVPPP

**Fig. 61.3** LAUP and UVPPP.

Unlike adults with OSA, affected children are often small and thin due to the increased work of breathing and increased metabolic demands.

They may in severe cases demonstrate failure to thrive. However, increasing levels of obesity among children and teenagers may in the future lead to more obesity-related OSA in these age groups.

## Clinical presentation

Most children are brought in by parents who are worried by the child's breathing patterns during sleep. Most will mention snoring but also periods where there is cessation of breathing. Obstruction may vary and worsen if there is tonsillitis or upper respiratory tract infection. In children OSA does not cause daytime somnolence. Paradoxically OSA in children may cause bedwetting, night sweating, daytime hyperactivity and even conduct disorders.

Parents often describe other problems attributable to adeno-tonsillar hypertrophy such as blocked nose, rhinorrhoea, mouth breathing, etc.

## Diagnosis

- *Clinical examination.* There is usually obvious tonsillar enlargement and nasal blockage.
- *Sleep study* (more often a home study). It is common practice to obtain a confirmatory sleep study prior to treatment. This is mainly for risk stratification purposes. Children shown to have severe OSA preoperatively have an increased risk of anaesthetic complications after operation. They should not receive sedative premedication or opioid analgesics and should be nursed on a high dependency unit (or ITU) with oxygen saturation monitoring postoperatively.

## Management

In the vast majority of cases, paediatric OSA is cured by adeno-tonsillectomy. OSA is becoming one of the most common indications for this procedure.

Lumps in the neck are common and may represent a variety of pathological entities. These may range from simple reactive lymphadenopathy to malignant disease. Neck lumps can occur in all age groups. It is therefore essential to apply a thorough and methodological approach to their diagnosis. This is covered in Chapter 49.

## ANATOMY

Conventional anatomy teaching splits the neck into anterior and posterior triangles for descriptive purposes (Fig. 62.1). The boundary between the two is the sternomastoid muscle. Unfortunately many neck lumps occur along the jugular chain of lymph nodes which is underneath the sternomastoid and are therefore strictly speaking in neither the anterior nor the posterior triangle. Additionally increased use of imaging (CT/MRI) for staging of malignant neck disease demands a more accurate system of nomenclature.

The Memorial Sloan Kettering classification is slightly more complicated but more anatomically sound and easily applied to imaging findings (Fig. 62.2)

## DIFFERENTIAL DIAGNOSIS
(See p. 211)

It is first worth remembering that the neck is enveloped in skin and subcutaneous tissues and therefore 'normal' skin lumps such as sebaceous cysts and lipomas may occur in the neck as well. The surgical sieve is thoroughly covered on p. 211 but it is admittedly difficult to remember because of the number of conditions. A simpler alternative is to consider all neck lesions as a) midline or b) lateral neck masses.

### Midline neck masses

- Submental lymphadenopathy.
- Plunging ranula (see p. 262).
- Thyroglossal cyst (see p. 281).
- Thyroid mass (see p. 282).

### Lateral neck masses

- Salivary gland enlargement (see p. 263).
- Branchial cyst.
- Cystic hygroma.
- Carotid body tumour.
- Lymphadenopathy.
- Thyroid mass.
- Rarities – laryngocoele, pharyngeal pouch, dermoids.

## BRANCHIAL CYST

Branchial abnormalities are the result of failure of fusion along the line of the second branchial cleft. The branchial arches replicate the gill bars seen in fishes; in between them are the branchial clefts. In higher

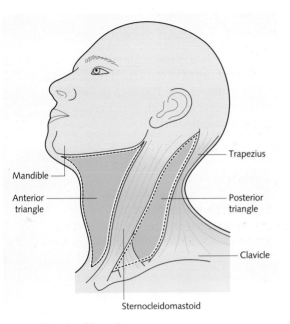

Fig. 62.1 Triangles of the neck.

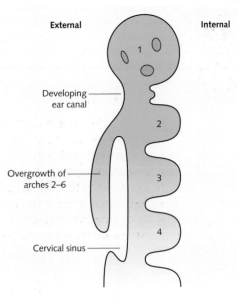

Fig. 62.3 Embryology of branchial anomalies.

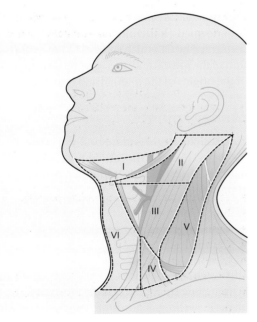

Fig. 62.2 Cervical lymph node levels.

animals these are overgrown in utero to form the smooth outline of the neck (Fig. 62.3). Failure of closure at the lower end of the cleft produces a branchial sinus. This is a small punctum seen at the lower end of the sternomastoid muscle which sometimes discharges mucus. A branchial fistula represents failure of fusion along the whole cleft and connects the skin of the neck with the pharynx. Closure of the upper and lower parts of the cleft and failure of fusion in the middle leads to a branchial cyst, the most common type of abnormality.

## Clinical presentation

These congenital lesions tend to present in late adolescence or early adulthood. Commonly they are asymptomatic smooth soft swellings emerging from under the upper part of the sternomastoid muscle. Sometimes they present as a result of secondary infection, usually at the time of respiratory infection, and are hot red and tender. The infection presumably spreads haematogenously.

Beware the diagnosis of branchial cyst in the middle-aged adult smoker. Cystic degeneration in a malignant lymph node is well described and may only be diagnosed after excision.

## Diagnosis

Diagnosis is based mainly on clinical history and examination. It is common to perform an ultrasound scan which can confirm the diagnosis. Any thickened or irregular areas in the cyst wall may be further sampled by ultrasound guided FNAC.

## Management

Surgical excision under general anaesthetic is the treatment of choice for these lesions.

## CYSTIC HYGROMA

This is another congenital lesion of the neck. It is commonly visible in utero and is the result of overgrowth of dilated lymphangiomatous vessels. Some lesions present later but always before 2 years. Unlike some haemangiomatous lesions they do not regress after birth and because of the cosmetic deformity they may cause are usually excised surgically.

### Clinical presentation

Many of these lesions are noted on routine anomaly scans during pregnancy. Some may be large enough to cause concern regarding airway post-delivery. They are most common on the neck (75%), usually around the craniocervical junction. They appear as large, soft, ill-defined, fluctuant masses which may transilluminate. Most are asymptomatic; if near the eye, however, they may cause amblyopia.

### Diagnosis

This is usually clinical. Supplementary evidence about other tissues involved is best done with MRI. This may, however, require a general anaesthetic.

### Management

Unilocular cystic areas may respond to injection with a sclerosant such as OK432. More commonly surgical excision is required. This may be performed soon after birth for simple lesions. However, if there is evidence of neurovascular involvement, e.g. facial nerve, then surgery may be delayed until the child is bigger (2 years). The aim of surgery is removal of all of the lesion if possible while avoiding neurovascular damage. This may require a full neck dissection in a small infant and is not for the inexperienced or occasional neck surgeon.

## CAROTID BODY TUMOUR

This lesion is a paraganglionoma of the carotid sinus. It is formed in the neural tissue of the carotid body chemoreceptor. It is seen in the elderly and is more common at altitude (presumably as a result of increased stimulation).

Rule of 10s: 10% are familial, 10% bilateral, 10% malignant and 10% secrete catecholamines.

### Clinical features

These tumours most often present as slow-growing firm masses in the upper part of the neck ('potato tumours'). They are said to be mobile horizontally but not vertically and they may have a bruit.

### Diagnosis

The diagnosis is often not suspected until ultrasound is performed (hopefully before FNAC!). It may be confirmed by CT which shows a lesion at the bifurcation of the carotid and angiography showing splaying of the origins of the internal and external carotids.

### Management

Most lesions are excised surgically; it is usually possible to peel them off the carotid vessels. In elderly frail patients observation or radiotherapy may be more appropriate.

## CERVICAL LYMPHADENOPATHY

This catch-all title hides a vast range of diagnoses. Lymph node enlargement is the most common cause of neck swelling. Causes of lymphadenopathy are listed in Fig. 62.4.

### Anatomy of the cervical lymphatic chain

Lymph from the various tissues of the head and neck drains initially to superficial lymph node groups and thence to the deep cervical chains which surround

**Fig. 62.4** Causes of lymphadenopathy

Reactive lymphadenopathy – infection or inflammation anywhere within the head and neck but especially ears, nose, paranasal sinuses, oral cavity, teeth, tonsils

Infective lymphadenitis:
Viral – EBV, HIV, herpes simplex
Bacterial – TB, atypical TB, cat scratch disease
Spirochaetal – syphilis
Parasitic – toxoplasmosis

Inflammatory lymphadenitis:
Sarcoidosis, rheumatoid arthritis, SLE

Neoplastic:
Metastatic squamous carcinoma
Lymphoma
Leukaemias
Thyroid and salivary metastases
Others, e.g. gastric adenocarcinoma, lung

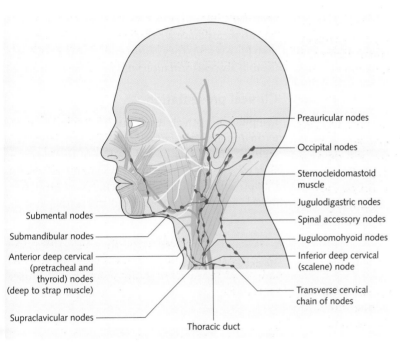

**Fig. 62.5** Cervical lymph nodes.

Preauricular nodes
Occipital nodes
Sternocleidomastoid muscle
Jugulodigastric nodes
Spinal accessory nodes
Juguloomohyoid nodes
Inferior deep cervical (scalene) node
Transverse cervical chain of nodes

Submental nodes
Submandibular nodes
Anterior deep cervical (pretracheal and thyroid) nodes (deep to strap muscle)
Supraclavicular nodes
Thoracic duct

the internal jugular veins (Fig. 62.5). The deep cervical chain on the right side ends in the junction of the internal jugular and subclavian veins; on the left side it joins the thoracic duct.

## GRANULOMATOUS LYMPHADENOPATHY

This is granulomatous inflammation with characteristic epithelioid giant cells occurring within the

Never forget that intrathoracic, breast, abdominal and even pelvic malignancy may present initially with a supraclavicular lymph node, especially on the left side – a so-called Virchow's node.

lymph nodes. It is of course a histological diagnosis. Conditions causing granulomatous lymphadenitis include tuberculosis (tuberculous adenitis), atypical mycobacterial infection, cat scratch disease and sarcoidosis.

## Tuberculous adenitis

TB infection still remains common and is actually increasing in prevalence in Western countries. Mycobacterial adenitis represents reactivation of dormant tubercle bacillae in the lymph glands It is more common in immigrants from the Asian subcontinent, the immunosuppressed and lower socioeconomic groups. It is most often seen in adults. BCG vaccination confers protection but is not 100% effective.

### Clinical presentation

TB adenitis typically appears as bilateral, progressive, often massive lymphadenopathy, usually in the supraclavicular region or the posterior triangle. There may be multiple lymph nodes affected and they may be 'matted' together and quite firm. Affected lymph nodes may show suppuration (collar stud abscess) but characteristically there is little inflammatory response; the lack of erythema, heat and pain has led to the term 'cold abscess'.

### Diagnosis

TB is difficult to diagnose due to the fastidious nature of the mycobacterium. It may take up to 6 weeks to grow in culture:

- *CXR.* Upper lobe fibrosis or other signs of previous pulmonary TB.
- *Purified protein derivative (PPD) or tuberculin testing.* A negative reaction makes TB unlikely.
- *US and FNAC.* Sufficient material may be gained for microbiology or identification of acid fast tubercle bacilli (AFBs) by this route. However, finding tubercle bacilli is rare and impatience often sets in while waiting for culture results; this leads to more invasive procedures being undertaken.
- *Open node biopsy.* If there is a high clinical suspicion of TB then open node biopsy may be undertaken. Half the node should be sent for culture and half for histology (looking for AFBs, granulomata, giant cells and caseation).

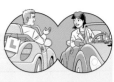

If there is any suspicion of squamous carcinoma open biopsy is contraindicated (see later). Perform a FNAC first.

### Management

Management is with anti-tuberculous chemotherapy continued for 6 months.

## Atypical mycobacterial infections

Infection caused by other mycobacteria such as *Mycobacterium avium-intracellulare* is less severe than that seen with typical TB; however, it may also be less responsive to antimicrobial therapy. Unlike typical TB, 'atypicals' have a tendency to infect young children (1–6 years). They cause cervical lymphadenopathy and abscess formation with few systemic features.

### Clinical presentation

Lymphadenopathy is usually unilateral and confined to the pre-auricular, submandibular and submental regions. There may be induration of the overlying skin which often looks 'brawny'. Frank abscess formation with fluctuance may occur. There is often no pyrexia and the lesion feels cold and is not painful.

In any child with an obvious neck abscess who is playing happily and lets you examine the area without complaint think of atypical mycobacterial infection.

### Diagnosis

- FNAC (see TB above).
- Excision biopsy of a node may be required for diagnosis.

### Management

- Prolonged antimicrobials are required based on sensitivities.
- Occasionally areas of skin involvement need to be excised to allow resolution.

## Cat scratch disease

This is usually a mild self-limiting infection of children. It is caused by the bacterium *Bartonella henselae* which is passed from cats to humans in bites or scratches.

## Clinical presentation

There is usually a lump at the site of inoculation which settles spontaneously. After 2–3 weeks this is followed by tender bilateral cervical lymphadenopathy and a mild fever. The lymph node enlargement may persist for 2–4 months and then resolves.

## Diagnosis

The diagnosis is often based on the history of cat exposure along with serological testing. Occasionally it is revealed on excision biopsy and histological demonstration of characteristic granulomata.

## Management

Management is supportive.

## TOXOPLASMOSIS

The causative organism is *Toxoplasma gondii* passed to human by ingestion of infected cat faeces or under-cooked meat.

## Clinical presentation

It may cause a generalized lymphadenopathy in an otherwise well child. The lymphadenopathy is bilateral, occasionally tender and may persist for months.

## Diagnosis

The diagnosis is based on serology for specific antibody estimation or polymerase chain reaction (PCR).

## METASTATIC SQUAMOUS CARCINOMA

Squamous carcinoma is the most common type of upper aero-digestive tract malignancy. Like all squamous carcinomas it tends to spread to local lymph node areas rather than produce distant metastases.

Spread is relatively predictable for each primary site and mostly occurs in a stepwise fashion, involving adjacent lymph node groups one after the other. Depending on the location of the metastatic lymph node one can predict the likely primary site (Fig. 62.6). Likely head and neck primary sites include larynx, oral cavity, tonsil, nasopharynx and laryngopharynx.

It is worthwhile remembering that some intrathoracic, abdominal and even testicular cancers may present with supraclavicular lymphadenopathy (Virchow's node). FNAC will help to differentiate many of these adenocarcinomas.

Around 10% of all upper aero-digestive tract SCCs present with metastatic lymph nodes and no clinically visible tumour on inspection, the so-called occult primary.

## Clinical presentation

There is progressive painless unilateral (at first) lymphadenopathy. The patient is usually in their 6th or 7th decade and they are nearly always a smoker. The lymphadenopathy is characteristically rock hard. There may be obvious symptoms of the primary cancer, e.g. hoarseness, dysphagia, alternatively the primary sites may be asymptomatic. Weight loss and generalized cachexia may occur. Marked cachexia is most often seen with oesophageal and gastric malignancies.

## Diagnosis

- US – key features suggesting malignancy (though not necessarily SCC) are:
  - Size >1.5 cm
  - Shape. Normal =rugby ball shaped. Cancer = football shaped.
  - Chaotic blood flow on Doppler imaging
  - Loss of normal lymph node anatomy.
- FNAC – may be diagnostic in the majority of cases and helps differentiate other pathologies, e.g. lymphoma, adenocarcinoma.
- Examination of entire upper aero-digestive tract – flexible and rigid endoscopy.
- CT scanning may be useful in suggesting a primary site and in staging disease.
- Positron emission tomography (PET) shows malignant disease and may be useful in identifying a primary site where this is not clinically obvious.

**Fig. 62.6** Lymph drainage pathways.

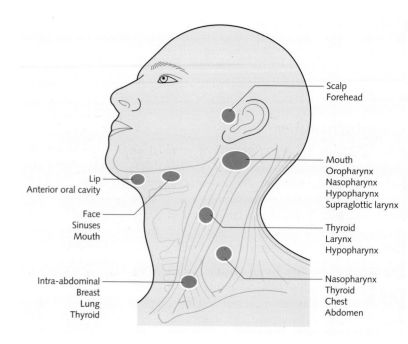

Scalp
Forehead

Mouth
Oropharynx
Nasopharynx
Hypopharynx
Supraglottic larynx

Thyroid
Larynx
Hypopharynx

Nasopharynx
Thyroid
Chest
Abdomen

Lip
Anterior oral cavity

Face
Sinuses
Mouth

Intra-abdominal
Breast
Lung
Thyroid

Open node biopsy in squamous malignancy is contraindicated. It may seed tumour into the skin and it also interferes with the predictable lymph drainage patterns on which neck dissection is based. It therefore increases the risk of a more major resection and reconstruction and decreases the chance of cure.

## Management

The management involves eradication of neck disease in combination with the treatment of the primary site. It may involve radiotherapy or more commonly surgery. Neck dissection is the therapeutic removal of all or part of the cervical lymphatic chain. It is often done at the same time as resection of the primary tumour. There are three main types of operation (Fig. 62.7).

1. Radical neck dissection removes all the lymph nodes of the anterior and posterior triangles plus the sternomastoid, accessory nerve and internal jugular vein. It causes marked postoperative shoulder morbidity with reduced movement and pain.
2. Modified radical neck dissection. Usually leaves the SCM, accessory and jugular intact.

3. Selective neck dissections. Remove the lymph node drainage areas for a particular drainage site while leaving most other structures intact, e.g. supra-omohyoid neck dissection for an oral malignancy.

## LYMPHOMA

Lymphomas are malignancies of the haematopoietic system and particularly the B and T lymphocytes. They may involve lymph nodes (nodal) and also extranodal sites (e.g. liver and bone marrow). The most common presenting complaint is cervical lymphadenopathy. They are often split into Hodgkin's (HL) and non-Hodgkin's lymphoma (NHL). After squamous carcinomas lymphomas represent the second most common type of malignancy in the head and neck. They are particularly common in immunosuppressed patients.

### Clinical features

Lymphoma can affect all age groups from childhood onwards. HL has a bimodal age distribution, the first peak being in the range of 15–35 years. NHL increases in frequency with age, many patients being elderly. Males are affected more frequently than females (3:1).

Although both Hodgkin's and non-Hodgkin's lymphomas cause neck masses, they are more common

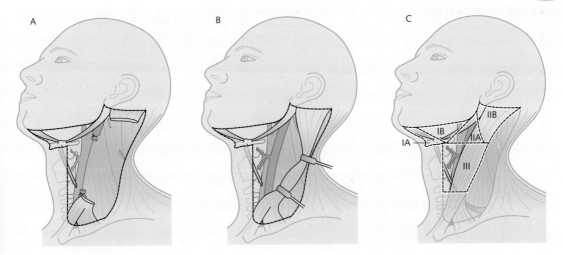

**Fig. 62.7** Types of neck dissection. (A) Radial neck dissection. (B) Modified radial neck dissection. (C) Selective neck dissection.

in the former. Classically there is rapidly increasing painless lymphadenopathy. Common sites are supraclavicular and lower deep cervical nodes. The nodes may be multiple and are described as rubbery hard. Alcohol sometimes causes the nodes to become painful. NHL may cause enlargement within Waldeyer's ring (e.g. unilateral tonsillar enlargement).

In any patient with a neck lump remember to ask about the 'B' symptoms of fever, weight loss, night sweats and pruritis. Full examination may reveal lymphadenopathy at other sites and occasional hepatosplenomegaly.

## Diagnosis

- US and FNAC. Cytology is still important even when lymphoma is suspected clinically. Before proceeding to open node biopsy a FNAC should be carried out to exclude a squamous carcinoma (see above).
- Open node biopsy. Full diagnosis and staging relies upon a thorough histological examination of the architecture in an affected lymph node. Excision biopsy of an entire node is therefore required.
- CT. It is common practice to perform a staging CT of the head, neck, chest, abdomen and pelvis.
- 'Lymphoma panel'. Other investigations such as LFTs, LDH and bone marrow aspiration are normally undertaken once the diagnosis has been established by biopsy. They are used to stage the disease.

## Management

The management of lymphomas is complex and is outside the scope of this book. It is usually either with external beam radiotherapy or chemotherapy. Excellent cure rates are achievable for many subtypes of lymphoma.

### Objectives

You should be able to:

- Say how different airway problems can affect children at different ages.
- Say what stridor is.
- Describe laryngomalacia.
- Give a brief account of paediatric vocal cord palsy and its presentation.
- Discuss subglottic stenosis in the child.
- Discuss the two main causes of infective stridor.
- Discuss croup.
- Discuss epiglottitis.
- Most importantly, describe the emergency management of children with croup or epiglottitis.

The common problems in paediatric ENT surgery include tonsillar and adenoidal problems, otitis media and hearing loss. These are covered in the relevant chapters alongside the adult conditions.

Problems with the paediatric airway are by no means common. They are, however, extremely important. The rest of this chapter will be devoted to them. See also Chapter 50, Stridor.

## PAEDIATRIC AIRWAY PROBLEMS

Unlike the adult airway, which is at its narrowest at the level of the vocal folds, the paediatric airway is narrowest in the subglottic area at the level of the cricoid cartilage. At birth the airway in a normal neonate has a diameter of 5–7 mm; in preterm or low birth weight babies it may be even less than this.

A 1 mm increase in oedema circumferentially causes a 44% narrowing of the subglottis (Fig. 63.1). However, if we consider air flow, this reduces by 80%. The paediatric airway is therefore tenuous at the best of times and airway collapse may happen quickly with disastrous consequences.

### Stridor

Stridor is monophonic musical airway noise produced by partial obstruction of the upper airway. It is a sign that must always be taken seriously, especially in the child. The character of the stridor may determine the location of the obstruction. If it is at or above the vocal cords the noise is usually inspiratory, if in the intrathoracic trachea the stridor is expiratory, and if in-between, e.g. cervical trachea, it may be both (biphasic).

### Causes of paediatric stridor

#### From birth/early infancy
- Laryngomalacia.
- Subglottic stenosis (congenital and acquired).
- Congenital laryngeal abnormalities (cysts, haemangiomas, webs, etc.).
- Recurrent laryngeal nerve (RLN) palsy.

#### Childhood
- Inhaled foreign body.
- Croup.
- Epiglottitis.
- Papillomatosis.

### Laryngomalacia

Laryngomalacia is the most common cause of stridor in infancy. It is essentially a developmental disorder affecting the cartilaginous structures of the larynx which makes it more 'floppy' than usual. The epiglottis and supraglottic structures have a tendency to collapse inwards on inspiration (Fig. 63.2).

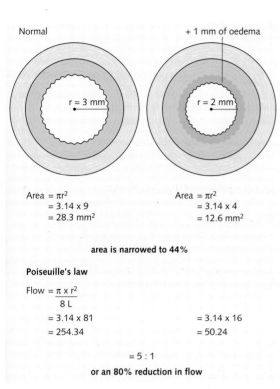

Normal

r = 3 mm

Area = πr²
     = 3.14 x 9
     = 28.3 mm²

+ 1 mm of oedema

r = 2 mm

Area = πr²
     = 3.14 x 4
     = 12.6 mm²

**area is narrowed to 44%**

**Poiseuille's law**

Flow = $\dfrac{\pi \times r^2}{8 L}$

     = 3.14 x 81                = 3.14 x 16
     = 254.34                   = 50.24

= 5 : 1

**or an 80% reduction in flow**

**Fig. 63.1** Physiology of airway obstruction.

## Clinical presentation

Laryngomalacia usually causes mild inspiratory stridor. The symptoms come on a few weeks after birth and mostly resolve by around 1 year. The stridor is worse when the baby is supine and when they are upset. A few babies have more severe problems with severe stridor, difficulty feeding and failure to thrive.

## Diagnosis

Flexible naso-endoscopy is easily tolerated in the neonate. It allows a beautiful view of the larynx and demonstrates the inward collapse of the airway in inspiration that is the hallmark of laryngomalacia.

## Management

Most cases require only reassurance that the child will grow out of the problem. The rare severe cases may be dealt with surgically by the operation of ary-epiglotto-plasty, which divides the tight ary-epiglottic folds and stops the epiglottis from being sucked into the airway.

## Subglottic stenosis

Narrowing in the region of the cricoid cartilage is called subglottic stenosis (Fig. 63.3). It occurs as both a congenital and an acquired type. It used to be

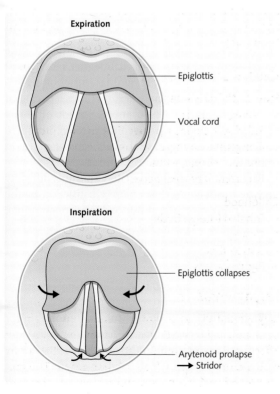

**Expiration**

Epiglottis

Vocal cord

**Inspiration**

Epiglottis collapses

Arytenoid prolapse
→ Stridor

**Fig. 63.2** Laryngomalacia.

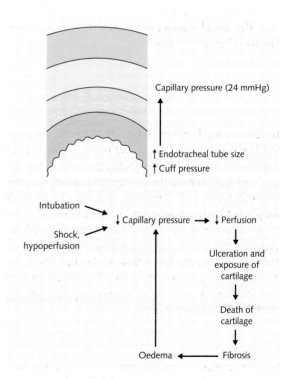

Capillary pressure (24 mmHg)

↑ Endotracheal tube size
↑ Cuff pressure

Intubation → ↓ Capillary pressure → ↓ Perfusion

Shock,
hypoperfusion

Ulceration and
exposure of
cartilage

Death of
cartilage

Oedema ← Fibrosis

**Fig. 63.3** Aetiology of subglottic stenosis.

thought that most cases were congenital in origin. It is now recognized that most are in fact the result of endotracheal intubation in a preterm infant.

Various factors are implicated in the aetiology of acquired subglottic stenosis. These include trauma and pressure from an endotracheal tube, infection, gastric reflux, and generalized hypoxia and shock. The most important factor in reducing the number of these problems has been a reduction in the size of endotracheal tubes used in neonates and the realization that it is better to accept a smaller tube with an air leak than to run the risk of subglottic stenosis.

### Clinical presentation

Congenital lesions may present with stridor shortly after delivery. They usually improve with growth. Acquired stenosis should be suspected in any child who presents with stridor and a previous history of intubation. Frequently these children do not present until they are older. There is often a history of recurrent stridor with upper respiratory tract infection; this is often misdiagnosed as croup.

### Diagnosis

Formal diagnosis really requires microlaryngoscopy under general anaesthesia to assess the subglottic area. Often the information is gained from the anaesthetist who is unable to pass an age-appropriate endotracheal tube into the trachea.

### Management

Many mild cases will settle with further growth. More severe cases may require surgical widening of the airway, a laryngotracheal reconstruction (LTR). The aim is to avoid prolonged tracheostomy.

## Paediatric vocal cord palsy

Bilateral vocal cord palsy may present in the neonate. There is usually stridor commencing shortly after birth, an abnormal cry and choking episodes. The paralysis may be transient and is often blamed on birth trauma. However, in some children it is associated with more widespread abnormalities of the brain and brainstem such as the Arnold–Chiari malformation.

### Diagnosis

- Flexible naso-endoscopy often reveals the problem.
- MRI of the brain and brainstem is carried out to look for underlying abnormality.

### Management

- *Tracheostomy* is usually required to secure the airway. This is a more hazardous procedure in the neonate than the adult and runs a risk of haemorrhage and damage to other surrounding structures, e.g. a pneumothorax.
- *Observation.* Many cases will resolve within 18 months. If there has been no improvement at 2 years the abnormality is likely to be permanent.
- *Surgery.* For the small number of children who do not recover function the aim of surgery is to remove the tracheostomy. Various procedures are used to 'lateralize' one vocal fold and improve the airway. This may have a deleterious effect on the voice.

## Foreign body in the airway

In any child with sudden-onset respiratory difficulty you must consider a foreign body. If there is a risk of this the child should undergo bronchoscopy under general anaesthetic.

### Clinical presentation

The child is usually less than 5 years old. Often the actual event may go unnoticed; however, parents will describe the following coughing and choking fits with some accuracy. There is sometimes a period of stridor and there may be cyanosis. Paradoxically by the time the child is assessed they frequently seem quite well. Rarely there are obvious signs of increased respiratory effort and audible stridor.

Late presentations do occur and the initial difficulty may be misdiagnosed as croup. Obstruction by the foreign body may later produce a lobar pneumonia, with hypoxia, fever and rigors. The site of obstruction is most often in the right main bronchus.

### Diagnosis

It is imperative that you have a high degree of suspicion in all children with respiratory distress.

Radiography may be helpful. Posterior-anterior (PA) and lateral chest films are required in both expiration and inspiration. In the early stages there may be hyperinflation of the affected lobe. Later collapse and lobar consolidation occur. The foreign body itself may also be visible.

## Management

Foreign bodies are removed via rigid bronchoscopy under a general anaesthetic.

## Infective causes of stridor

Infectious diseases account for a high proportion of cases of paediatric stridor. They tend to happen in early childhood and may occur in epidemics. The two most common causes are croup and epiglottitis.

## Croup (laryngo-tracheo-bronchitis)

This is a variable illness caused by infection with a parainfluenza virus or respiratory syncytial virus. It is most often a mild condition and only around 5% of patients are hospitalized.

### Clinical presentation

The child is usually aged between 18 months and 2 years. There is often a 2–3 day history of preceding URTI.

The main feature of croup is the characteristic cough. It is barking and often sounds like a seal.

Coughing fits may be followed by episodes of high-pitched inspiratory stridor. These are rarely severe enough to cause respiratory distress. The child is usually well between coughing/stridor attacks. The illness may last for 1–2 weeks.

### Diagnosis

The key to the diagnosis lies in hearing the characteristic cough.

### Management

- *Humidification*. Steam inhalation is unproven but usually advised.
- *Steroids*. More severe cases are treated with systemic corticosteroids with or without nebulized adrenaline.
- *Intubation*. Very rarely respiratory distress necessitates endotracheal intubation.

## Epiglottitis

This is a much more serious condition and is potentially lethal if mismanaged. It is seen in children and adults. It is caused by infection with *Haemophilus influenzae* type B (HIB). Owing to the immunization programme it is now rare in children. Infection of the structures of the supraglottis causes pain, difficulty swallowing and airway obstruction of rapid onset.

### Clinical presentation

Affected children are often aged between 1 and 5 years. This is an illness with a rapid onset. There is often throat pain and the child drools saliva. Stridor is prominent and is often severe and accompanied by obvious respiratory distress. The child sits upright with their chin protruding and uses their accessory muscles of respiration. They look unwell and are markedly pyrexial.

### Diagnosis

The diagnosis is based on the history and clinical features.

### Management

If you suspect that a child has epiglottitis do not try to examine the mouth or the airway. Try to prevent the child from becoming upset as crying may precipitate airway occlusion. *This is an emergency!*

Epiglottitis is an emergency:

- Do not examine the airway or otherwise upset the child. Let them sit on a parent's lap.
- Give humidified $O_2$ by getting the parent to hold it beneath the child's chin.
- Call for help from a senior anaesthetist, paediatrician and ENT surgeon.
- The child should be transferred quickly and quietly to a safe area (usually the operating theatre) where they are intubated with a surgeon standing by to perform an emergency tracheostomy if required.
- Once the airway is secured treatment is with high dose intravenous antibiotics.

**Objectives**

By the end of this chapter you will know very little more about history taking than you did at the start. That is because it is almost impossible to teach history taking in a book. You should listen, use Fig. 64.1 to guide your enquiries, and practise.

A detailed history is of paramount importance, as in all aspects of medicine. Despite what you may think, it is good listening that most often provides the diagnosis. It is important to the patient to describe their symptoms in their own words, but it is equally important for you to guide them appropriately and to clarify the history if necessary. The history should follow the same scheme as for a standard surgical clerking. This should include the following headings:

- Patient details.
- Presenting complaint.

**Fig. 64.1** Symptoms to ask about in history taking

| Ears | Hearing loss, discharge, tinnitus, vertigo, otalgia, facial weakness, headache |
|------|--------------------------------------------------------------------------------|
| Nose/paranasal sinuses | Nasal blockage, rhinorrhoea, sneezing, loss of smell, facial pain, bleeding, facial numbness, headache |
| Nasopharynx | Nasal blockage, snoring, unilateral hearing loss, epistaxis |
| Oral cavity | Pain, dysarthria, swallowing difficulty, snoring |
| Pharynx/upper oesophagus | Dysphagia, choking, pain, weight loss, hoarseness, haematemesis |
| Lower oesophagus | Dysphagia, odynophagia, reflux, heartburn, weight loss |
| Larynx | Hoarseness, stridor, cough, haemoptysis, dysphagia |
| Salivary gland | Swelling with meals, pain, bad taste, facial weakness |
| Thyroid | Swelling, pain, dysphagia, stridor, hoarseness, hypo- and hyperthyroid symptoms |

- History of presenting complaint.
- Past medical history including drug history.
- Systematic enquiry.
- Family and social history.

## SYSTEMATIC ENQUIRY IN THE ENT PATIENT

For each different area within the head and neck there are symptoms that suggest disease in that area. Once you have decided from the history which area or areas you are interested in, then focus on these areas by asking about the relevant symptoms. Doing this well comes with practice. At first I would suggest taking a copy of Fig. 64.1 as a guide and asking about everything . Once you become more experienced you will be able to zoom in on what is likely to be relevant and what is not.

It is always wise in an ENT history to ask about other related areas. For example, in a patient with ear problems ask about the nose and sinuses, etc.

Obviously there are more symptoms than shown in Fig. 64.1 but these are covered in more detail with the individual disorders.

# Examination of the ENT patient

## Objectives

You should be able to develop your own format for examining:

- The ears and hearing.
- The vestibular system.
- The nose and sinuses.
- The oral cavity.
- The neck.
- The thyroid gland.

For many students, examination of the ears, nose or throat is something they dread. Lack of familiarity with the terrain breeds fear. As in all branches of medicine practice pays dividends. Examiners will usually forgive a wrong diagnosis but are less tolerant of clumsy, inappropriate or, worst of all, painful examination technique. Practise examining these areas in all the patients you see whether surgical or medical and you will soon become competent.

Even when you are focusing on small areas, try to assess the patient as whole and do not forget that ENT patients may have systemic disease masquerading as head and neck pathology.

## GENERAL EXAMINATION TIPS

Most examinations in ENT involve looking down deep, dark, often mysterious holes. Good lighting is essential. The cornerstone of the ENT armamentarium is the head mirror. It is likely that in the near future improvements in fibreoptic and battery-powered head lights will consign mirrors to the museum. However, at the present time they are still in widespread use and you will need to learn how to use one (Fig. 65.1). The light source is positioned just behind and to one side of the patient. Position the head mirror on your head so that your right eye is looking out through the hole. Next look at the area in question, point the light source at your mirror, and then, by tilting the mirror, you should be able to reflect the light on to the right spot. (If you think that is difficult remember they used candles in the old days!)

One question that every student asks when preparing for clinical exams is 'should I talk while examining the patient or not?' There is nothing wrong with providing a running commentary as long as it is the right one! A good tip is to talk while examining and then at the end to summarize your findings formally. This allows you the chance to mention everything you find while being able to withdraw any more fanciful statements you may have made in the heat of the moment.

## EXAMINATION OF THE EAR

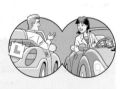

In an exam use the following format (it is explained in greater detail below):

- Introduce yourself.
- Ask: Which is your better hearing ear? Do you have any pain or tenderness?
- Test the hearing clinically.
- Tuning fork tests.
- Examine the ear with a head mirror.
- Examine the ear with an otoscope.
- Offer to examine the post-nasal space and perform a clinical examination of the cranial nerves (in an exam this will rarely be required).

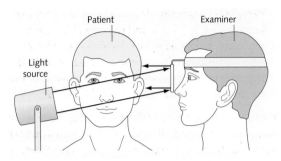

Fig. 65.1 Using the head mirror.

## Test the hearing clinically

Clinical hearing tests have mostly been replaced by widely available audiometric tests. You may still be asked to assess the hearing clinically in an exam. This takes a lot of practice to do smoothly. Explain to the patient what you are about to do. 'I am going to test your hearing. I will say some words/numbers into your ear. If you can hear them I would like you to repeat them back to me.'

- Sit to one side of the patient and test the better ear first. For the left ear use your right hand to reach behind the head and gently rub the tragus of the opposite ear to prevent any sounds being heard in the non-test ear. Use your other hand to shield your mouth so the patient cannot lip read.
- Two-syllable words (called spondees), e.g. 'cowboy', 'bluebell', or alternatively numbers are used. Numbers are easier in the heat of an exam.
- Pronounce the words at whispered voice level (WV), conversational level (CV), and loudly (LV) and at varying distances from the test ear (15 cm and 60 cm).
- Start with the most difficult (WV 60 cm, then WV 15 cm, CV 60 cm, CV 15 cm). Keep going until the patient repeats the spondee correctly on two occasions Record the best result for each ear.

| Interpreting the results | 60 cm | 15 cm |
|---|---|---|
| WV | 30 dBHL* – normal | 30–70 dBHL |
| CV | 30–70 dBHL | 30–70 dBHL |
| LV | >70 dBHL | >70 dBHL |

* Decibels hearing level.

## Tuning fork tests

In the assessment of hearing a 512 Hz tuning fork is used (it is written on the neck of the fork). The tone produced (middle C) is supposed to be readily heard by the human ear while at the same time producing minimal vibration, which may be sensed by proprioception even when the sound is not heard.

Practise sounding the fork either by gently 'twanging' the fork or by striking it gently on your elbow or the side of your shoe (the patient's head is not a substitute!).

Remember that normally sounds that are transmitted through the air (air conduction or AC) are heard better than those transmitted through bone (bone conduction or BC). So AC>BC.

There are two commonly used tests that you need to be familiar with: Weber's lateralizing test and Rinne's test (Figs 65.2, 65.3).

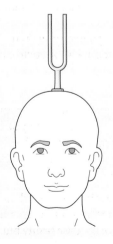

Fig. 65.2 Weber's lateralizing test. Radiates to the better ear in sensorineural hearing loss and to the worse ear in conductive hearing loss.

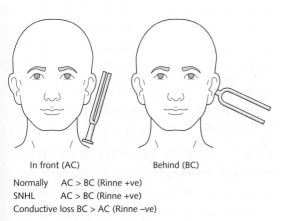

In front (AC)          Behind (BC)

Normally      AC > BC (Rinne +ve)
SNHL          AC > BC (Rinne +ve)
Conductive loss BC > AC (Rinne –ve)

**Fig. 65.3** Rinne's test.

## Weber's lateralizing test

To perform Weber's test sit in front of the patient and explain what you are about to do. 'I am going to place this tuning fork on top of your head. Tell me if you hear it louder in your left ear, your right ear or whether the sound is in the middle.'

- Gently sound the tuning fork and place it in the midline of the head at the vertex as shown (see Fig. 65.2). Normal (binaural) hearing results in a sound that that is heard in the middle. In a sensorineural loss (as you would expect) the sound is louder in the good ear.
- Where it gets slightly tricky is that when you have a conductive hearing loss, the affected ear hears bone-conducted sounds (BC) better than normally, and so Weber's test radiates to the bad ear.
- Try the test on yourself and then stick a finger in your ear to produce a conductive loss.

## Rinne's test

Rinne's test is easy! Again sit in front of the patient. Explain the test. 'I am going to put this tuning fork in front of your ear and then behind your ear. Listen to both the sounds and tell me which is the louder. In front or behind.'

- Testing each ear in turn, sound the tuning fork and place it first around 3 cm from the meatus and then place the base firmly but gently on the mastoid process behind the ear (see Fig. 65.3). If necessary prompt the patient with 'in front or behind?'

- Remember normally air conduction is better than bone (AC>BC). This is still the case if there is a sensorineural hearing loss. However, in an ear with a conductive loss, bone conduction, which bypasses the normal vibrating mechanisms of the ear, is better than air conduction (BC>AC).

In order to make sense of these tests they need to be considered together. Weber's test tells you whether there is a difference between the ears, and Rinne's' test whether that difference is due to a conductive or sensorineural hearing loss (Fig. 65.4).

## Inspection of the ear

You will need to use a battery-operated head light or head mirror/light combination to see adequately. The patient should be seated. You should sit with your eyes at the same level as the patient's ear. First look briefly from the front assessing symmetry – you may need to get the patient to move their hair out of the way. Next inspect the ears in turn from the side (see Fig. 65.5). Look for any redness and oedema of the outer ear. Inspect the skin in front of the ear looking for scars, sinuses or swellings.

Never miss the scar of an old mastoidectomy operation – bend the pinna forwards and look very carefully.

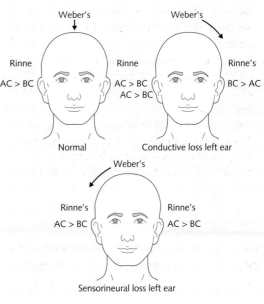

**Fig. 65.4** Putting the tests together.

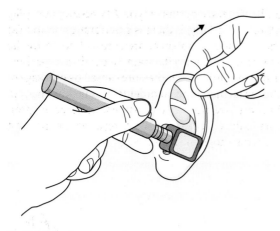

Fig. 65.5 Using the otoscope. Otoscopic examination of the right ear.

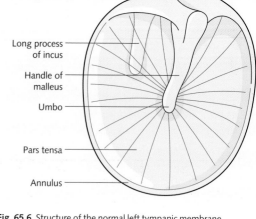

Fig. 65.6 Structure of the normal left tympanic membrane.

Examine the pinna looking for swelling, erythema or visible discharge from the canal. Grasping the pinna gently, fold it forward to inspect the skin behind the ear; again look for erythema, scars, sinuses or swellings.

## Otoscopy

Familiarize yourself with the otoscope – they really aren't as complicated as you think. They essentially comprise a light source and a magnified eyepiece to which are connected specula of various sizes. Hold it like a pen, in the left hand for the left ear and vice versa (Fig. 65.5).

Now the difficult bit: try and identify the features of the tympanic membrane (TM). Find the handle of the malleus and then work upward towards the pars flaccida; next trace the edge of the TM, known as the annulus, all the way around (Fig. 65.6). Observe the colour and concavity of pars tensa of the TM and note the location and size of any perforations, sucked in areas or discharge.

Seeing wax and crusty material deep down in the ear canal and on the tympanic membrane is abnormal. Lurking beneath it there may well be a large cholesteatoma. The only way to be sure is to use microsuction to remove the debris and re-inspect the ear.

# AUDIOMETRIC TESTS

## Pure tone audiometry (PTA)

This is what is commonly known as a hearing test. The PTA utilizes electronically generated sounds of varying frequency and intensity played to the patient either via air conduction using headphones or via bone conduction using a vibrating device on the mastoid. It relies upon the patient to respond when they hear a sound usually by pressing a button. It is thus not easily performed on young children. A population-based standard of hearing is used as a comparison, 0 decibels hearing level (dBHL) being perfect hearing. Obviously the worse the hearing loss the higher the intensity of the sound (in dBHL) before it is heard. As with tuning fork tests, air conduction should be better than bone conduction (AC>BC); if there is a conductive hearing loss BC may exceed AC and a consequent 'conductive gap' may be seen (Fig. 65.7).

## Tympanometry

This is an objective test of middle ear function. Its great advantage is it requires little by way of patient cooperation. Tympanometry seems complicated but is really quite simple. It measures the compliance or 'stretchability' of the tympanic membrane (i.e. its ability to move with changes in pressure; Fig. 65.8).

Think of the TM as a drum skin. It is most stretchable when it has not yet been stretched; in the

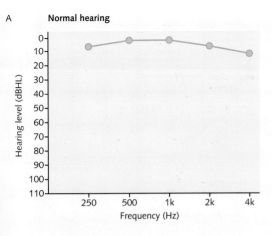

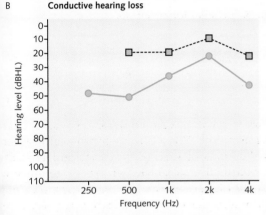

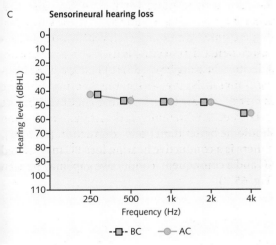

-□- BC    —●— AC

**Fig. 65.7** Pure tone audiogram.

and a flat trace occurs, a type 2 tympanogram (Fig. 65.8B). Similarly, if there is a perforation in the TM then changes in outer ear pressure will not move the TM, again creating a flat trace. In the third type there is negative middle ear pressure caused by blockage of the Eustachian tube. In order to get the drum back to its most 'stretchable' we must first decrease the pressure in the outer ear, thus creating a negative peak on the tympanogram (Fig. 65.8C).

## Other tests of hearing

> The ideal test of hearing should be objective, readily available and easily performed by non-specialists. This is particularly true if we consider screening tests for hearing loss in neonates and children.

Oto-acoustic emissions (OAE) testing is now readily available in a portable form and is increasingly popular for this purpose. A probe placed in the ear canal acts as a sound generator and a microphone records the minute changes in current generated by movement of hair cells in the cochlea in response to sounds.

Brainstem electrical response audiometry (BERA) is an objective assessment of the auditory pathways and is also used for screening of children. Electrodes on the scalp measure the minute electrical signals generated in the hearing pathways.

## EXAMINATION OF THE DIZZY PATIENT

### Examine the ears

The initial aim is to exclude pathology of the ears and therefore clinical examination of the ears and hearing should proceed as detailed above. Careful attention should be paid to the tympanic membrane in order to exclude suppurative middle ear disease as a cause. Pure tone audiometry should be performed in all patients as it is a good screening test for eighth nerve pathology.

normal ear the compliance is greatest when the pressure either side of it is equal, thus creating the peak of the type 1 tympanogram (Fig. 65.8A). If the middle ear fills with fluid (glue ear) the TM becomes stiff as the fluid cannot be compressed or stretched,

**Fig. 65.8** Tympanometry.

**Tympanometry**

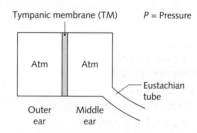

Tympanic membrane (TM)    P = Pressure

Atm    Atm

Eustachian tube

Outer ear    Middle ear

A  **Type I (normal) – the TM is most 'stretchable' when it hasn't been stretched**

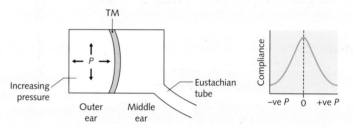

TM

Increasing pressure

← P →

Outer ear    Middle ear

Eustachian tube

Compliance

−ve P    0    +ve P

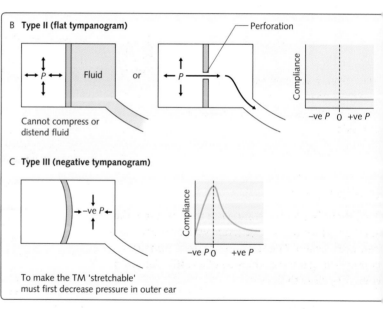

B  **Type II (flat tympanogram)**

Perforation

← P →    Fluid    or    ← P →

Cannot compress or distend fluid

Compliance

−ve P    0    +ve P

C  **Type III (negative tympanogram)**

→ −ve P ←

Compliance

−ve P 0    +ve P

To make the TM 'stretchable' must first decrease pressure in outer ear

## Neurological examination

A full neurological examination is very important in the patient who presents with vertigo. It is especially important to fully examine the cranial nerves.

Look particularly for nystagmus, testing all positions of gaze, remembering of course that nystagmus at the extremes of gaze may be a normal finding. Signs of trigeminal nerve dysfunction may be an early indicator of cerebellopontine angle pathology, the most sensitive early test being loss of the corneal reflex. Also look carefully for facial weakness resulting from eighth nerve dysfunction

# Clinical tests of vestibular function

## Observation of gait

This is a very useful functional assessment. Uncompensated vestibular lesions may result in the patient veering towards the affected vestibule. It is also useful to look for the characteristic gait abnormalities of other conditions, e.g. hemiplegia, Parkinsonism, peripheral neuropathy, etc. Ask the patient to walk heel to toe towards you while looking up at your face.

## Unterberger's test

The patient is asked to walk on the spot with their eyes closed and their arms outstretched for 30 seconds. If they rotate around more than 30° or move forward or backwards more than 1 m the test is abnormal, indicative of vestibular dysfunction.

Think of each vestibule like an aeroplane engine. If one engine is underperforming then the plane (patient) tends to veer to that side.

## Romberg's test

The patient is asked to stand with their feet together and their hands by their side, first with eyes open and then eyes closed. The test, if positive, results in the patient falling towards the side of a vestibular lesion when they close their eyes.

## Dix–Hallpike test

This is the diagnostic test for benign paroxysmal positional vertigo. The test is positive if nystagmus and vertigo are produced by a rapid change in the patient's position (Fig. 65.9).

## Medical examination

Cardiovascular examination may also be useful in the patient with dizziness. In particular the finding of an arrhythmia, postural drop in blood pressure or carotid bruit may lead to a non-otological diagnosis as an explanation for dizziness.

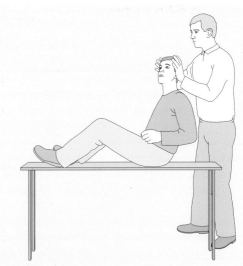

A　Patient sitting, head rotated 45° to one side

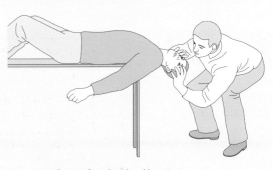

B　Rapidly transferred to 'head hanging' with test ear 45° down

**Fig. 65.9** The Dix-Hallpike test.

## EXAMINATION OF THE NOSE

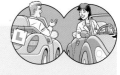

In an exam use the following format:

- Introduce yourself.
- Position yourself. Head light on. Eyes at level of patient's nose. Knees together and to one side of patient's knees.
- Inspect the external nose from in front and from the side.
- Perform a spatula misting test.
- Use a Thuddicum's speculum to examine the nose.
- Offer to use an endoscope (rarely required).
- Offer to examine the mouth, neck and assess facial sensation (rarely required).

## External examination

Examination of the nose begins with a formal inspection of the external nasal structure, keeping in mind the underlying skeletal and cartilaginous elements (Fig. 65.10). Examine from the front looking at the nasal skin, and at the nasal structure for asymmetry or other deformity. Then look from either side looking at the profile of the nasal skeleton and its projection. Finally, with the patient's head tilted slightly back, look from below at the base of the nose, the columella and the nasal apertures, it may be possible to see an obvious septal deviation at this stage.

Before proceeding to examine the inside of the nose it is usual to make a rough assessment of the patency of the nasal airways. There are two main methods. The first is to occlude each nostril from below with the thumb of one hand and ask the patient to breathe in gently through their nose. This is then repeated with the opposite nostril and opposite hand and the two sides compared.

The second method is the spatula misting test. Hold a chrome tongue spatula beneath the nostrils while the patient breathes through the nose. Misting of the metal surface reveals the airflow through each side. More formal assessment of nasal airflow is now available (see special tests later).

## Intranasal examination

Fibreoptic nasal endoscopes are now readily available and give an excellent view of the entirety of the internal nose. However, it is unlikely that you will be asked to use one and you will have to familiarize yourself with the less useful and more fiddly head light and nasal speculum examination shown below.

You will need a head light or head mirror. With the patient seated in front of you and their head tilted slightly back, the Thuddicum's nasal speculum is held as shown and the blades gently inserted into the nasal aperture (Fig. 65.11). It should be possible to inspect the nasal septum and particularly Little's area. With a little persistence you will see first the inferior turbinate laterally and above it the middle turbinate. Look carefully at the mucosa of the septum and turbinates – is it swollen, wet, or polypoid in nature? Polyps, if present, are often visible in the middle meatus between middle and inferior turbinates; they can be distinguished from the turbinates by their whitish, translucent appearance and often their lack of sensitivity to pressure.

An alternative method is to use a rigid nasal endoscope. These instruments can be carefully passed into the nose and give an excellent view. They may also be passed into the post-nasal space where the structures of the nasopharynx, including the Eustachian tube, orifices should be readily apparent.

## Special investigations

### Tests of nasal patency

There are many investigations designed to objectively record nasal blockage. Perhaps the most useful is nasal inspiratory peak flow (NIPF) which is readily measured and may show improvement with therapy. Acoustic rhinometry utilizes a technique similar to 'sonar'; sound waves are recorded as they bounce off structures within the nose. Blockage can be recorded, sides compared and the effects of therapy monitored.

**Fig. 65.10** The nasal skeleton.

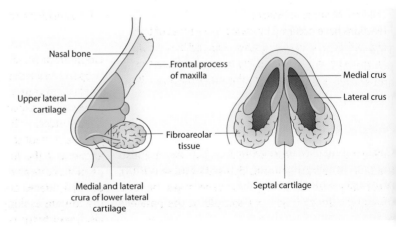

Nasal bone

Frontal process of maxilla

Medial crus

Lateral crus

Upper lateral cartilage

Fibroareolar tissue

Medial and lateral crura of lower lateral cartilage

Septal cartilage

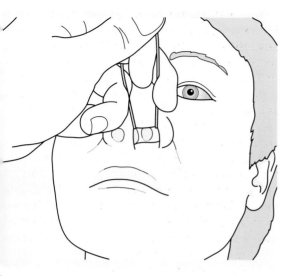

**Fig. 65.11** Using a Thuddicum's nasal speculum.

## Allergy testing

One of the most common nasal disorders is allergic rhinitis. The simplest test for allergy is the skin prick test. This involves the delivery of a small amount of allergen into the epidermis of the forearm using a needle. Ten potential allergens and two controls are conventionally used. Commonly used allergens include grasses, pollens, house dust mite, moulds, cat and dog fur. A positive test result is revealed as the typical wheal and flare reaction classically seen in a type 1 hypersensitivity reaction.

Due to its nature this test is unsuitable for very small children. Major anaphylactic reactions have occurred following these types of test and, although very rare, resuscitation facilities should be available. It is also necessary to stop antihistamine medication prior to testing as this may result in a false negative test result.

Several in vitro tests of hypersensitivity are also available. The most commonly used of these is *RAST* (*radioallergosorbant testing*) which measures the level of allergen specific IgE in a sample of the patient's serum.

Other tests used in nasal disease are listed below:

| Test | Used to test for … |
| --- | --- |
| Serum ACE (angiotesin converting enzyme) | Sarcoidosis |
| Serum ANCA (anti-neutrophilic cytoplasmic antigen) | Wegener's granulomatosis |
| Mucociliary biopsy | Mucociliary dysfunction, e.g. primary ciliary dyskinesia |
| Mucociliary clearance rate (of saccharine placed beneath turbinate) | Mucociliary dysfunction |
| Nitric oxide (nasal and pulmonary levels) | Rhinosinusitis |

## EXAMINATION OF THE ORAL CAVITY

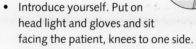

In an exam follow this format:
- Introduce yourself. Put on head light and gloves and sit facing the patient, knees to one side.
- Examine the lips externally.
- Ask the patient to open their mouth.
- Examine the mucous membranes systematically using a tongue spatula to retract the cheeks. Examine the tongue, labial, buccal and palatal mucosa. Remember if you see pathology always palpate the area.
- Examine the teeth. Note obvious disease and loose teeth.
- Examine the salivary glands.

Good illumination is essential to examine the mouth properly and either a head light or head mirror can be used for this purpose. Sit facing the patient and put on gloves. First inspect the outer aspects of the lips looking for ulcers or lumps. Next look inside the mouth. Get the patient to protrude their tongue; pay careful attention to the dorsal surface; note the normal surface papillae. Note any ulcers, white patches (leukoplakia) or depapillated areas. Examine the under-surface of the tongue looking specifically at the mucosa, and also identify the orifices of the submandibular ducts

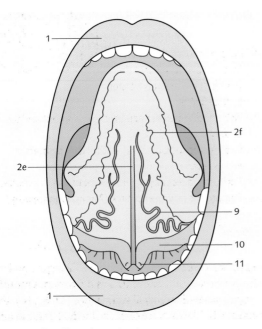

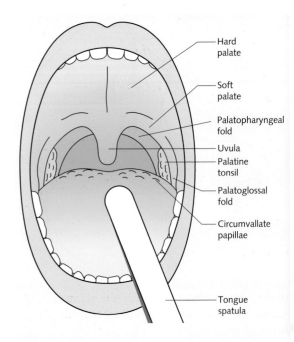

**Fig. 65.12** The sublingual area.

**Fig. 65.13** Examination of the tonsils.

as they empty either side of the lingual frenulum at the sublingual papillae (Fig. 65.12). Now examine the lateral borders of the tongue looking carefully for any abnormalities. If any ulcers or white patches are detected it is extremely useful to palpate them. The hard, 'craggy' feel of a malignant ulcer is completely different to the soft feel of aphthous oral ulceration.

It is important to look at the teeth and a dental mirror may be used to facilitate this. Be aware of the common annotation systems. Look at each tooth in turn for signs of decay (caries) and assess mobility by gently grasping the tooth and rocking it from side to side. At the same time look at the supporting gingivae for signs of inflammation (periodontitis).

The oral mucosa is often the site of disease ranging from inflammation through to neoplasia. It is very important to systematically examine the entirety of the oral mucosa. Look carefully at the buccal sulci and the hard and soft palates. Finally examine the tonsillar fossae and posterior tongue. A tongue depressor is useful for this (Fig. 65.13). Note the size, texture and symmetry of the tonsils. Enlargement is usually noted using the grading shown in Fig. 65.14.

Finally it is the submandibular and parotid salivary glands. The duct orifices lie on the sub-lingual papillae and opposite the upper second molar tooth. Note the quantity and quality of the saliva expressed looking carefully for suppuration. With a gloved finger placed inside the lingual sulcus and the other hand

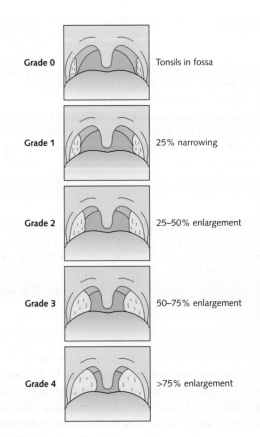

**Fig. 65.14** Grading of tonsil enlargement.

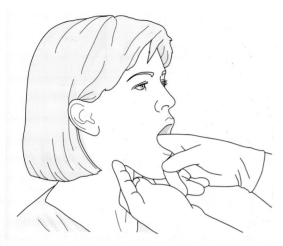

**Fig. 65.15** Bimanual palpation of the submandibilar gland.

under the mandible externally the submandibular glands may be bimanually palpated (Fig. 65.15).

## EXAMINATION OF THE LARYNX

When examining the patient with laryngeal symptoms it is important to bear in mind that extra-laryngeal disease may be the cause. It is important that you pay attention to any general signs of malignancy that may be present. Carefully examine the neck looking for thyroid disease or lymphadenopathy. Look also for scars from previous thyroid or neck surgery.

While you are introducing yourself to the patient ask them a question and take the opportunity to listen to their voice. Is it normal, hoarse or breathy? Ask the patient to take a deep breath in and out (listen for stridor) and to cough; a good cough is a reliable sign of good vocal cord adduction.

### Clinical examination of the larynx

The advent of the fibreoptic naso-endoscope makes the examination of the larynx easier for both patient and clinician alike. However, this technology is not available everywhere. It is important that you are able to examine the larynx by the more traditional method of indirect laryngoscopy.

In a exam follow this format:
- Introduce yourself. Ask the patient 'how are you?' Listen to their voice.
- Ask them to take a deep breath in and out and to cough.
- Expose and look carefully at the neck for scars, lumps, etc.
- Perform indirect laryngeal examination with a mirror.
- Palpate the larynx and neck (? lymphadenopathy).

### Indirect laryngoscopy (Fig. 65.16)

Wear a head light or a head mirror. Sit facing the patient with your eyes at the same level as the patient's mouth. Using a warmed laryngeal mirror (see Fig. 65.16), the tongue is held in a piece of gauze by the left hand and the mirror is gently inserted to lie against the soft palate. This should give you a mirror image view of the larynx. This takes practice but the sooner you start ….

### Fibreoptic naso-endoscopy (FNE)

This is fortunately much easier. The lubricated endoscope is passed via the nostril (some patients may require a spray of topical local anaesthetic). It passes below the inferior turbinate and via the nasopharynx to lie just above the larynx. It gives an excellent view of the vocal folds, larynx, tongue base and pharynx. It also allows functional assessment and can remain in place as the patient talks, sings, coughs and swallows.

Further specialized examination and investigation of the larynx is discussed in Chapter 59.

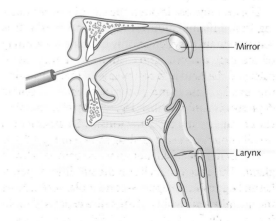

**Fig. 65.16** Indirect laryngoscopy.

## EXAMINATION OF THE NECK

It is extremely common in both clinical practice and medical examinations to be asked to examine the neck. You should develop a technique that is thorough and efficient. Unfortunately this, as usual, means that you will have to practise.

Follow the usual clinical process of inspection, palpation, auscultation.

In an exam follow this format:
- Introduce yourself and sit in front of the patient.
- Expose the neck down to the clavicles.
- Inspect in front and from the side.
- If you see a lump describe it in the usual terms (site, size, shape, etc.) and get the patient to swallow (to see if it moves, i.e. thyroid mass) and stick out their tongue (thyroglossal cyst).
- Then move behind the patient and palpate the neck, talking as you go.
- If you find a thyroid mass, give the patient a drink of water and get them to swallow while you palpate.
- If you find lymph nodes offer to examine axillae, groins, liver and spleen.
- Also say that you would perform a full head and neck and endoscopic examination to ascertain if there was a primary site.

Inspect the neck from in front and from either side. Note any skin lesions, scars or visible masses.

When palpating the neck for lumps (mainly lymphadenopathy) it is extremely important to develop a system. I would suggest starting at the angle of the mandible and then working down the sternomastoid muscle to the clavicle; then come up from the thyroid to the submental and submandibular area. Finally examine the posterior triangle from top to bottom, not forgetting the occipital nodes and the preauricular nodes (Fig. 65.17).

Most often the pathology that you will be seeking will be a mass in the neck. You should describe it as you would any mass, i.e. in terms of its site, size, shape, surface, etc. Depending on the position and likely aetiology of the mass then further manoeuvres may be appropriate. If you suspect a thyroid mass, movement with swallowing should be elicited; a thyroglossal cyst should move with tongue protrusion, a cystic hygroma should transilluminate, and a carotid body tumour should be pulsatile and may have a bruit.

If you find what you suspect is a neck swelling assess whether it is solitary or whether there is generalized lymphadenopathy. If you think there is generalized cervical lymph node enlargement, especially if it is suggestive of lymphoma (large, sometimes massive swelling which is usually multiple, often bilateral and characteristically rubbery to the touch), then tell the examiner you would like to examine the rest of the lymphoreticular system (other lymph node groups and liver and spleen). If it is solitary, suspicious or frankly cancerous (large, rock hard non-tender swelling), then explain that you would like to examine all of the drainage sites, i.e. perform a full head and neck examination including flexible endoscopy

## EXAMINATION OF THE THYROID GLAND

Again this frequent clinical problem is reflected as an equally frequent examination question.

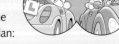

In an exam, if asked to examine the thyroid gland follow this plan:
- Introduce yourself and sit in front of the patient.
- Check the thyroid status.
- Look at the eyes and assess retraction, exophthalmos and lid lag.
- Inspect the neck.
- If there is a mass (and there nearly always is) then describe what you see. Ask the patient to swallow.
- Move behind the patient and palpate the thyroid. If there is a mass describe it. While palpating get them to swallow and assess movement.
- If there is a mass:
  - Palpate the neck carefully for lymphadenopathy (see above)
  - Auscultate for a bruit
  - Assess if it is retrosternal
  - Offer to examine the larynx for cord palsy.

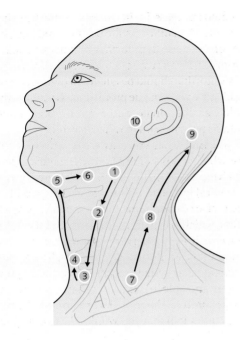

**Fig. 65.17** Schema for examination of the neck.

**Fig. 65.17** Schema for examination of the neck.

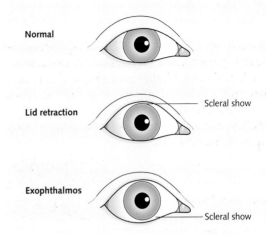

**Fig. 65.19** Dysthyroid eye disease.

## Assessment of thyroid function

Observe the patient, looking for the signs of thyroid dysfunction (Fig. 65.18).

Examine the hands; look for sweating and tremor. Palpate the radial pulses. Look at the small muscles of the hand and the fingers for wasting. Look carefully at the eyes and observe for the signs of dysthyroid eye disease (Fig. 65.19). Get the patient to follow your finger, ask them to report any double vision and at the same time observe for loss of ocular motility and lid lag. If there is gross exophthalmos it is worthwhile mentioning to the examiner that you would formally test the acuity and pupillary reflexes (don't worry – they won't make you do it!).

Offer to check the ankle jerk reflexes (again, don't worry – the examiner will politely decline).

## Examine the thyroid gland

Before rushing round behind the patient to examine their thyroid it is worth taking a few seconds to observe the thyroid area from the front. Bear in mind the local anatomy (Fig. 65.20). Look for any swelling or scars.

**Fig. 65.18** Signs of thyroid dysfunction

|  | Hyperthyroidism | Hypothyroidism |
|---|---|---|
| General appearance | Thin, agitated, sweaty | Obese, sluggish, peaches and cream complexion |
| Hair |  | Sparse coarse hair, loss of outer 1/3 eyebrows |
| CVS | Tachycardia, AF | Bradycardia |
| Hands | Small muscle wasting, tremor Thyroid acropachy | Puffy hands, 'spade like appearance' |
| Eyes | Exophthalmos, upper lid retraction, ophthalomoplegia | (NB 'Burnt out' Graves' disease have eye signs but are hypothyroid) |
| CNS | Agitation, restlessness Brisk reflexes | Slow movements, hallucination, dementia Slow-relaxing reflexes |

**Fig. 65.20** Local relations of the thyroid gland.

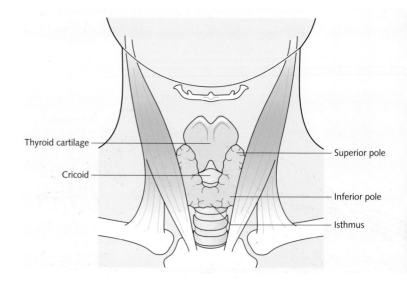

Thyroid cartilage

Cricoid

Superior pole

Inferior pole

Isthmus

Next stand behind the patient and palpate the thyroid gland while at the same time observing the contour of the patient's neck from above. Normally the thyroid is impalpable. Try to determine whether there is any generalized or localized enlargement. If you can feel a mass note its size, surface characteristics and texture. Try to ascertain if it is solitary or whether there are multiple lumps within the gland. Once you have identified a mass you need to confirm that it is within the thyroid gland. The thyroid being enveloped in pretracheal fascia moves on swallowing. Offer the patient a glass of water and ask them to hold a sip of it in their mouth. Again palpate the mass from behind and ask the patient to swallow – you should feel a thyroid mass elevate on swallowing. Auscultate over the mass with your stethoscope; you may find a bruit in hyperthyroidism (if you are lucky). If the mass is large you should attempt to locate its lower border; the easiest way to do this is to feel for the trachea below the thyroid and also try and insert a fingertip between the lower border of the gland and the sternum or clavicle. If you cannot then the thyroid is likely to extend retrosternally; you may be asked to percuss the upper thorax to try and determine its extent. Do not percuss the neck – it is not nice!

If you find a thyroid mass (and if you have not, then what have you been doing all this time?) it is essential that you do not forget to systematically check for associated cervical lymphadenopathy as detailed above.

A thyroid mass with palpable neck nodes is cancer until proven otherwise.

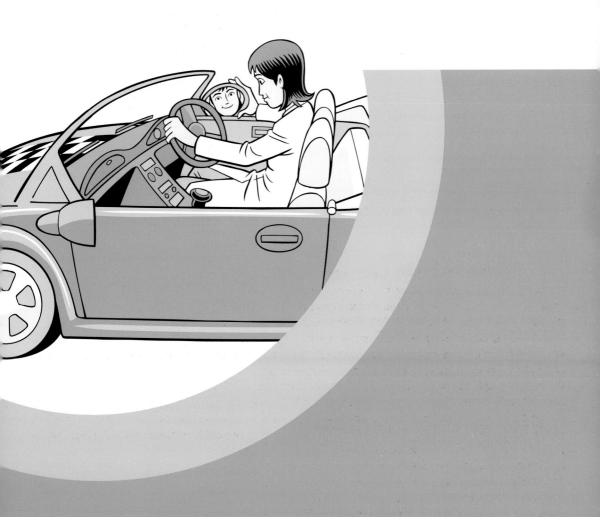

# SELF-ASSESSMENT

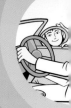

# Multiple-choice questions (MCQs)

Indicate whether each answer is true or false.

## Ophthalmology

1. **Conjunctivitis is associated with:**
   a. Dull, deep pain keeping patient awake at night.
   b. Itchy eyes.
   c. Posterior synechiae and irregular pupil.
   d. Scratchy, pink eyes.
   e. Sticky eyes.

2. **The following are associated with painful loss of vision:**
   a. Angle closure glaucoma.
   b. Anterior uveitis.
   c. Central retinal vein occlusion.
   d. Scleritis.
   e. Subconjunctival haemorrhage.

3. **Signs that are related to blunt ocular trauma include:**
   a. Hyphaema.
   b. Iritis.
   c. Traumatic mydriasis.
   d. Retinal tear.
   e. Vitreous haemorrhage.

4. **An inferior blow out fracture should be suspected when the following are present:**
   a. Crepitus.
   b. Enopthalmos.
   c. Numbness over ipsilateral eyebrow.
   d. Pain on eye movement.
   e. Diplopia on downgaze or upgaze.

5. **Common causes of gradual visual loss include:**
   a. Angle closure glaucoma.
   b. Blepharitis.
   c. Cataract.
   d. Posterior capsular opacification following cataract surgery.
   e. Refractive error.

6. **Symptoms related to gradual visual loss include:**
   a. Central scotoma.
   b. Floaters.
   c. Glare.
   d. Haloes.
   e. Nyctalopia.

7. **Painless loss of vision occurs following:**
   a. Acute angle closure glaucoma.
   b. Cataract.
   c. Central retinal vein occlusion.
   d. Primary open angle glaucoma.
   e. Diabetic maculopathy.

8. **Common causes of painful, sudden visual loss include:**
   a. Arteritic ischaemic optic neuropathy (giant cell arteritis).
   b. Central retinal vein occlusion.
   c. Keratitis.
   d. Scleritis.
   e. Wet age-related macular degeneration.

9. **Causes of binocular diplopia include:**
   a. Cranial nerve palsy (third, fourth or sixth).
   b. Iridectomy.
   c. Orbital cellulitis.
   d. Myasthenia gravis.
   e. Thyroid eye disease.

10. **Causes of proptosis include:**
    a. Lymphoma.
    b. Myasthenia gravis.
    c. Preseptal cellulitis.
    d. Thyroid eye disease.
    e. Wegener's granulomatosis.

11. **Causes of ptosis include:**
    a. Blepharitis.
    b. Cataract surgery.
    c. Horner's syndrome.
    d. Myasthenia gravis.
    e. Thyroid eye disease.

12. **Causes of epiphora due to compromise of lacrimal drainage include:**
    a. Allergic conjunctivitis.
    b. Facial nerve palsy.
    c. Medial ectropion.
    d. Nasolacrimal duct obstruction.
    e. Pterygium.

13. **Cataract is caused by:**
    a. Diabetes.
    b. Intrauterine infections.

c. Steroids.
d. Trauma.
e. Uveitis.

14. **Chloramphenicol antibiotic is used for the following conditions:**

    a. Corneal abrasion.
    b. Anterior uveitis.
    c. Herpetic keratitis.
    d. Perforating corneal injury.
    e. Recurrent corneal erosion syndrome with acute exacerbation.

15. **The following occur in primary open angle glaucoma:**

    a. Always raised intraocular pressure.
    b. Homonymous inferior quadrantanopias.
    c. Nerve fibre layer defect.
    d. Paracentral arcuate scotoma.
    e. Swollen optic disc.

16. **The following symptoms are suggestive of angle closure glaucoma:**

    a. Earache.
    b. Haloes of light.
    c. Nausea and vomiting.
    d. Photopsia.
    e. Rash on ipsilateral side of forehead.

17. **Treatments for glaucoma include:**

    a. $\alpha_2$ adrenergic agonist.
    b. β-blockers.
    c. Laser peripheral iridotomy.
    d. Prostaglandin analogues.
    e. Surgical trabeculectomy.

18. **Ocular diabetic changes lead to:**

    a. Macular oedema.
    b. New vessels elsewhere.
    c. Rubreosis.
    d. Tractional retinal detachment.
    e. Vitreous haemorrhage.

19. **A 39-year-old type 2 diabetic attends diabetic retinopathy screening. The following conditions require referral to the local ophthalmologist:**

    a. Background diabetic retinopathy with decrease in vision.
    b. Background diabetic retinopathy with macular changes.
    c. Background diabetic retinopathy with normal vision.
    d. Pre-proliferative retinopathy.
    e. Proliferative diabetic retinopathy.

20. **A myope has a sudden increase in floaters, photopsia and no visual field loss. His visual acuity is 6/5 in his affected eye. Likely differential diagnoses are:**

    a. Angle closure glaucoma.
    b. Posterior vitreous detachment.
    c. Retinal detachment – macular off.
    d. Retinal detachment – macular on.
    e. Superior retinal tear without retinal detachment.

21. **Giant cell arteritis can lead to:**

    a. Cupped optic disc.
    b. Double vision.
    c. Jaw claudication.
    d. Second eye involvement.
    e. Swollen optic disc.

22. **HIV infection can lead to the following ophthalmic manifestations:**

    a. Behçet's disease.
    b. Cytomegalovirus (CMV retinitis).
    c. Herpes zoster ophthalmicus (shingles).
    d. Kaposi's sarcoma.
    e. Necrotizing scleritis.

23. **Anterior uveitis is associated with the following:**

    a. Ankylosing spondylitis.
    b. Arteritic anterior ischaemic optic neuropathy.
    c. Cytomegalovirus retinitis.
    d. Rheumatoid arthritis.
    e. Ulcerative colitis.

24. **Causes of leukocoria include:**

    a. Coat's disease.
    b. Congenital cataract.
    c. Retinoblastoma.
    d. Retinopathy of prematurity.
    e. Rubella intrauterine infection.

25. **A baby suspected of amblyopia should have the following examinations performed:**

    a. Colour vision.
    b. Cover test.
    c. Cycloplegic refraction.
    d. Dilated eye examination.
    e. Visual fields.

26. **The following cause a cloudy cornea at birth:**

    a. Congenital glaucoma.
    b. Congenital rubella.
    c. Forceps assisted delivery.
    d. Neurofibromatosis.
    e. Von Hippel–Lindau disease.

27. **Causes of swollen discs include:**

    a. Anterior ischaemic optic neuropathy (arteritic).
    b. Proliferative diabetic retinopathy.
    c. Optic disc drusen.
    d. Papilloedema.
    e. Severe thyroid eye disease.

28. **The following optic disc associations are correct:**

    a. Disc cupping and glaucoma.
    b. Disc drusen and age-related macular degeneration.
    c. New vessels at disc and central retinal vein occlusion.
    d. Pale disc and optic neuritis.
    e. Swollen disc and optic nerve tumour.

**29. The optic nerve function, in cases of suspected optic neuropathy, can be assessed by the following:**

a. Acuity.
b. Extraocular eye movements.
c. Visual fields.
d. Red colour desaturation.
e. Relative afferent pupil defect (RAPD).

**30. Relative afferent pupil defect (RAPD) can be tested in the following situations:**

a. Anisocoria, where pupils are unequal but both are reactive to light.
b. Fixed and dilated left pupil, left eye 6/60 vision and a reactive right pupil.
c. Prosthetic or artificial eye and one reactive pupil.
d. Pupils are equal and reactive to light (PEARL).
e. Right eye 6/9 vision, right dilated pupil, and a reactive left pupil.

# Dermatology

**31. Which *one* of the following conditions is commonly associated with erythema multiforme?**

a. Lichen simplex.
b. Eczema.
c. Herpes simplex.
d. Scleroderma.
e. Rosacea.

**32. Which *one* of the following is *not* a characteristic feature of systemic lupus erythematosus:**

a. Photosensitivity.
b. Butterfly rash.
c. Vasculitis.
d. Alopecia.
e. Morphoea.

**33. Erythema nodosum is associated with:**

a. Inflammatory bowel disease.
b. Sarcoidosis.
c. Eczema.
d. Oral contraceptive pill.
e. Tuberculosis.

**34. Acne is characterized by:**

a. Comedones, papules, pustules and cysts.
b. Colonization by *Propionibacterium acnes*.
c. Increased sebum excretion.
d. Rhinophyma.
e. Scarring.

**35. These dermatological terms are correctly described:**

a. Poikiloderma: hyperpigmenatation, telangiectasia and atrophy.
b. Macule: a small raised lesion, less than 5 mm in diameter.
c. Milium: a small keratin-containing cyst.
d. Lichenification: thickening of the skin with increased skin markings.
e. Carbuncle: a collection of boils.

**36. The following lesions are benign:**

a. Freckle.
b. Viral wart.
c. Squamous papilloma.
d. Seborrhoeic keratosis.
e. Dysplastic naevus.

**37. The following are features of basal cell carcinoma:**

a. More than 50% of cases metastases.
b. The most common skin cancers in fair skin.
c. The edge is typically rolled-up and pearly.
d. Ulceration can occur.
e. Can be caused by arsenic ingestion.

**38. Nail changes can be found in the following conditions:**

a. Psoriasis.
b. Fungal infections.
c. Severe illness.
d. Lichen planus.
e. Urticaria.

**39. Hair loss can be caused by:**

a. Severe illness.
b. Melasma.
c. Drugs.
d. Ringworm.
e. Traction.

**40. Topical steroids can cause the following complications:**

a. Striae.
b. Perioral dermatitis.
c. Tinea incognito.
d. Cushing's syndrome.
e. Vasculitis.

**41. Cutaneous manifestations of diabetes mellitus include:**

a. Eczema.
b. Necrobiosis lipoidica.
c. Granuloma annulare.
d. Leg ulcers.
e. Xanthomas.

**42. The following are risk factors for *Candida albicans* infection on the skin:**

a. Pregnancy.
b. Diabetes mellitus.
c. Use of topical corticosteroids.
d. Repeated washing.
e. Obesity.

**43. Treatments of acne vulgaris include:**

a. Topical antibiotics.
b. Topical benzoyl peroxide.
c. Retinoids.
d. Methotrexate.
e. Anti-androgens.

44. **Psoriasis can present in the following characteristic patterns:**
    a. Palmoplantar pustulosis.
    b. Erythroderma.
    c. Guttate.
    d. Plaque.
    e. Perioral dermatitis.

45. **Complications of atopic eczema include:**
    a. Eczema herpeticum.
    b. Lichen planus.
    c. Growth retardation.
    d. Bacterial infections.
    e. Cataracts.

46. **The following drugs can cause a lichen planus-like rash:**
    a. Captopril.
    b. Gold.
    c. Penicillamine.
    d. Paracetamol.
    e. Quinine.

47. **The common causes of erythroderma include:**
    a. Psoriasis.
    b. Eczema.
    c. Pityriasis vesicolour.
    d. Drug-related.
    e. Pityrisis rubra pilaris.

48. **The following dermatoses can be improved by sunlight:**
    a. Eczema.
    b. Psoriasis.
    c. Pityriasis rosea.
    d. Porphyria cutanea tarda.
    e. Mycosis fungoides.

49. **The common skin flora includes:**
    a. *Neisseria.*
    b. *Staphylococcus.*
    c. *Streptococcus.*
    d. *Corynebacterium.*
    e. *Propionibacterium.*

50. **The following statements are true regarding viral rashes:**
    a. The Coxsackie virus is the cause of hand, foot and mouth disease.
    b. Koplik's spots are a feature of chickenpox.
    c. Umbilicated pearly-pink papules are found in molluscum contagiosum.
    d. Varicella virus causes chicken pox and shingles.
    e. The slapped-cheek appearance is found in fifth's disease.

51. **Which *one* of the following is *not* a typical clinical feature of venous insufficiency in the leg?**
    a. Hyperpigmentation.
    b. Lipodermatosclerosis.
    c. Eczema.
    d. Ulceration.
    e. Pain.

52. **Hyperpigmenatation can be caused by the following:**
    a. Addison's disease.
    b. Drug-induced.
    c. Chronic liver disease.
    d. Vitiligo.
    e. Post-inflammatory.

53. **The following statements are true regarding pemphigus vulgaris:**
    a. Treatment includes systemic steroids.
    b. The trunk is affected more than the limbs.
    c. Direct immunofluorescence reveals autoantibodies deposited along the basement membrane.
    d. The blisters are easily ruptured.
    e. Nikolsky's sign is positive in this condition.

54. **Drug eruptions can include:**
    a. Photosensitivity.
    b. Hyperpigmentation.
    c. Urticaria.
    d. Vasculitis.
    e. Cellulitis.

55. **The types of melanomas include:**
    a. Nodular.
    b. Superficial spreading.
    c. Lentigo malignant.
    d. Guttate.
    e. Acral lentiginous.

56. **The risk factors for the development of squamous cell carcinoma include:**
    a. Sun exposure.
    b. Radiation.
    c. Arsenic.
    d. Chronic ulceration.
    e. Prolonged exposure to topical emollients.

57. **Seborrhoeic warts may be identified by the following clinical characteristics:**
    a. Stuck-on appearance.
    b. Well-defined edge.
    c. Not greater than 1 cm in diameter.
    d. Warty surface.
    e. Individual or many lesions.

58. **Cutaneous manifestations of internal malignancy include:**
    a. Generalized pruritus.
    b. Acanthosis nigricans.
    c. Dermatomyositis.
    d. Ichthyosis.
    e. Dermatofibromas.

**59. The following treatments can be used to treat the linked skin conditions:**

a. Cryotherapy for seborrhoeic warts.
b. Curettage for basal cell carcinomas.
c. Electrocautery for small haemangiomas.
d. Surgical excision for melanoma.
e. Systemic steroids for skin tags.

**60. The features of tinea capitis include:**

a. Kerion.
b. Alopecia.
c. More common in Afro-Caribbean children.
d. Always caused by *Candida albicans*.
e. Can become widespread in schools.

**61. Prednisolone can be used to treat:**

a. Eczema.
b. Bullous pemphigoid.
c. Discoid lupus.
d. Acne.
e. Vasculitis.

**62. Causes of hirsutism include:**

a. Acromegaly.
b. Polycystic ovary syndrome.
c. Cushing's syndrome.
d. Lichen planus.
e. Hyperprolactinaemia.

**63. Hypopigmenatation can be caused by:**

a. Post-inflammatory.
b. Vitiligo.
c. Leprosy.
d. Cryotherapy.
e. Minocycline.

## Ear, Nose and Throat

**Best of five. For each of the following questions, select the *single best answer* from the five options given.**

**64. Which *one* of the following statements is true? Laryngeal cancer:**

a. Is most often an adenocarcinoma.
b. Is strongly associated with consumption of alcohol.
c. Is best treated with chemotherapy.
d. Most frequently affects the vocal fold.
e. Always presents with hoarseness.

**65. Which *one* of the following statements is true? Otalgia:**

a. Is common in otitis media with effusion.
b. Often follows the ear discharge seen in acute otitis media.
c. Is common in Ménière's disease.
d. Is often bilateral.
e. May be caused by a postcricoid carcinoma.

**66. Which *one* of the following statements is true? Nasal polyps:**

a. Are rare in childhood.
b. Systemic steroids are contraindicated.
c. If unilateral need no further action.
d. Are commonly associated with recurrent acute sinusitis.
e. Are cured by surgical removal.

**67. Which *one* of the following statements is true? Cholesteatoma:**

a. Is caused by excess fat deposition in the middle ear.
b. Is most often associated with pre-existing disease of the pars tensa.
c. May cause sensorineural hearing loss.
d. Is often eradicated by a prolonged course of antibiotics.
e. Is uncommon.

**68. Which *one* of the following statements is true regarding tympanometry?**

a. It is rarely performed in children.
b. It measures the area of the ear drum.
c. It is frequently normal in otitis media with effusion.
d. Compliance may be reduced in otosclerosis.
e. It shows a flat trace in normal subjects.

**69. Which *one* of the following statements is true regarding oral cancer:**

a. It is an uncommon problem worldwide.
b. It presents with painful persistent oral ulceration.
c. It frequently metastasizes to bone.
d. If it is associated with spread to cervical lymph nodes the survival drops by 20%.
e. The biggest risk factor is tobacco.

**70. Which *one* of the following statements is true? Obstructive sleep apnoea (OSA) in adults:**

a. May cause daytime somnolence.
b. Causes early morning waking.
c. Is commonly due to adenotonsillar hypertrophy.
d. Is best treated surgically.
e. Is seen most often in obese females.

**71. Which *one* of the following statements is true regarding recurrent acute tonsillitis?**

a. It is most commonly a bacterial infection.
b. It is most common in infants between 2 and 5 years of age.
c. If untreated it leads to peritonsillar abscess formation.
d. If it occurs more than six times per year the patient may benefit from tonsillectomy.
e. It is the most common reason for tonsillectomy in the UK.

**72. Which *one* of the following statements is true? Bell's palsy:**

a. Is often associated with mastoid pain.
b. Is caused by herpes zoster infection of the seventh nerve.

c. May cause hypoacusis.
d. Is treated with high dose antibiotics.
e. Leads to a permanent paralysis in the majority of cases.

73. Which *one* of the following statements is true regarding nasal bone fractures?

a. They are common in children.
b. Radiographs are useful in diagnosis.
c. They should be assessed 3–4 weeks following the injury to allow soft tissue swelling to settle.
d. They are the most common type of facial bone fracture.
e. If associated with a widened intercanthal distance they should be treated by urgent manipulation.

74. Which *one* of the following statements is true? In Ménière's disease there is:

a. Loss of consciousness.
b. Conductive hearing loss.
c. Fluctuating sensorineural hearing loss.
d. Headache.
e. Positional vertigo.

75. Which *one* of the following statements is true? Vocal cord nodules:

a. Are more common in male smokers.
b. May be pre-malignant.
c. Occur on the posterior part of the vocal cords.
d. Are commonly unilateral.
e. May be treated with speech therapy.

76. Which *one* of the following statements is true regarding differentiated thyroid cancer?

a. Follicular adenoma may be diagnosed by cytology.
b. It is most often seen as a hot nodule on scintigraphy.
c. It is more common in men.
d. It may occur in a multinodular goitre.
e. It may be treated with external beam radiotherapy.

77. Which *one* of the following statements is true? Hereditary haemorrhagic telangiectasia (HHT):

a. Is transmitted in an autosomal recessive manner.
b. Only rarely results in epistaxis.
c. Results in arterial malformation affecting mucous membranes.
d. Is sometimes treated with closure of the nares.
e. Is rarely associated with anaemia.

78. Which *one* of the following statements is true? Laryngomalacia:

a. Causes stridor from birth.
b. Causes biphasic stridor.
c. Requires urgent surgery.
d. Causes stridor that may be positional.
e. Results in failure to thrive in most cases.

79. Which *one* of the following statements is true? Otitis media with effusion:

a. Is caused by chronic middle ear infection.
b. Results in frequent earache.
c. Occurs most often in the 3–7 year age group.
d. Produces a sensorineural hearing loss.
e. Has minimal impact on educational attainment.

80. Which *one* of the following statements is true? Thyroglossal cysts:

a. Are usually located above the hyoid bone.
b. Are uncommon in children.
c. Do not move with swallowing.
d. Are attached to the foramen caecum.
e. Do not recur after excision.

81. Which *one* of the following statements is true? Acute bacterial sinusitis:

a. Is usually secondary to disease of the osteomeatal complex.
b. Is commonly due to **Staph.** aureus.
c. Is contagious.
d. Occurs commonly in nasal polyposis.
e. Is best diagnosed using facial radiographs.

82. Which *one* of the following statements is true? Lichen planus:

a. Affects the soft palate most often.
b. Occurs in children.
c. Is associated with skin lesions on the extensor surface of the forearms.
d. Causes painful ulceration.
e. In its erosive form may be pre-malignant.

83. Which *one* of the following statements is true? Otosclerosis:

a. Is more common in men.
b. Primarily affects the incudostapedial joint.
c. May improve in pregnancy.
d. Results in immobility of the stapes.
e. Does not produce a sensorineural hearing loss.

84. Which *one* of the following statements is true? Branchial cysts:

a. Are a first branchial cleft anomaly.
b. Are derived from the ultimo-branchial apparatus.
c. Should be treated with suspicion in smokers.
d. Are often associated with a middle ear effusion.
e. Are most often seen to arise near the lower third of the sternocleidomastoid muscle.

85. Which *one* of the following is an accepted risk factor for head and neck cancer?

a. Exposure to sunlight.
b. Consumption of salted fish.
c. Smoking.
d. Herpes simplex virus infection.
e. Heavy consumption of alcohol.

323

86. Which *one* of the following statements is true?
Allergic rhinitis:

a. Shows decreased serum eosinophil levels.
b. May be treated with topical corticosteroids.
c. Is mediated by a Gell and Coombs type IV reaction.
d. Is best treated with topical vasoconstrictors.
e. Is common in the elderly.

87. Which *one* of the following statements is true?
Tonsillectomy:

a. Is most often carried out in the setting of acute tonsillitis.
b. Is commonly performed as a day-case procedure.
c. Carries a 2–7% risk of postoperative haemorrhage.
d. Does not usefully treat OSA in children.
e. Is often carried out under local anaesthetic.

88. Which *one* of the following statements is true regarding salivary gland tumours?

a. Overall 40% are malignant.
b. 80% affect the submandibular gland.
c. They are more common in the upper lip than the lower.
d. They are most often adenoid cystic carcinomas.
e. They should be diagnosed by open biopsy.

89. Which *one* of the following statements is true regarding tracheostomy?

a. It opens the trachea at the first ring.
b. Patients cannot speak.
c. Cuff pressures of 40 mmHg are acceptable.
d. Tubes must be changed after 8 hours to prevent blockage.
e. It may be performed using the Seldinger technique.

90. Which *one* of the following statements is true regarding fractures of the temporal bone?

a. They are associated with a haemotympanum.
b. Facial palsy is more common following transverse than longitudinal fracture.
c. They are increasing in incidence.
d. They commonly involve the trigeminal nerve.
e. They seldom cause hearing loss.

91. Which *one* of the following statements is true regarding atypical TB of the head and neck?

a. It affects immunocompromised and elderly patients.
b. It affects young children.
c. It usually causes posterior triangle lymphadenopathy.
d. Chest symptoms are common.
e. It can cause painful indurated lesions of the skin.

92. Which *one* of the following statements is true?
Epistaxis:

a. Is often helped by ice packs applied to the forehead.
b. May benefit from ligation of branches of the ophthalmic artery.

c. Most commonly arises from the posterior part of the nose.
d. Following trauma, often requires nasal packing.
e. Is commonly treated by endovascular embolization.

93. Which *one* of the following statements is true?
Benign paroxysmal positional vertigo (BPPV):

a. Causes a visible horizontal nystagmus at rest.
b. Is a mild self-limiting condition.
c. Causes episodic dizziness on standing.
d. May be diagnosed by a positive Dix–Hallpike test.
e. May be diagnosed by a positive Epley manoeuvre.

94. Which *one* of the following is not associated with Reinke's oedema?

a. Human papillomavirus.
b. Hypothyroidism.
c. Laryngopharyngeal acid reflux.
d. Smoking.
e. Female gender.

95. Which *one* of the following is not associated with recurrent oral ulceration?

a. Microcytic anaemia.
b. Behçet's syndrome.
c. Stress.
d. Cigarette smoking.
e. Coeliac disease.

96. Which *one* of the following statements is true?
Tinnitus:

a. May be musical.
b. If pulsatile is always of no significance.
c. Is associated with hearing loss in many cases.
d. Is easily treated.
e. May benefit from the oral administration of betahistine.

97. Which *one* of the following statements is true?
Choanal atresia:

a. Is more commonly bilateral than unilateral.
b. Usually presents at 3–4 months with failure to thrive.
c. Is diagnosed most often by CT scan.
d. If bilateral may cause cyanosis on feeding.
e. Affects boys more commonly than girls.

98. Which *one* of the following statements is true regarding laryngeal papillomatosis?

a. The presence of cellular atypia on biopsy is a worrying sign.
b. It may be cured with laser surgery.
c. It affects the structures of the supraglottis most commonly.
d. It is due to herpes simplex virus infection.
e. Transmission may be prevented by caesarean section.

# Short-answer questions (SAQs)

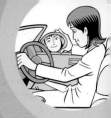

## Ophthalmology

1. A 35-year-old female smoker has abnormal thyroid function blood tests. Describe the signs and symptoms for thyroid eye disease.

2. A 55-year-old male is having difficulty painting and has recently been advised not to drive by his optician. Describe the benefits and risks of modern cataract surgery.

3. A 60-year-old male has two brothers with glaucoma. Outline the four components of an eye examination in this suspected glaucoma patient.

4. A 52-year-old woman develops loss of central vision in her right eye. Compare and contrast age-related macular degeneration and diabetic maculopathy.

5. A mother observes that her newborn daughter has a grey-looking eye. Describe the importance of diagnosing a congenital cataract or cloudy cornea at birth.

6. Differentiate between five common types of optic discs.

7. A 29-year-old female is having difficulty seeing the colour red with her left eye and has left ocular pain on eye movements. Describe five methods of assessing her optic nerve function.

## Dermatology

8. What are epidermal and dermal changes of the skin?

9. What are the characteristic clinical features of lichen planus?

10. What prognostic factor is important in malignant melanoma?

11. What are the common factors that can exacerbate psoriasis?

12. What features would worry you about a mole?

13. What skin conditions are associated with chronic sun exposure?

## Ear, Nose and Throat

14. A 56-year-old mechanic complains of hearing loss. What tests of hearing can you use to assess this? Think about clinical and laboratory tests.

15. A 23-year-old student has troublesome allergic rhinitis. She has had skin prick testing which showed a positive reaction to house dust mite. Outline your management advice.

16. A 34-year-old male patient has a mass in his thyroid gland. He wants to know what the chances are that it is malignant. What factors in the history and examination increase the risk of malignancy?

17. A hyperactive but otherwise healthy 5-year-old snores and seems to stop breathing in her sleep. What do you think is the likely diagnosis? What investigations would you perform? And what would be the likely treatment in this age group?

18. A 45-year-old male patient has had dizziness 'where the room spins around' when he turns over in bed; this lasts a few seconds then resolves. What are the three common causes of vertigo? What is the likely diagnosis here and why? What test is used for this condition and how is it treated?

19. Why do thyroglossal cysts develop?

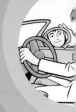

**For each scenario described below, choose the \*single\* most likely match from the list of options.** *Each option may be used once, more than once, or not at all.*

## Ophthalmology

### 1. Concerning red eye and changes in vision:

A. Acute angle closure glaucoma
B. Allergic conjunctivitis
C. Anterior uveitis
D. Bacterial conjunctivitis
E. Cataract
F. Central vein occlusion
G. Herpetic keratitis
H. Microbial keratitis
I. Primary open angle glaucoma
J. Viral conjunctivitis

*Instruction:* For each scenario described below, choose the **single** most likely diagnosis from the above list of options. Each option may be used once, more than once or not at all.

1. A 54-year-old man known to have diabetes and hypertension presents with sudden painless loss of vision.

2. A 19-year-old woman presents with yellow–green sticky eyes and visual acuity of 6/6 bilaterally.

3. A 10-year-old boy with asthma has bilateral pink, itchy, watery eyes.

4. A 22-year-old man presents with bilateral red, watery, scratchy eyes and enlarged pre-auricular lymph nodes. He had flu-like symptoms 1 week ago.

5. A 60-year-old woman presents with sudden painful loss of vision, photophobia, haloes and poorly reacting pupil.

### 2. Concerning eyelids and double vision:

A. Blepharitis
B. Chalazion
C. Distichiasis
D. Dysthyroid eye disease
E. Ectropion
F. Entropion
G. Epiphora
H. Herpes zoster ophthalmicus
I. Orbital cellulitis
J. Nasolacrimal duct obstruction

*Instruction:* For each scenario described below, choose the **single** most likely diagnosis from the above list of options.

1. A 23-year-old woman presents with a painless pea-sized lump in the eyelid.

2. A 54-year-old man has epiphora and everted lower eyelids caused by lid laxity.

3. A 15-year-old boy presents with painful restricted eye movements, reduced vision, diplopia and pyrexia.

4. A 65-year-old man presents with acne rosacea and pink, irritated, crusty eyelid margins.

5. A 53-year-old woman has upward rolled eyelashes rubbing against the cornea as a result of an inverted lower eyelid.

### 3. Concerning the cornea and cataracts:

A. Acanthamoeba keratitis
B. Anterior uveitis
C. Bacterial conjunctivitis
D. Cataract
E. Cystoid macular oedema
F. Endophthalmitis
G. Herpetic keratitis
H. Microbial keratitis
I. Phacomorphic glaucoma
J. Posterior capsular opacification

*Instruction:* For each scenario described below, choose the **single** most likely diagnosis from the above list of options.

1. A 63-year-old woman had cataract surgery 3 years ago and has experienced a gradual painless loss of vision over the last 12 months.

2. A 55-year-old man presents with a sudden painful loss of vision and hypopyon 6 days after cataract surgery.

3. The patient is a 22-year-old female contact lens wearer who washes her lenses every night with tap water. She swam yesterday with contact lenses and swimming goggles and today has developed a very painful left eye. The affected eye looks slightly pink.

4. A 61-year-old Asian patient develops, 5 weeks after cataract surgery, a red, photophobic, watery eye.

Postoperative steroid drops ran out 2 weeks ago. There is no hypopyon and the affected eye has visual acuity of 6/6.

5. A 29-year-old female contact lens wearer develops a red, painful eye . She looks in the mirror and can see a white spot on the cornea.

# 4. Concerning retinal conditions:

A. Dry age-related macular degeneration
B. Hypertensive retinopathy
C. Central retinal vein occlusion
D. Posterior vitreous detachment
E. Retinal detachment – macula off
F. Retinal detachment – macula on
G. Superior retinal tear
H. Transient monocular blindness (non-embolic)
I. Vitreous haemorrhage
J. Wet age-related macular degeneration

*Instruction:* For each scenario described below, choose the **single** most likely diagnosis from the above list of options.

1. A 49-year-old man presents with a sudden painless loss of vision and visual acuity of hand movements. Ocular findings include rubreosis and retinal haemorrhages in four quadrants.

2. A 23-year-old man has a sudden increase in floaters and photopsia. There is no loss of peripheral visual field. The retina appears flat, but tobacco dust was noted clinically by the referring optician.

3. A 32-year-old man presents with a sudden increase in floaters, photopsia and an inferior loss of field, and visual acuity of 6/24.

4. A 25-year-old woman has a monocular grey patchy loss followed by recovery of vision over 5 minutes.

5. A 39-year-old woman presents with a sudden increase in floaters, photopsia and a nasal loss of visual field, and visual acuity of 6/5.

# 5. Concerning medical ophthalmology and uveitis:

A. Ankylosing spondylitis
B. Crohn's disease
C. Endophthalmitis
D. Giant cell arteritis
E. Intermediate uveitis
F. Juvenile idiopathic arthritis
G. Rheumatoid arthritis
H. Sarcoidosis
I. Sjögren's syndrome
J. Toxoplasma chorioretinitis

*Instruction:* For each scenario described below, choose the **single** most likely diagnosis from the above list of options.

1. A 40-year-old woman has a dry mouth, blurry vision and intermittently scratchy eyes.

2. A 53-year-old woman has a severely painful eye, such that she cannot sleep. Her hands have swan-neck finger deformities and proximal tender swollen joints.

3. A 24-year-old woman with previous optic neuritis and suspected multiple sclerosis develops painless misty vision due to increased vitreous floaters.

4. A 31-year-old man with chronic lower back ache develops a red, painful, photophobic right eye.

5. A 75-year-old man with a sixth nerve palsy and a swollen optic disc.

# 6. Concerning paediatric ophthalmology and strabismus:

A. Amblyopia
B. Anisometropia
C. Cloudy cornea
D. Congenital cataract
E. Congenital glaucoma
F. Esotropia
G. Exotropia
H. Leukocoria
I. Neonatal conjunctivitis
J. Retinopathy of prematurity

*Instruction:* For each scenario described below, choose the **single** most likely diagnosis from the above list of options.

1. A 5-year-old girl with her left eye turning inwards or convergent squint.

2. A newborn baby with a white pupillary reflex; the mother had primary toxoplasmosis during the pregnancy.

3. A 9-week premature baby, weighing 1100 g, who is being ventilated on a special care baby unit.

4. A 6-year-old boy with one eye looking outwards or divergent squint.

5. A 7-year-old girl has visual acuity of right 6/18 and left 6/5. Her right eye does not improve on pinhole testing. Both ocular examination and eye movements are normal.

# 7. Concerning neuro-ophthalmology:

A. Fourth nerve palsy
B. Giant cell arteritis
C. Homonymous hemianopia
D. Horner's syndrome
E. Orbital blow out fracture
F. Papilloedema
G. Pituitary tumour
H. Relative afferent pupil defect

I. Sixth nerve palsy

J. Third nerve palsy

*Instruction:* For each scenario described below, choose the **single** most likely diagnosis from the above list of options.

1. A 53-year-old patient with poorly controlled diabetes has sudden painless diplopia, maximal on looking to his right, and not noticed at all when reading.

2. A 71-year-old patient has left-sided hemiparesis and sensory inattention.

3. A 76-year-old man has a recent history of headaches, nausea and vomiting. On examination he has bilateral swollen optic discs and an elevated opening pressure on lumbar puncture.

4. A 24-year-old man is hit by a squash ball on his eyebrow.

5. A 54-year-old woman has bitemporal visual field defects.

# Dermatology

## 8. Concerning skin rashes:

A. Lichen planus

B. Plaque psoriasis

C. Pityriasis rosea

D. Erythema multiforme

E. Lichen sclerosus

F. Contact dermatitis

G. Rosacea

H. Bullous pemphigus

I. Guttate psoriasis

J. Pityriasis vesicolor

*Instruction:* For each scenario described below, choose the **single** most likely diagnosis from the above list of options.

1. A 20-year-old man presents with numerous macules of varying sizes on his upper trunk and arms. Their surface has a fine scaling and they are not itchy.

2. A 26-year-old woman has many round pink patches that seem to be arranged parallel to the ribs. She also mentions that there was a much larger pink patch that appeared a few days before most of the rash appeared.

3. A middle-aged man presents with a sudden eruption of a widespread and very itchy rash. The individual lesions are purple, flat topped papules and have white lines on their surface.

4. A teenager presents with an acute symmetrical, red, scaly, widespread rash. Someone has described the lesions as being 'like raindrops'. He recently had a sore throat.

5. A 60-year-old woman comes to clinic with tense blisters several centimetres in length on her limbs. She also mentions that she had red, itchy patches several weeks before these blisters appeared.

6. A middle-aged woman presents with white, wrinkled plaques on her body. Her vulva is itchy and sore.

## 9. Concerning skin infections:

A. Viral warts

B. Molluscum contagiosum

C. Orf

D. Herpes zoster

E. Herpes simplex

F. Erthythema infectiosum

G. Measles

H. Hand, foot and mouth disease

I. Scabies

J. Intertrigo

*Instruction:* For each scenario described below, choose the **single** most likely diagnosis from the above list of options.

1. A farmer, after handling sheep for a number of weeks, presents with a single, quickly enlarging nodule on one of the fingers of his right hand.

2. A middle-aged man, during his recovery from pneumonia, develops a sudden eruption of pain and tenderness to a localized part of his trunk. This is limited to one side of his body.

3. A 16-year-old girl appears in clinic with a sudden crop of tender and painful small vesicles around her lips. She has had this rash several times before.

4. A 6-year-old girl is brought to clinic with numerous tiny dome-shaped papules all over her body. There are small indentations in the centre of the lesions.

5. A mother brings her 3-year-old boy to clinic because he has developed redness to his checks, as if someone has slapped him.

6. A homeless man presents with intense itching that does not affect his head. He is also pruritic in his finger webs. His friends had the same symptoms.

## 10. Concerning skin changes in systemic disease:

A. Scurvy

B. Necrobiosis lipoidica

C. Granuloma annulare

D. Acanthosis nigricans

E. Erythema nodosum

F. Sweet's disease

G. Hirsutism

H. Pellagra

I. Pretibial myxoedema

J. Thrombophlebitis

*Instruction:* For each scenario described below, choose the **single** most likely diagnosis from the above list of options.

1. A homeless man presents with large areas of bruising but denies any significant trauma to account for them. He has not been eating well.

2. A 30-year-old man with Crohn's disease has multiple tender red nodules on his lower legs.

3. An obese lady complains that the skin in her armpits is darkening and thickening.

4. A middle-aged lady notices that she is increasingly anxious and losing weight. The skin on her shins is raised and shiny.

5. Yellow–red plaques are found on the shins of a diabetic young woman.

6. Round firm plaques appear on a 25-year-old man on the dorsum side of his hands. They were skin coloured and asymptomatic. He was not diabetic.

## 11. Concerning skin lesions:

A. Milium
B. Keloid
C. Lipoma
D. Seborrhoeic wart
E. Dermatofibroma
F. Epidermal cyst
G. Actinic keratosis
H. Skin tags
I. Viral wart
J. Pyogenic granuloma

*Instruction:* For each scenario described below, choose the correct lesion from the above list of options.

1. A middle-aged man would like a single soft non-tender nodule on his back removed. It is movable over the underlying skin.

2. A young woman presents with a rapidly growing red and fragile nodule on tip of her finger. It bleeds easily and she remembers pricking her finger during gardening a few days earlier.

3. A 20-year-old woman develops a non-changing, small, firm, skin-coloured papule on her lower leg. She remembers that it appeared after an insect bite and it has been present for at least 3 years.

4. An elderly gentleman has developed a number of brown wart-like lesions on his back and face. They are sometimes itchy.

5. A 78-year-old man has multiple small scaly lesions on his scalp and face. There is underlying redness where the scale is.

6. A young Afro-Caribbean man has developed a protuberant and firm linear plaque on his sternum. It began to develop after he had sustained trauma to this area.

## 12. Concerning sebaceous disorders:

A. Rosacea
B. Perioral dermatitis
C. Hidradenitis suppurativa
D. Acne
E. Hyperhidrosis
F. Seborrhoeic dermatitis
G. Asteatotic dermatitis
H. Sebaceous hyperplasia
I. Angiokeratoma
J. Melasma

*Instruction:* For each scenario described below, choose the **single** most likely diagnosis from the above list of options.

1. A young woman who is an eczema sufferer has used topical steroids regularly on her face. She has recently developed multiple papulopustular lesions around her chin and lips.

2. A teenager has multiple papules and pustules, along with open and closed comedones all over her face.

3. A 50-year-old woman presents with numerous papules and pustules on her face. She has noticed that her eyes are gritty and her nose has enlarged.

4. An obese woman is suffering from multiple inflamed nodules and abscesses affecting both her axillae and her groin.

5. A 74-year-old man presents with multiple red patches scattered on his body. They are round and very itchy.

6. A 65-year-old man has dandruff and greasy scaling on his face, especially around his nose and forehead.

## 13. Concerning erythroderma:

A. Psoriasis
B. Drug allergy
C. Pemphigus foliaceus
D. Contact dermatitis
E. Pityriasis rubra pilaris
F. Lymphoma
G. Mycosis fungoides
H. Sezary syndrome
I. Stasis eczema
J. Morphea

*Instruction:* For each scenario described below, choose the **single** most likely cause for the erythroderma in the patient from the above list of options.

1. Fixed red patches that are not particularly itchy and do not completely improve with topical steroids.

2. Widespread confluent erosions on the patient's back. The scalp and upper chest are also affected.

3. Some areas of the body are not affected, forming islands of normal skin. The palms are thickened.

4. Onset of erythroderma occurs after the patient took carbamazepine a few weeks earlier.

5. An elderly woman has dry, red, itchy skin on both her shins.

6. The patient has previously had nail pitting, onychylosis and thick scaly plaques on his elbows.

## 14. Concerning leg ulcers:

A. Venous
B. Arterial
C. Tuberculosis
D. Diabetes mellitus
E. Pyoderma gangrenosum
F. Squamous cell carcinoma
G. Syphilis
H. Leprosy
I. Buerger's disease
J. Vasculitis

*Instruction:* For each scenario described below, choose the **single** most likely cause for the patient's leg ulcer from the above list of options.

1. A 55-year-old man has a rash on his lower legs that could be described as multiple purpuric papules. He also has haematuria.

2. An elderly lady has had a non-changing ulcer for over 15 years, until a few months ago, when it enlarged and is now fungating.

3. A 75-year-old man is a smoker with high blood pressure. He also has intermittent claudication and his ulcer is painful.

4. This leg ulcer is over the patient's medial malleolus and he has varicose veins.

5. The ulcer has an undermined purple ulcer with surrounding erythema. The patient also has ulcerative colitis.

6. The patient also has several patches of well-defined light-coloured areas on his body with decreased sensation.

## 15. Concerning pigmentation:

A. Vitiligo
B. Melasma (chloasma)
C. Addison's disease
D. Minocycline-induced
E. Peutz–Jeghers syndrome
F. Albinism
G. Pityriasis versicolor
H. Poikiloderma
I. Freckles
J. Phenylketonuria

*Instruction:* For each scenario described below, choose the **single** most likely cause of changes in skin pigment from the above list of options.

1. A young man experiences darkening of his skin while being treated for acne.

2. A pregnant woman becomes concerned that she has developed symmetrical confluent brown patches on her face.

3. A young woman has developed several lighter round patches on her skin. She also has thyroid disease and alopecia areata.

4. A man has developed hyperpigmentation in his palmar creases. He is also weak and feels dizzy when standing.

5. A 25-year-old man notices that he cannot develop a sun tan on certain areas on his back, although he can on the rest of his body. His back is covered with hypopigmented macules. Prior to this he had red macules covered in fine scale on these lighter areas.

6. A young man has become concern about numerous brown macules on his lips and on the inside of his mouth. His father and brother have a similar problem.

## 16. Concerning the terminology of skin lesions:

A. Cyst
B. Plaque
C. Vesicle
D. Nodule
E. Macule
F. Papule
G. Wheal
H. Pustule
I. Erosion
J. Ulcer

*Instruction:* For each description below, choose the **single** term from the above list of options that best describes the lesion

1. An elevated lesion that is less than 5 mm in diameter.

2. A plateau-like raised area on the skin.

3. A compressible small round or plateau-like lesion that can be itching. It tends not to last for more than 24 hours.

4. A defect in the skin that only affects the epidermis.

5. A localized area in the skin that has changed in colour and is not raised or depressed.

6. A small blister measuring less than 5 mm in diameter.

## 17. Concerning skin pre-malignant and malignant disorders:

A. Basal cell carcinoma
B. Keratocanthoma
C. Squamous cell carcinoma
D. Dermatofibrosarcoma
E. Bowen's disease (intra-epidermal carcinoma)
F. Kaposi's sarcoma

G. Actinic keratosis
H. Atypical naevus
 I. Lentigo maligna
J. Lymphoma

*Instruction:* For each scenario described below, choose the **single** most likely diagnosis from the above list of options.

1. A large well-defined scaly plaque, usually found on the lower legs of elderly patients. It may have a similar appearance to that of a psoriatic plaque.

2. This skin cancer occurs in a longstanding area of ulceration and scarring.

3. A 67-year-old lady presents with a nodule on her neck that has a pearly edge, telangiectasia and central crusting.

4. An elderly gentleman presents with a rapidly enlarging nodule on his scalp. It has a dome shape with a central crater.

5. A slowly enlarging, uniformly flat brown macule on the face.

6. The mole is 9 mm in diameter and has an irregular edge.

# Ear, Nose and Throat

## 18. Concerning hearing loss:

A. Otitis media with effusion
B. Ménière's disease
C. Nasopharyngeal carcinoma
D. Otitis externa
E. Vestibular schwannoma
F. Presbyacusis
G. Congenital hearing loss
H. Otosclerosis
 I. Wax impaction

*Instruction:* The following patients all have hearing loss. Choose the **single** most appropriate diagnosis from the above list.

1. A 55-year-old man develops sudden onset vertigo preceded by left-sided tinnitus and hearing loss. Audiograms show a unilateral sensorineural hearing loss. A gadolinium enhanced MRI scan is normal.

2. A 4-year-old boy is referred by the paediatrician with speech delay. Audiograms show bilateral conductive hearing losses; tympanometry shows flat traces.

3. A 35-year-old female patient is concerned about gradual hearing loss. Examination of her ears is normal. Tuning fork tests are performed which show that Weber's test radiates to her left ear, Rinne's is positive on the right and negative on the left. Tympanograms are normal.

4. A 72-year-old female patient is finding it increasingly difficult to follow conversations. Ear examination is normal. Audiograms show a symmetrical high-frequency sensorineural hearing loss.

## 19. Concerning neck lumps:

A. Metastatic squamous carcinoma
B. Thyroglossal cyst
C. Lymphoma
D. Pleomorphic adenoma
E. Branchial cyst
F. Carotid body tumour
G. Reactive lymphadenopathy
H. Papillary carcinoma

*Instruction:* The following patients all have neck lumps. Choose the **single** most appropriate diagnosis from the above list.

1. A 27-year-old man has a 3 month history of a swelling in the upper part of the lateral neck; the swelling is painless and slowly enlarging. Ultrasound shows a fluid filled unilocular structure at the anterior border of the upper third sternomastoid.

2. A 57-year-old female smoker presents with a 2 month history of hoarseness and a painless lateral neck swelling. Examination reveals a hard 3 cm swelling in level III. Laryngoscope shows a fungating supraglottic mass. Biopsy of the larynx shows keratin pearls.

3. A slow-growing painless mass at the angle of the mandible in a 50-year-old man. Ultrasound shows a circumscribed mass in the lower pole of the parotid gland.

4. A 70-year-old woman presents with a firm mass just below the angle of the mandible. It has a bruit.

## 20. Concerning nasal blockage:

A. Allergic rhinitis
B. Inverted papilloma
C. Juvenile angiofibroma
D. Nasal polyposis
E. Deviated nasal septum
F. Adenoidal hypertrophy
G. Choanal atresia
H. Nasopharyngeal carcinoma
 I. Physiological nasal cycle

*Instruction:* The following patients all have nasal blockage. Choose the **single** most appropriate diagnosis from the above list.

1. A 6-year-old girl with nasal blockage and purulent nasal discharge. Flexible endoscopy shows a mass arising from the posterior wall of the nasopharynx.

2. A 35-year-old male banker attends complaining of nasal blockage affecting alternate sides of his nose. One side is blocked for around 4 hours and then it switches sides. Examination is normal.

3. A 42-year-old man complains of unilateral nasal blockage for the last 2 years. Examination with an endoscope shows a polypoid lesion arising from the right middle meatus. A CT of his sinuses confirms a unilateral mass with widening of the maxillary sinus osteum.

4. An 18-year-old female patient complains of nasal blockage and rhinorrhoea which is constant and there for the last 12 months. Examination shows pale oedematous inferior turbinates.

## 21. Concerning stridor:

A. Epiglottitis
B. Unilateral vocal cord palsy
C. Croup
D. Subglottic carcinoma
E. Laryngomalacia
F. Squamous carcinoma – glottic
G. Bilateral vocal cord palsy
H. Subglottic stenosis
I. Tracheomalacia

*Instruction:* The following patients all have stridor. Choose the **single** most appropriate diagnosis from the above list.

1. You are asked to see a 6-year-old child in casualty. He has a cough and mild pyrexia. Following a coughing fit he has an inspiratory stridor.

2. A 40-year-old lady has just had a total thyroidectomy for a goitre. You are called to the ward postoperatively as she has an inspiratory stridor and is desaturating. Her wound looks normal and she is talking in short sentences.

3. A 60-year-old male smoker and heavy drinker attends A&E. He is markedly pyrexial and looks unwell. He has pain on swallowing and is spitting out his saliva. His neck is tender and he has audible stridor.

4. You are asked to assess a 3-month-old child who has been admitted to PICU with a chest infection and has required intubation. He has failed to extubate on two occasions, becoming stridulous and distressed. He was born prematurely and had respiratory distress at birth requiring prolonged intubation.

## 22. Concerning dizziness:

A. Pre-syncope
B. Benign paroxysmal positional vertigo
C. Vestibulitis
D. Ménière's disease
E. Cholesteatoma
F. Vestibular schwannoma
G. Vertebrobasilar insufficiency
H. Cardiac arrhythmia
I. Acute mastoiditis

*Instruction:* The following patients all have dizziness. Choose the **single** most appropriate diagnosis from the above list.

1. A 56-year-old woman had acute onset of rotational vertigo which lasted for around 1 week and was followed by 3 weeks of unsteadiness. You see her 6 weeks later. There are no other symptoms or signs.

2. A 70-year-old man has feelings of intermittent light headedness ('my head is swimming') lasting 30 minutes or so. On one occasion he has lost consciousness because of his dizziness.

3. You are asked to see a 25-year-old woman in A&E. She feels that her right ear is blocked and uncomfortable; she has tinnitus in that ear and has recently become very dizzy. She is very anxious. Basic observations, pulse, temperature, blood pressure are normal.

4. A 60-year-old male patient has recently had bouts of dizziness which are precipitated by looking upwards.

## 23. Concerning hoarseness:

A. Reinke's oedema
B. Vocal cord polyp
C. Recurrent laryngeal nerve palsy
D. Psychological
E. Vocal cord nodules
F. Laryngeal papilloma
G. Viral laryngitis
H. Reflux laryngopharyngitis
I. Squamous cell carcinoma
J. Functional dysphonia

*Instruction:* The following patients all have hoarseness. Choose the **single** most appropriate diagnosis from the above list.

1. A 45-year-old female smoker has been hoarse for months. Laryngoscopy shows bilaterally swollen inflamed vocal cords.

2. A 15-year-old boy is increasingly hoarse. Laryngoscopy shows an abnormal larynx with swellings affecting the supraglottis and vocal cords, almost obscuring the airway.

3. You are asked to see a 35-year-old woman with aphonia. Laryngoscopy shows a normal larynx with vocal cord adduction on coughing.

4. A 42-year-old market trader requests a consultation. He is a smoker and frequently hoarse. Laryngoscopy reveals bilateral sessile swellings at the anterior third of the vocal folds.

## 24. Concerning oral lesions:

A. Candidiasis
B. Squamous carcinoma
C. Adenoid cystic carcinoma
D. Lichen planus
E. Fibro-epithelial polyp
F. Hairy leukoplakia
G. Pemphigoid

H. Ranula

I. Pemphigus

*Instruction:* The following patients all have oral lesions. Choose the **single** most appropriate diagnosis from the above list.

1. A smooth raised sessile lump on the buccal mucosa.

2. Reticulated white patches affecting the tongue and buccal mucosa.

3. A large irregular ulcer affecting the buccal mucosa in an elderly non-smoker. The lesion is painful on palpation but feels soft. She is seeing an ophthalmologist for eye problems.

4. A raised painless white patch in the retromolar area of a 60-year-old smoker.

## 25. Concerning dysphagia:

A. Oesophageal cancer
B. Cerebrovascular accident
C. Candidal oesophagitis
D. Pharyngeal pouch
E. Globus pharyngeus

F. Achalasia
G. Plummer–Vinson syndrome
H. Myasthenia gravis

*Instruction:* The following patients all have dysphagia. Choose the **single** most appropriate diagnosis from the above list.

1. A 24-year-old intravenous drug abuser presents with a 3-day history of painful and difficult swallowing.

2. A 64-year-old woman has dysphagia, especially to solids. She finds that she feels food stick and sometimes she later regurgitates old food into her mouth. She has lost weight.

3. A 70-year-old man is admitted with dehydration and weight loss. He has had dysphagia which was initially to solid food but he now has difficulty even with liquids.

4. A 52-year-old woman has intermittent swallowing difficulty with nasal escape of liquid which she finds embarrassing. On further questioning she admits to feeling generally listless and she gets occasional double vision.

# Ophthalmology

**1. a. False**  The symptoms given are those of scleritis.
  **b. True**  Itchy eyes are associated with allergic conjunctivitis.
  **c. False**  The symptoms given are those of iritis.
  **d. True**  Scratchy, pink eyes are associated with viral conjunctivitis.
  **e. True**  Sticky eyes are associated with bacterial conjunctivitis.

**2. a. True**  Other features include semi-dilated pupil and corneal oedema.
  **b. True**  A photophobic or light-sensitive eye occurs as a result of the pupil moving in a sticky environment.
  **c. False**  No pain, but loss of vision occurs.
  **d. True**  A dull, severe pain, which prevents the patient from sleeping.
  **e. False**  No pain or loss of vision occurs.

**3. a. True**  Individual red blood cells and inferior blood level are visible on slit lamp examination of the anterior chamber.
  **b. True**  Individual white blood cells are visible on slit lamp examination of the anterior chamber.
  **c. True**  A dilated pupil following trauma can take many weeks to settle.
  **d. True**  Other retinal features include retinal detachment and commotio retinae.
  **e. True**  In a non-diabetic can be secondary to retinal tear and detachment.

**4. a. True**  Air from the nasal cavity spreads subcutaneously through an orbital fracture. Hence the feeling of bubble wrap popping under the skin.
  **b. True**  CT-orbit (3 mm fine cut) is usually requested, rather than facial X-ray, to aid subsequent surgical management. Orbital contents herniating downwards through fracture can be seen as 'tear-drop' sign.
  **c. False**  Infraorbital nerve supplies ipsilateral cheek, upper gums and teeth.
  **d. True**  Optic neuritis can also have this symptom.
  **e. True**  Due to restriction of eye muscles on affected side.

**5. a. False**  Primary open angle glaucoma can lead to slow visual field loss.
  **b. False**  Characteristically irritation and soreness rather than visual loss should occur.

**c. True**  1% of the world is blind from cataract, which is a curable or reversible form of blindness.
  **d. True**  30% of pseudophakes are likely to have PCO within 5 years of cataract surgery.
  **e. True**  Nuclear sclerotic cataracts can induce a myopic shift and hence a change in spectacle prescription.

**6. a. True**  'Positive' with macular pathology and 'negative' with optic nerve disease.
  **b. True**  Can be due to white blood cells (vitritis), red blood cells (haemorrhage) or wear and tear that can precede a posterior vitreous detachment or retinal tear.
  **c. True**  Posterior subcapsular cataracts can lead to glare.
  **d. False**  This symptom is suggestive of subacute angle closure glaucoma.
  **e. True**  Can be due to inherited eye diseases, particularly retinitis pigmentosa.

**7. a. False**  Ocular pain is usually present.
  **b. True**  Gradual, dull vision occurs.
  **c. True**  A sudden loss of vision and risk factors including hypertension and diabetes.
  **d. True**  Field defects and optic disc cupping occur without pain.
  **e. True**  Blurry central vision due to either retinal serous fluid or ischaemia.

**8. a. True**  Extraocular pain such as jaw claudication and temporal scalp tenderness can occur.
  **b. False**  A sudden, painless visual loss occurs.
  **c. True**  Infective (e.g. contact lens related microbial keratitis) or inflammatory aetiology (e.g. rheumatoid related sclerokeratitis) can lead to this scenario.
  **d. True**  Particularly in posterior scleritis, which characteristically keeps the patient awake.
  **e. False**  A sudden, painless central visual loss occurs.

**9. a. True**  A complete neuro-ophthalmic examination should be performed.
  **b. False**  A cause of monocular diplopia from in effect two pupils.
  **c. True**  Eye movements should be examined in suspected cases.
  **d. True**  Variable diplopia can occur.

e. True    Inferior and medial rectus extraocular muscles are commonly affected during inflammatory phase.

**10.** a. True    Neoplastic lesions within the orbit can cause axial and non-axial proptosis.

     b. False    Variable ptosis can occur with myasthenia.

     c. False    Orbital cellulitis is associated with proptosis.

     d. True    The commonest cause of proptosis, whether bilateral or unilateral.

     e. True    Orbital inflammatory disorders (e.g. Wegener's, sarcoidosis).

**11.** a. False    A chalazion of the upper eyelid can cause a mechanical ptosis.

     b. True    Due to overstretching of the eyelids from the lid speculum.

     c. True    A 1 mm partial ptosis occurs.

     d. True    Variable ptosis can occur.

     e. False    Lid retraction and lid lag usually occur.

**12.** a. False    A hyperlacrimation or reflex lacrimal hypersecretion occurs.

     b. True    Lower lid ectropion can occur due to lack of orbicularis oculi muscle tone.

     c. True    The lower lid punctum is not apposed to the globe so tears run on to the cheek.

     d. True    Can be congenital or acquired.

     e. False    A nasal conjunctival growth over the cornea towards the pupil. It occurs commonly in hot, sandy climates or people who work in dusty factories.

**13.** a. True    Increased hydration of the crystalline lens occurs.

     b. True    Congenital cataracts can develop following such infections.

     c. True    A side effect from systemic and topical steroid usage.

     d. True    Penetrating and non-penetrating ocular injuries can lead to cataract.

     e. True    Inflammation within the eye speeds up the process of cataract.

**14.** a. True

     b. False    Steroids are principally required.

     c. False    Antivirals are principally required.

     d. False    Eye shield and urgent referral. No topical medications, which may cause further wound gape and expulsion of intraocular contents.

     e. True    A poorly healed corneal abrasion may lead to a new abrasion and associated symptoms. Ocular lubricants may be required long term as prophylaxis.

**15.** a. False    Not always. Usually a raised intraocular pressure for that individual, which could be normal or low compared to others in the population.

     b. False    This field defect occurs with a parietal lobe lesion.

     c. True    Gangion cells, which make up the nerve fibre layer, are getting squashed at the optic nerve head.

     d. True    Nasal step or paracentral scotoma fields can occur.

     e. False    A cupped optic disc occurs.

**16.** a. False    Ocular pain occurs.

     b. True    Particularly a symptom of subacute angle closure glaucoma.

     c. True    A central nervous system mediated (vomiting centre) response.

     d. False    Photophobia occurs.

     e. False    Ipsilateral headache can occur. The rash is suggestive of herpes zoster ophthalmicus.

**17.** a. True    Tradenames include Alphagan and Iopidine.

     b. True    Previously a first line agent for open angle glaucoma. Tradenames include Timolol and Betagan. Not to be used in asthma and bronchitis patients.

     c. True    Particularly useful for angle closure and chronic narrow angle glaucoma.

     d. True    A first-line agent for open angle glaucoma. Tradenames include Xalatan, Travatan and Lumigan.

     e. True    Particularly useful for uveitis-related glaucoma.

**18.** a. True    A form of diabetic maculopathy.

     b. True    This sign occurs in proliferative diabetic retinopathy, at the border between normal and ischaemic (peripheral) retina.

     c. True    This sign occurs in proliferative diabetic retinopathy. New vessels on the iris.

     d. True    This complication can occur following proliferative diabetic retinopathy.

     e. True    This sudden painless loss of vision is due to bleeding from new vessels at disc or elsewhere.

**19.** a. True    Diabetic maculopathy warrants referral.

     b. True    Focal or macular grid laser may be required.

     c. False    A decrease in vision is required.

     d. True    Closer monitoring of the patient can be performed before further progression to proliferative diabetic retinopathy.

     e. True    The patient may require pan-retinal laser photocoagulation.

**20.** a. False    Photophobia, pain and not increased floaters are more likely with angle closure glaucoma.

     b. True    A possibility if the vision is good, but retinal tear must be excluded.

c. False   Good vision is not compatible with macular off retinal detachment.

d. True   Triad of increased floaters, photopsia and small (unnoticed) peripheral loss of vision are present.

e. True   Tobacco dust is a useful clinical sign in this situation.

**21.** a. False   Glaucoma leads to cupped disc.

b. True   Diplopia in an elderly patient warrants an urgent ESR blood test.

c. True   A pathonomonic sign.

d. True   An extracranial blood vessel can be affected, including the other eye.

e. True   A sign of arteritic anterior ischaemic optic neuropathy.

**22.** a. False   Oral and genital ulcers, panuveitis, arteritis, HLA-B51 positive blood test and hypopyon may occur.

b. True   Associated with a low CD4 white cell count (<100).

c. True   In young adults should alert to the possibility of HIV infection.

d. True   This pigmented lesion can hide in the conjunctival fornix under the eylids.

e. False   Can be caused by vasculitic conditions such as Wegener's granulomatosis or Rheumatoid arthritis.

**23.** a. True   Non-steroidal systemic treatment can prevent spinal deformities and prevent ocular inflammatory relapses.

b. False   Inflammatory rather than vasculitic aetiology.

c. False   A posterior uveitis occurs rather than just an anterior uveitis.

d. False   Scleritis, not uveitis.

e. True   An enteric cause and association of anterior uveitis.

**24.** a. True   A white reflex due to retinal exudation.

b. True   A white reflex and reduced red reflex due to lens media opacity.

c. True   The most sinister cause for a white reflex, which must not be forgotten.

d. False   Retinal changes with leukocoria occur in familial exudative vitreoretinopathy.

e. True   'ToRCH' screen – Toxoplasmosis, Rubella, Cytomegalovirus, Herpes simplex

**25.** a. False   Very difficult to perform with a baby. A very important test for a child or adult.

b. True   To elicit latent and manifest strabismus.

c. True   Refractive error, anisometropia, ametropia are common causes for amblyopia.

d. True   To exclude media opacity and retinal disease.

e. False   Very difficult to perform with a baby. Visual acuity must be attempted (e.g. forced choice preferential learning).

**26.** a. True   Clinical features include corneal haze, buphthalmos and Halb's striae.

b. True   Intrauterine infections can cause corneal and lenticular opacities.

c. True   Birth trauma can lead to breaks in Descemet's corneal layer.

d. False   A phakomatosis.

e. False   A hereditary disorder with skin, other organ, retina and neurological manifestations.

**27.** a. True   A feature of giant cell arteritis affecting extracranial blood vessels.

b. False   New vessels at optic disc occur.

c. False   Disc drusen cause a pseudo-swollen optic disc appearance.

d. True   Bilateral swollen optic discs with raised intracranial pressure (on lumbar puncture).

e. True   Optic neuropathy occurs due to swollen orbital (fat) tissue squashing the optic nerve.

**28.** a. True   Squashing of the optic disc changes its shape (in cross-section) from a saucer to a tea cup.

b. False   Macular drusen not disc drusen.

c. True   Ischaemic retina can cause new vessels at disc or on iris (rubreosis).

d. True   A pale disc implies an optic neuropathy over 2 months ago.

e. True   Can occur by compression of the optic nerve by glioma or meningioma.

**29.** a. True   Acuity should never be omitted when a casualty patient presents with an eye problem.

b. False   Eye movements test cranial nerves III, IV and VI, rather than II, the optic nerve.

c. True   Enlarged blind spot can occur in conditions like optic neuritis.

d. True   A very sensitive early warning sign of optic nerve dysfunction.

e. True   Cannot be performed if one eye has been removed or enucleated.

**30.** a. True   20% of the UK population have this feature and are normal (physiological anisocoria).

b. True   One working right pupil and two working optic nerves are present.

c. False   Two eyes and optic nerves are required for RAPD test. The ipsilateral optic nerve needs to be working, or seeing, when a fixed dilated pupil is present.

d. True   An RAPD may be still be present despite PEARL.

e. True   One working left pupil and two working optic nerves are present.

# Dermatology

**31.** c.

**32.** e.

**33.** a. True
b. True
c. False
d. True
e. True

**34.** a. True
b. True
c. True
d. False
e. True

**35.** a. True
b. False
c. True
d. True
e. True

**36.** a. True
b. True
c. True
d. True
e. False

**37.** a. False
b. True
c. True
d. True
e. True

**38.** a. True
b. True
c. True
d. True
e. False

**39.** a. True
b. False
c. True
d. True
e. True

**40.** a. True
b. True
c. True
d. True
e. False

**41.** a. False
b. True
c. True
d. True
e. True

**42.** a. True
b. True
c. True
d. False
e. True

**43.** a. True
b. True
c. True
d. False
e. True

**44.** a. True
b. True
c. True
d. True
e. False

**45.** a. True
b. False
c. True
d. True
e. True

**46.** a. True
b. True
c. True
d. False
e. True

**47.** a. True
b. True
c. False
d. True
e. True

**48.** a. True
b. True
c. True
d. False
e. True

**49.** a. False
b. True
c. True
d. True
e. True

**50.** a. True
b. False
c. True
d. True
e. True

**51.** e.

**52.** a. True
b. True
c. True
d. False
e. True

**53.** a. True
b. True
c. False
d. True
e. True

**54.** a. True
b. True
c. True
d. True
e. False

**55.** a. True
b. True
c. True
d. False
e. True

**56.** a. True
b. True
c. True
d. True
e. False

**57.** a. True
b. True
c. False
d. True
e. True

**58.** a. True
b. True
c. True
d. True
e. False

**59.** a. True
b. True
c. True
d. True
e. False

**60.** a. True
b. True
c. True
d. False
e. True

**61.** a. True
b. True
c. True
d. False
e. True

**62.** a. True
b. True
c. True
d. False
e. True

**63.** a. True
b. False
c. True
d. True
e. True

# Ear, Nose and Throat

**64.** d. Laryngeal cancer is most frequently a squamous cell carcinoma. It is strongly associated with tobacco usage and less strongly with heavy consumption of alcohol. The tumour most commonly arises form the structures of the glottis; however, supra-glottic and subglottic varieties exist and may not cause hoarseness until late in the disease process. Treatment is with surgery or radiotherapy; chemotherapy is increasingly combined with these modalities.

**65.** e. Otalgia may be caused by disease of the ear or its surrounding structures, or it may be referred from any of the nerves that innervate the ear. Post-cricoid tumours may cause referred otalgia via the vagus nerve. OME rarely causes pain. In acute otitis media the pain is due to the suppurative process beneath an intact tympanic membrane and therefore resolves following perforation. Ménière's disease does not cause otalgia.

**66.** a. Nasal polyps in childhood raise the possibility of cystic fibrosis or mucociliary clearance disorder. Patients with polyps rarely suffer from sinusitis symptoms. Nasal polyps are not curable but are best treated with corticosteroids topically or occasionally orally. Surgery is used following failure of medical therapy. Unilateral nasal polyps may represent an inverted papilloma or other tumours. They require further investigation with imaging and biopsy.

**67.** c. Cholesteatoma is relatively common (1:10 000 population per year). It is caused by proliferation of squamous epithelium in the middle ear cleft. It is thought that most cholesteatomas are preceded by retraction and pocket formation in the superior part of the tympanic membrane (attico-antral). Hearing loss can occur as a result of ossicular erosion (conductive) or later in the disease process by invasion of the cochlea (sensorineural). Treatment involves surgical removal of the cholesteatoma from within the middle ear and mastoid (mastoidectomy).

**68.** d. Tympanometry measures the compliance of the tympanic membrane. It is an objective test and is well tolerated by children in whom it is extremely useful. In OME tympanic membrane compliance is reduced and the trace is flat. A normal trace shows a peaked appearance. Compliance is also reduced in some cases of otosclerosis due to stiffening of the ossicular chain.

**69.** e. While relatively uncommon in the UK, oral cancer is very common in large parts of south Asia and China. The main risk is from tobacco consumption. Betel chewing is also a risk factor in Asian populations. The primary lesion is usually a progressive ulcer of the oral mucosa. The ulcers are frequently painless until they invade nerve tissue. Spread is to the cervical lymph nodes and decreases survival by 50%; bony metastasis is rare.

**70.** a. OSA is most commonly due to obesity and is more common in males. It causes disturbed sleep patterns with loss of the REM phase and resultant daytime sleepiness. Early morning wakefulness is suggestive of depression/anxiety. OSA is best treated with weight loss and CPAP (continuous positive airway pressure). Surgery is rarely indicated.

**71.** d. Recurrent acute tonsillitis is caused by both viruses and bacteria; clinically it is difficult to determine which is the cause. It is common in children of school age and young adults. Peritonsillar abscess is an uncommon complication of tonsillitis. OSA is now the most common indication for tonsillectomy.

**72.** a. Bell's palsy is a facial paralysis which is thought to be caused by herpes simplex infection of the seventh nerve. It causes facial paralysis, loss of taste sensation and hyperacusis along with decreased tear production. In most cases the paralysis is temporary. It is treated with steroids and antivirals.

**73.** d. Fractured nasal bones are rare in children and are most often seen in young adults. The diagnosis is a clinical one; radiographs are rarely helpful and are not routinely requested. The patient should be assessed around 1 week after injury to decide if manipulation of displaced nasal bones is required. Widening of the medial intercanthal distance suggests significant naso-ethmoidal injury. CT scans are required to confirm the diagnosis. Open reduction and reconstruction may be required for these injuries.

**74.** c. Ménière's disease comprises episodic ear fullness, tinnitus and roonal vertigo. Sensorineural hearing loss occurs and may fluctuate. Headache and loss of consciousness do not occur.

**75.** e. Vocal cord nodules are commonly bilateral and located on the anterior $1/3$ of the vocal fold. They are not pre-malignant. They are more common in young females and are related to occupation (singers, teachers, etc.). They and the vocal misuse which causes them is best treated with speech therapy.

**76.** d. Thyroid cancer is more common in women. It can present as a solitary nodule or as a nodule within a multinodular goitre. Follicular adenoma can only be confirmed on histology following surgical excision. These lesions are not sensitive to conventional radiotherapy.

**77.** d. HHT is transmitted in an autosomal dominant manner. It produces capillary malformations of mucosal surfaces. Commonly affected areas include the oral cavity, nose and GIT. Epistaxis is often recurrent and severe. Bleeding may be severe enough to cause anaemia. Recurrent epistaxis may be treated with surgical closure of the nasal cavity (Young's procedure).

**78.** d. Laryngomalacia usually results in mild stridor which commences around 6 weeks after birth and is often worse in the supine position. The problem usually gets better with growth and rarely requires surgical intervention. Failure to thrive occurs only in severe cases.

**79.** c. It is thought to be caused by relative Eustachian tube immaturity. OME causes a conductive hearing loss. Its most important effect is speech and language delay which may be detrimental to educational and even socioeconomic achievements.

**80.** d. Thyroglossal cysts are the most common congenital neck lumps in children. They are attached to the tongue base and thyroid and therefore move with tongue protrusion and swallowing. They are usually found below the hyoid bone. They notoriously recur following surgery.

**81.** a. Bacterial sinusitis usually follows functional obstruction of the osteomeatal complex by allergy or viral upper respiratory tract infection. It is not contagious. Surprisingly, it is not common in nasal polyposis. Diagnosis is based on history and examination. Facial radiographs are neither sensitive nor specific. CT is preferable.

**82.** e. Lichen planus causes white patches and occasional painless ulceration of the buccal mucosa, tongue and gingivae. It may be associated with scaly patches on the flexor surfaces of the forearms. It occurs mainly in older adults. The erosive form may be considered pre-malignant.

339

83. d. Otosclerosis is a disease of bone turnover which primarily affects the fistulae ante fenestrum of the oval window. It causes stapes fixation and a conductive hearing loss. Cochlear otosclerosis may also occur leading to a sensorineural hearing loss. The disease is more common in women and often worsens in pregnancy.

84. c. This developmental abnormality is thought to be derived from ectoderm from the first branchial arch. It presents as a cystic swelling anterior to the upper third of the sternomastoid. Malignant lymphadenopathy may present in a similar manner, therefore smokers with 'branchial cysts' should be thoroughly investigated. Any neck lump associated with a middle ear effusion should be regarded as a nasopharyngeal carcinoma until proven otherwise.

85. d. Smoking is the major risk factor for these malignancies in the UK. Alcohol, UV light and salt fish are all co-factors for various head and neck malignancies. Despite lots of research interest, herpes simplex is not an accepted risk factor.

86. b. Allergic rhinitis shows increased serum eosinophil levels. It is mediated by a type I hypersensitivity reaction. Vasoconstrictors may treat the symptoms but are contraindicated in what is a chronic condition as they may lead to rhinitis medicamentosa. Allergic diseases become less prevalent with age and are uncommon in the elderly.

87. c. The most common reasons for tonsillectomy include recurrent acute tonsillitis and OSA (in children). In the UK it is nearly always performed under GA and with an overnight stay. The presence of acute tonsillitis is a contraindication to surgery.

88. c. 80% affect the parotid gland. 80% are pleomorphic adenomas. Minor salivary gland tumours affect the upper lip more than the lower. Diagnosis is based on clinical history supplemented by FNA and ultrasound. Open biopsy should not be performed owing to the risk of tumour seeding.

89. e. Tracheostomy involves opening the trachea at the third or fourth tracheal ring. High entry may lead to stenosis. The operation may be done via a standard horizontal skin incision or percutaneously using the Seldinger technique. Cuff pressures should not exceed tissue capillary perfusion pressure (25 mmHg) or necrosis and subglottic stenosis may occur.

90. a. Fractures of the temporal bone are nearly always associated with blood under the ear drum. They are decreasing in incidence (seat belts). They usually result in hearing loss. Facial palsy is more common with longitudinal fractures.

91. b. Atypical TB affects young children. It causes pre-auricular cervical and submandibular lymphadenopathy, often with brawny skin involvement. The skin and lymph node lesions are usually painless. Chest symptoms are rare.

92. b. Epistaxis most commonly arises from the antero-inferior septum, Little's area. Less commonly it may arise from the posterosuperior part of the nose; ligation of the anterior and posterior ethmoid arteries (from the ophthalmic) may help to stop this. Ice packs have little effect. Traumatic epistaxis usually stops spontaneously. Embolization is a rarely used option of last resort.

93. b. BPPV causes episodic dizziness, usually when rolling over in bed. The symptoms may be short-lived but are often unpleasant. Diagnosis is based on the history and a positive Dix–Hallpike test, that is the presence of rotational nystagmus on hanging the head over the edge of a couch. The nystagmus lasts only 20 seconds or so and is not present at rest.

94. a. Reinke's oedema is swelling contained in the superficial lamina propria of the vocal folds (Reinke's space). It is generally precipitated by irritants and there may be a hormonal link. HPV is not associated.

95. d. Recurrent oral ulceration is said to be less common among smokers. It may be caused by haematinic deficiencies and is seen in Behçet's in combination with genital and ocular ulcers. Idiopathic or aphthous ulceration is often brought on by stress. Coeliac disease may present with recurrent oral ulceration.

96. c. Tinnitus is the perception of noise from the auditory system in the absence of stimulation. Musical tinnitus is a misnomer – this is an auditory hallucination and requires referral to a psychiatrist. Pulsatile tinnitus may be the presenting symptom of a vascular tumour within the ear neck or skull base. Tinnitus is most often associated with hearing loss. Medication is of no proven benefit and treatment may be difficult.

97. d. Choanal atresia is more common in girls than in boys and results from failure of the posterior choanae to develop properly. Unilateral disease is more common than bilateral. Infants are obligate nasal breathers, therefore bilateral atresia may cause problems soon after birth, especially when feeding. Diagnosis may be confirmed by failure to pass a nasogastric tube through the nose. CT scans are used to plan surgical treatment.

98. e. Laryngeal papillomatosis is caused by infection with human papillomavirus (HPV). This is thought to be vertically transmitted from the birth canal of an infected mother. Children and young adults are most commonly affected with lesions most often in the glottis. It is a difficult disease to treat. Serial laser or microdebrider resection is the mainstay of therapy but is not curative.

# Ophthalmology

1. Thyroid eye disease symptoms include scratchy or gritty eyes, redness, conjunctival and eyelid swelling, diplopia (particularly on upgaze), cosmetic appearance (prominent eyes) and, in advanced cases, visual loss. Thyroid eye disease signs include proptosis, conjunctival injection, lid retraction, lid lag (on down gaze) and, in advanced cases, optic neuropathy (e.g. decreased acuity, red desaturation, swollen optic disc).

2. Main benefits are improvements in vision and glare symptoms. Patients often state that their colour vision has also improved dramatically. The microsurgical procedure is usually performed under local or topical anaesthesia, as a day case, without corneal sutures. Complications, which ideally should be mentioned during consent, include endophthalmitis (0.1% risk) and suprachoroidal haemorrhage (0.1% risk). The risk of retinal detachment increases dramatically if there is a posterior capsular rupture during surgery, with vitreous loss. High myopia and pre-existing lattice degeneration also increase the risk. Up to 30% of patients within 5 years will develop posterior capsule opacification, which will require YAG laser capsulotomy.

3. The four components of an eye examination relevant to the glaucoma patient include: intraocular pressure (IOP), anterior chamber angle, optic nerve ('optic disc') and visual field.

   a. Standard IOP is measured using the Goldmann tonometer to gently flatten the tear film on the cornea. A drop of topical anaesthetic with flourescein is initially placed on the cornea.

   b. The anterior chamber angle is the space between the cornea and iris. Aqueous fluid drainage from the eye is via the angle and can be obstructed by the iris itself (e.g. angle closure glaucoma) or by abnormal blood vessels (e.g. rubeosis).

   c. The optic nerve structure can be seen in two dimensions with a direct ophthalmoscope and in three dimensions with a slit lamp owing to a binocular view. A normal optic disc looks relatively flat like a plate or saucer, whereas a squashed optic nerve head, due to raised intraocular pressure, leads to the appearance of a tea cup or a cupped optic disc.

   d. The functional consequence of optic nerve damage is documented by visual field testing. Paracentral or arcuate scotomas which respect the horizontal mid-line are suggestive of glaucomatous visual field loss rather than neurological, where the vertical meridian is respected.

4. Age-related macular degeneration (ARMD) is a disorder of the retinal pigment epithelium (RPE), which acts as the trash can for photoreceptors. The waste products that are not recycled overspill and form drusen. These are usually centred around the fovea in the centre of the macular region. 'DRY' ARMD: Patients present with a gradual painless reduction in vision, often over many years. Characteristically drusen (soft), pigment clumping and macular atrophy. 'WET' ARMD: A sudden loss or distortion of vision occurs due to the formation of a subretinal neovascular membrane (SRNVM) or to haemorrhage or subretinal fluid (SRF) or leakage. Diabetic maculopathy is due to either ischaemia, from poor circulation at the fovea, or leakage from damaged capillaries, causing retinal thickening or oedema and formation of hard exudates or circinates. The patient may be asymptomatic or present with a gradual deterioration of vision. The location of circinate exudates tends to be centred eccentric to the fovea, whereas macular drusen tend to be centred over the fovea.

5. A cloudy cornea or cataract can lead to blindness or amblyopia (i.e. 'lazy eye'). Visual acuity develops during early childhood, usually until 8 years of age. If the ocular images are not aligned in childhood, then the brain concentrates on the better seeing eye at the expense of the other eye. The result is suppression of visual development of the misaligned eye or amblyopia.

6. Congenital cataract is an important cause of amblyopia due to stimulus deprivation. It may present with a cloudy pupil or leukocoria at screening following birth. Investigation and treatment of any underlying treatable cause should be performed. Chromosomal abnormalities, metabolic abnormalities and intrauterine infections can all cause congenital cataract. Congenital glaucoma, forceps delivery or birth trauma and congenital rubella can all cause a cloudy cornea.

7. The five main types of optic discs, which should not be confused or mistaken, are: normal, new vessels at disc, cupped (glaucoma), pale (optic atrophy) and swollen.

   a. The normal optic disc comprises a central optic cup and an outer optic disc. The pink zone between the cup and disc is called the neuroretinal rim (NRR). About 1.5 million ganglion cells, which start at the retinal surface, pass along the retina and turn 90° to exit the eye via the NRR of the optic disc. Retinal arteries, from the central retinal artery, enter the eye and climb over the NRR and pass along the retina, while retinal veins originating from the retinal surface climb over the NRR, turn 90° and leave along the optic nerve, similar to the ganglion cells.

b. New vessels at disc occur mainly in two conditions: proliferative diabetic retinopathy and following ischaemic central retinal vein occlusion. In both of these conditions retinal ischaemia causes additional new blood vessels to grow which are fragile and can leak and bleed to cause vitreous and/or pretinal haemorrhage.

c. Raised intraocular pressure for an individual can cause squashing of the optic nerve head. The change in morphology from a flat saucer shape (i.e. normal optic disc) to a tea cup shape (i.e. cupped optic disc) occurs in glaucoma.

d. A pale optic disc refers to the NRR changing its colour from pink to white. It does not refer to optic disc cupping, where the central optic cup may appear to be enlarged and white in colour. It takes about 2 months for a pale optic disc to develop and indicates an optic neuropathy, which can be from many causes (e.g. infective, inflammatory, neoplastic, etc.).

e. A swollen optic nerve head has an ill-defined optic disc and cup. There may be flame haemorrhages on the NRR and engorged blood vessels, particularly the venules at the optic nerve head. There can be many 'surgical sieve' causes: vascular, infective, inflammatory, neoplastic, etc. It can occur unilaterally in central retinal vein occlusion or bilaterally in papilloedema.

f. The five main ways of measuring this lady's left optic nerve function include:

AFFRO - **A**cuity, **F**ields, **R**elative afferent pupil defect (RAPD), **R**ed colour and **O**ptic disc appearance. She is suspected to have optic neuritis. One would expect the acuity to have decreased from 6/5 to 6/9 initially and then drop down within a week to counting fingers and then improve towards 6/9 again within 2 months. Not all patients have a full recovery of their vision. An enlarged blind spot accounts for a central type of scotoma noted by these patients. A left RAPD would be expected to confirm inflammation of the meninges surrounding the optic nerve. Red colour desaturation is highly sensitive for indicating an optic neuropathy or poor optic nerve function. Ishihara colour plate testing would also be poor on the affected left eye. The optic nerve head may appear normal, if retrobulbar optic neuritis, or swollen, if inflammation is right up to the eyeball. The pain on eye movement occurs due to stretching of the inflamed meninges, which is analogous to the sleeve of a shirt sliding when moving the hand left or right.

# Dermatology

8. See Fig. 15.1.

9. Lichen planus is characterized by small, flat-topped, purple, polygonal, puriritic papules. A fine lacy white pattern may be present known as Wickham's striae. They commonly occur on the flexor parts of the limbs.

10. The most important prognostic indicator for malignant melanoma is how deep the lesion has invaded into the skin:

| | |
|---|---|
| ≤0.75 mm | > 95 % 5-year survival |
| >0.75–1 mm | 80 % 5-year survival |
| >3.5 mm | 50 % 5-year survival |

11. The common trigger factors for psoriasis are: stress, excess alcohol, certain medications such as β-blockers and lithium, and infection.

12. The following features would raise concern about a mole:
- Rapid increase in size
- Change in colour
- Asymmetry
- Irregular margins
- Bleeding
- Itching
- Satellite lesions

13. Actinic keratosis, seborrhoeic keratosis, Bowen's disease, basal cell carcinoma, squamous cell carcinoma, melanomas.

# Ear, Nose and Throat

14. There are clinical test of hearing you can do in the consulting room. These include whispered, conversational and loud spondees and tuning fork tests. The main tuning fork tests are Weber's lateralising test and Rinne's test. More formal audiological testing relies upon the pure tone audiogram. Other tests include otoacoustic emissions (OAEs) and brain-stem-evoked response audiometry). Tympanometry, although not strictly speaking a test of hearing, is usually performed as it gives useful information about the state of the middle ear and therefore the cause of any hearing loss.

15. There are three main components in the management of allergic rhinitis:
   a. Allergen avoidance:
      i. Minimize soft furnishings in bed room
      ii. Hypoallergenic duvet mattress and pillow covers.
      iii. Boil wash of all bedding weekly
   b. Medical therapy tailored to symptoms
      i. Inhaled nasal steroids
      ii. Systemic 3rd generation anti-histamine
      iii. Others, e.g. anti-histamine eye drops
   c. Surgical therapy, although this is rarely indicated for simple allergic rhinitis. Occasional turbinate

reduction surgery if severe refractory nasal blockage.

Extra points for mentioning allergen immunotherapy (used for severe disease unresponsive to medication)

6. Risk of malignancy is increased with:

- Patient factors:
    Age (<20 or >65 years)
    Male sex
    Exposure to ionising radiation
    Family history thyroid cancer

- History:
    Rapid growth
    Hoarseness

- Examination:
    Hard fixed texture
    Cervical lymphadenopathy
    Vocal cord paralysis

17. This is a classic age group and history for obstructive sleep apnoea. Further investigation would be based on the history and examination (looking for the most likely causes, e.g. adeno tonsillar enlargement). Diagnosis depends on a sleep study (polysomnography or in children the less demanding home sleep study). For moderate to severe OSA in this age group the standard treatment is surgical removal of the tonsils and adenoids, this usually results in a rapid improvement in symptoms.

18. Three common causes of vertigo:

- Benign paroxysmal positional vertigo (BPPV)
- Menieres disease
- (Viral) labyrinthitis

The history here suggests BPPV. Brief severe episodes of rotatory vertigo caused by change in position (the key to diagnosis is the timing of the episodes). The diagnostic clinical test for BPPV aims to replicate vertigo and thus nystagmus with a rapid change in head position, the Dix-Hallpike Test. If positive it is followed by the treatment, the Epley particle repositioning manoeuvre which via a series of head and body movements aims to rotate the offending debris from the posterior semicircular canal. Surgical ablation of the posterior canal is also used for disease that is unresponsive to Epley manoeuvres.

19. The thyroid gland begins its development at around the 17th day of gestation as an out-pouching from the primitive stomatodeum ( mouth). It leaves the foramen caecum at the junction of the anterior and posterior tongue, and descends through the neck as the thyroglossal duct . It eventually comes to lie anterior to the trachea at around 3 weeks. During its descent "rests" of thyroid cells may be left behind. At a later date, usually early adulthood, these may form cystic lesions. These can occur anywhere from the tongue base to the lower neck but are most common around the hyoid bone close to the midline.

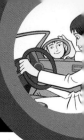

## Ophthalmology

### 1. Concerning red eye and changes in vision:

1. F   Risk factors for central retinal vein occlusion include hypertension and diabetes.
2. D   Chloramphenicol is widely used for this condition.
3. B   Hay fever sufferers and contact lens wearers have papillae and itchy eyes.
4. J
5. A   Nausea and vomiting may also occur.

### 2. Concerning eyelids and double vision:

1. B   Established chalazion requires incision and curettage.
2. E
3. I   Spread of infection to periorbital soft tissues leads to pyrexia.
4. A   Acne rosacea can flare up with alcohol intake.
5. F

### 3. Concerning the cornea and cataracts:

1. J   30% of people can develop capsular opacification within 5 years of cataract surgery.
2. F   Peak incidence of endophthalmitis occurs within 2 weeks of cataract surgery.
3. A   Saline is therefore preferred for contact lens cleaning regimes.
4. B   Patients should taper down steroid drops to avoid rebound anterior uveitis.
5. H   A corneal bacterial infection is most likely.

### 4. Concerning retinal conditions:

1. C   Two major causes of rubreosis include central retinal vein occlusion, and proliferative diabetic retinopathy.
2. G   Tobacco dust suggests presence of retinal tear, which may later lead to a retinal detachment.
3. E   Decreased visual acuity suggests macula has detached.
4. H   Embolic monocular blindness is usually black loss of vision.
5. F   No decrease in visual acuity suggests macula has not detached.

### 5. Concerning medical ophthalmology and uveitis:

1. I   Dry eye and dry mouth symptoms are suggestive of this condition.
2. G   Scleritis is associated with rheumatoid arthritis.
3. E   A subgroup of intermediate uveitis have pars planitis, which can be secondary to demyelination and thus be an aid to the diagnosis of multiple sclerosis.
4. A   Anterior uveitis can be associated with joint problems such as ankylosing spondylitis.
5. D   Urgent ESR and CRP blood tests should be requested. Ask for symptom of jaw claudication, which is pathognomonic for this life-threatening condition.

### 6. Concerning paediatric ophthalmology and strabismus:

1. F
2. D   Intrauterine infection can lead to congenital cataract.
3. J   Retinal laser may be required to those babies who have threshold disease.
4. G
5. A   Patching and refraction for spectacles are important prior to age 8 to minimize and avoid amblyopia.

### 7. Concerning neuro-ophthalmology:

1. I   Sixth nerve palsies are overcome by convergence when reading.
2. C   Right parietal lobe lesion is related to sensory inattention whereas left temporal lobe lesion may be associated with expressive dysphasia.
3. F   Do not to describe one swollen disc as papilloedema.
4. E   The shock waves converge posteriorly along the orbital walls and may cause an inferior blow out fracture.
5. G   An optic chiasm lesion is suggestive of a pituitary tumour or meningioma.

## Dermatology

### 8. Concerning skin rashes:

1. J   Pityriasis vesicolor. Usually there are no symptoms with this rash. The lesions are less sharply defined and the scaling is thinner compared with guttate psoriasis.

2. C Pityriasis rosea. The lesions are classically described as arranged in a 'Christmas tree' distribution. The large patch is known as the herald patch.

3. A Lichen planus. The white lines are known as Wickham's striae.

4. I Guttate psoriasis.

5. H Bullous phemphigus. These red patches are as pre-bullous lesions.

6. E Lichen sclerosus. In the male, it can cause phimosis and urethral stricture.

## 9. Concerning skin infections:

1. C Orf. It can be associated with secondary infection and erythema multiforme.

2. D Herpes zoster. In most cases, this rash occurs in people who have had chicken pox (varicella). It can appear when patients are immunocompromised.

3. E Herpes simplex.

4. B Molluscum contagiosum.

5. F Erthythema infectiosum. This rash is also known as fifth disease and has the slapped cheek sign.

6. I Scabies.

## 10. Concerning skin changes in systemic disease:

1. A Scurvy is due to vitamin C deficiency and can affect those who do not eat fresh fruit and vegetables.

2. E Erythema nodosum can be associated with a number of conditions.

3. D Acanthosis nigricans. Its aetiology may be related to a number of endocrine conditions, and to obesity and malignancy.

4. I Pretibial myxoedema.

5. B Necrobiosis lipoidica.

6. C Granuloma annulare.

## 11. Concerning skin lesions:

1. C Lipoma.

2. J Pyogenic granuloma.

3. E Dermatofibroma.

4. D Seborrhoeic wart.

5. G Actinic keratosis.

6. B Keloid.

## 12. Concerning sebaceous disorders:

1. B Perioral dermatitis. This improves with a prolonged course of oral tetracyclines but her rash may worsen when she stops her topical steroid.

2. D Acne.

3. A Rosacea. There are no comedones in this condition and it can cause rhinophyma.

4. C Hidradenitis suppurativa.

5. G Asteatotic dermatitis.

6. F Seborrhoeic dermatitis. This condition tends to occur where the sebaceous glands are most active.

## 13. Concerning erythroderma:

1. G Mycosis fungoides.

2. C Pemphigus foliaceus.

3. E Pityriasis rubra pilaris.

4. B Drug allergy.

5. I Stasis eczema. The spread of the eczema to other parts of the body is known as an IDE reaction.

6. A Psoriasis. There are typical nail changes associated with psoriasis.

## 14. Concerning leg ulcers:

1. J Vasculitis.

2. F Squamous cell carcinoma.

3. B Arterial.

4. A Venous. Venous ulcers can also affect the lateral malleolus, less often than the medial side, and can be painful but not usually as severe as arterial ulcers.

5. E Pyoderma gangrenosum. This can associated with inflammatory bowel disease, rheumatoid arthritis and myeloma.

6. H Leprosy.

## 15. Concerning pigmentation:

1. D Minocycline-induced.

2. B Melasma. The oral contraceptive pill can also cause this.

3. A Vitiligo.

4. C Addison's disease.

5. G Pityriasis vesicolor.

6. E Peutz–Jeghers syndrome. This condition is autosomal dominant and can be associated with bowel problems.

## 16. Concerning the terminology of skin lesions:

1. F Papule.

2. B Plaque.

3. G Wheal.

4. I Erosion.

5. E Macule.

6. C Vesicle.

## 17. Concerning skin pre-malignant and malignant disorders:

1. E Bowen's disease. The scale tends not to be as thick as that found in psoriasis.

2. C Squamous cell carcinoma.

3. A Basal cell carcinoma.

4. B Keratocanthoma.

5. I Lentigo maligna. When the abnormal cells penetrate the dermis, it then becomes lentigo maligna melanoma.

6. H Atypical naevus.

# Ear, Nose and Throat

## 18. Concerning hearing loss:

1. B Ménière's disease. Vertigo with tinnitus and hearing loss suggest vestibulocochlear dysfunction. From the list of available conditions vestibular schwannoma and Ménière's disease could both cause these symptoms and signs. A vestibular schwannoma would of course be visible on a gadolinium-enhanced MRI scan.

2. A Otitis media with effusion. Given that the child is only 4 years old the number of possibilities is limited. They would include otitis media with effusion (glue ear), congenital sensorineural hearing loss and wax impaction (extremely unlikely to cause a speech delay). The audiograms show a conductive loss with flattened tympanograms (reduced middle ear compliance) making OME the most likely diagnosis.

3. H Otosclerosis. An adult patient with conductive hearing loss in her left ear (from the tuning fork tests). The external ear and ear drum are normal which leaves only otosclerosis and middle ear effusion as likely diagnoses. Tympanometry is the key here; a normal tympanogram excludes a middle ear effusion.

4. F This elderly patient has gradual onset sensorineural loss in both ears. This is characteristic of age-related hearing loss or presbyacusis.

## 19. Concerning neck lumps:

1. E Branchial cyst. Slow growing painless swelling in the lateral neck in this age group could represent lymphoma, pleomorphic adenoma or a branchial cyst. The ultrasound appearances indicate a branchial cyst.

2. A Squamous cell carcinoma. In any patient with a neck lump and hoarseness, but especially in a smoker, one must consider malignancy. Either squamous cell carcinoma or lymphoma could present like this. The appearance of the larynx is suspicious of a supraglottic squamous cell carcinoma; keratin pearls in biopsy confirm this.

3. D Parotid mass. There is only one listed here, pleomorphic adenoma.

4. F Bilateral swellings and a bruit suggest carotid body tumour (10% bilateral).

## 20. Concerning nasal blockage:

1. F Nasal blockage in a schoolchild can be caused by allergy, adenoidal hypertrophy or rarely choanal atresia. A fleshy mass in the nasopharynx is of course the adenoids.

2. I Bankers get stressed! Examination is normal, it can only be a physiological nasal cycle.

3. B Unilateral blockage and visible polyps. This could represent nasal polyposis or inverted papilloma. CT findings of widening of the ostium and lack of changes in the other side suggest inverted papilloma. Nasal polyposis is nearly always bilateral.

4. A Classical allergic symptoms; oedematous mucosa in a young person equates to allergic rhinitis.

## 21. Concerning stridor:

1. C This child has a cough and a pyrexial illness. The stridor follows a coughing fit. The only infective diseases listed here are croup and epiglottitis. The history is classical for croup.

2. G The clue is the operation, total thyroidectomy. Unilateral cord palsy due to recurrent laryngeal nerve damage causes hoarseness but rarely breathing difficulty. Bilateral recurrent laryngeal nerve damage causes the cords to lie in an adducted position causing stridor but a relatively normal voice.

3. A This is a tricky one. He obviously has an infection. However, you may assume that both epiglottitis and croup are only seen in children. Wrong! Epiglottitis is more commonly seen in adult smokers and drinkers as most children have had *Haemophilus influenzae* vaccination.

4. H An infant with stridor and apparently recurrent chest infections. The possibilities are laryngomalacia and subglottic stenosis, both of which cause narrowing of the airway and subsequent respiratory difficulty if there is an upper respiratory tract infection. The history of neonatal intubation suggests subglottic stenosis secondary to the damaging effects of the endotracheal tube.

## 22. Concerning dizziness:

1. C Classic story for acute vestibulitis. Could possibly be vestibular schwannoma but the lack of hearing loss makes this less likely.

2. H Beware the dizzy patient with loss of consciousness! The cause lies outside the vestibular apparatus.

3. D   Aural fullness, worsening tinnitus and rotational vertigo are all symptoms of Ménière's disease. The symptoms can, of course, be caused by acute mastoiditis but this would be an unusual presentation and the lack of systemic features make it unlikely.

4. G   Yes it is positional but benign paroxysmal positional vertigo is usually precipitated rotational movements such as rolling over in bed. Dizziness with neck extension is a symptom of vertebrobasilar insufficiency.

## 23. Concerning hoarseness:

1. A   This is Reinke's oedema caused by laryngeal irritation. It nearly always affects both vocal folds causing generalized swelling rather than discrete masses.

2. F   Papillomata can affect the larynx in children leading to hoarseness and occasionally stridor. Nodules may also occur but are confined to the vocal cords.

3. D   Adduction on coughing is normal and indicates normal neurological input to the vocal cords.

4. E   A classic 'voice abuser' with classic vocal cord nodules.

## 24. Concerning oral lesions:

1. E   Fibro-epithelial polyps are soft sessile masses which affect the cheeks and tongue and are like skin tags affecting the oral mucosa.

2. D   Lichen planus causes white patches affecting cheeks and tongue.

3. G   A vesiculo-bullous disorder of the elderly that frequently affects the eye. Pemphigus also causes bullae and erosions, but most often with extensive skin involvement.

4. B   One of the most common sites for oral cancer is the retromolar area along with the tongue and tonsil. The lesions are frequently painless.

## 25. Concerning dysphagia:

1. C   This is strictly speaking odynophagia and is often a sign of inflammatory disease rather than malignancy. The drug habit of the patient should suggest immunocompromise, making candidal oesophagitis a possibility.

2. D   Pharyngeal pouches present in elderly patients with dysphagia and regurgitation. Weight loss does occur but is not as severe or abrupt as with malignant disease.

3. A   Progressive dysphagia with weight loss is cancer until proven otherwise. Both oesophageal and gastric malignancies can cause these symptoms.

4. H   This history strongly suggests neurological disease; the intermittent symptoms and frequent fatigue are typical of myasthenia gravis.

## Section I: Ophthalmology

Forrester, J. V., Dick, A. D., McMenamin, P. & Lee, W. R. 2002. *The Eye: Basic Sciences and Practice*, 2nd edn. London: W.B. Saunders

Khaw, P. T., Shah, P. & Elkington, A. R. 2004. *ABC of Eyes*, 4th edn. London: BMJ Books

Olver, J. & Cassidy, L. 2005. *Ophthalmology at a Glance*. 2nd edn. London: Blackwell Publishing

## Section II: Dermatology

### Chapter 15

Graham-Brown, R. & Burns, T. 2002. *Lecture Notes on Dermatology*, 8th edn. London: Blackwell Science

Buxton, P. K. 2003. *ABC of Dermatology*, 4th edn. London: BMJ Publishing

### Chapter 16

Du Vivier, A. 2002. *Atlas of Clinical Dermatology*, 3rd edn. London: Churchill Livingstone

Hunter, J. A., Savin, J. A. & Dahl, M. 2002. *Clinical Dermatology*, 3rd edn. London: Blackwell Science

### Chapter 17

Du Vivier, A. 2002. *Atlas of Clinical Dermatology*, 3rd edn. London: Churchill Livingstone

Fitzpatrick, T. B., Johnson, R. A., Wolff, K. & Suurmond, D. 2001. *Color Atlas and Synopsis of Clinical Dermatology: Common and Serious Diseases*, 4th edn. McGraw-Hill

### Chapter 18

Buxton, P. K. 2003. *ABC of Dermatology*, 4th edn. London: BMJ Publishing

Gawkrodger, D. J. 1997. *Dermatology: An Illustrated Colour Text*, 2nd edn. London: Churchill Livingstone

### Chapter 19

MacKie, R. M. 2003. *Clinical Dermatology*, 5th edn. London: Oxford University Press

Gawkrodger, D. J. 1997. *Dermatology: An Illustrated Colour Text*, 2nd edn. London: Churchill Livingstone

### Chapter 20

Du Vivier, A. 2002. *Atlas of Clinical Dermatology*, 3rd edn. London: Churchill Livingstone

Graham-Brown, R., Burns, T. 2002. *Lecture Notes on Dermatology*, 8th edn. London: Blackwell Science

### Chapter 21

Primary Care Dermatology Society and British Association of Dermatologists. 2003. *Guidelines for the Management of atopic eczema*. February 2003

Ellis, C., Luger, T., Abeck, D. et al. 2001. International Consensus Conference on Atopic Dermatitis II (ICCAD II): clinical update and current treatment strategies. *British Journal of Dermatology* **148**(Suppl. 63):3–10

National Prescribing Centre. 1998. The use of emollients in dry skin conditions. *MEREC Bulletin* 9:45–48

### Chapter 22

Bourke, J., Coulson, I. & English, J. 2001. Guidelines for care of contact dermatitis. *British Journal of Dermatology* **145**:877–885

### Chapter 23

Koo, J., Lee, E., Lee, C. S. & Lebwohl, M. 2004. Psoriasis. *Journal of American Academy of Dermatology* **50**:613–622

Lebwohl, M. 2003. Psoriasis. *Lancet* 361:1197–1204

Du Vivier, A. 2002. *Atlas of Clinical Dermatology*, 3rd edn. London: Churchill Livingstone

Graham-Brown, R. & Burns, T. 2002. *Lecture Notes on Dermatology*, 8th edn. London: Blackwell Science

### Chapter 24

Wojnarowska, F., Kirtschig, G., Highet, A. S., Venning, V. A. & Khumalo, N. P. 2002. Guidelines for the management of bullous pemphigoid. *British Journal of Dermatology* **147**:214–221

Harman, K. E., Albert, S. & Black, M. M. 2003. Guidelines for the management of pemphigus vulgaris. *British Journal of Dermatology* **149**:926–937

### Chapter 25

Buxton, P. K. 2003. *ABC of Dermatology*, 4th edn. London: BMJ Publishing

Hunter, J. A., Savin, J. A. & Dahl, M. 2002. *Clinical Dermatology*, 3rd edn. London: Blackwell Science

Du Vivier, A. 2002. *Atlas of Clinical Dermatology*, 3rd edn. London: Churchill Livingstone

### Chapter 26

www.merck.praxis.md pigmented skin lesions (accessed 09/Feb/2004)

Roberts, D. L. L., Anstey, A. V., Barlow, R. J. & Cox, N. H. 2002. UK guidelines for the management of cutaneous melanoma. *British Journal of Dermatology* **146**:7–17

## Chapter 27

Cox, N. H., Eedy, D. J. & Morton, C. A. 1999. Guidelines for the management of Bowen's disease. *British Journal of Dermatology* **141**:633–641

Telfer, N. R., Colver, G.B. & Bowers, P. W. 1999. Guidelines for the management of basal cell carcinoma. *British Journal of Dermatology* **141**:415–423

Motley, R., Kersey, P., Lawrence, C., British Association of Dermatologists, British Association of Plastic Surgeons, Royal College of Radiologists & Faculty of Clinical Oncology. 2002. Multiprofessional guidelines for the management of the patient with primary cutaneous squamous cell carcinoma. *British Journal of Dermatology* **146**:18–25

## Chapter 28

Buxton, P. K. 2003. *ABC of Dermatology*, 4th edn. London: BMJ Publishing

Gawkrodger, D. J. 1997. *Dermatology: An Illustrated Colour Text*, 2nd edn. London: Churchill Livingstone

## Chapter 29

Freedbery, I. M., Eisen, A. Z., Wolff, K., Austen, K. F., Goldsmith, L. A. & Katz, S. I. (eds). 2003. *Fitzpatrick's Dermatology in General Medicine*, 6th edn. New York: McGraw-Hill,

Rook, A., Wilkinson, D.S., Ebling, F. J. S., Champion, R. H. & Burton, J. L. (eds). 1998. *Textbook of Dermatology*, 6th edn. Oxford: Blackwell Scientific Publications

## Chapter 30

Du Vivier, A. 2002. *Atlas of Clinical Dermatology*, 3rd edn. London: Churchill Livingstone

Wakelin, S. 2001. *Systemic Drugs in Dermatology*. London: Manson Publishing

## Chapter 31

Veien, N. K. 1998. The clinician's choice of antibiotics in the treatment of bacterial skin infections. *British Journal of Dermatology* **139**:30–36

## Chapter 32

Sterling, J. C., Handfield, S. & Hudson, P. M. 2001. Guidelines for the management of cutaneous warts. *British Journal of Dermatology* **144**:4–11

Hunter, J. A., Savin, J. A & Dahl, M. 2002. *Clinical Dermatology*, 3rd edn. London: Blackwell Science

## Chapter 33

Rook, A., Wilkinson, D. S., Ebling, F. J. S., Champion, R. H. & Burton, J. L. (eds). 1998. *Textbook of Dermatology*, 6th edn. Oxford: Blackwell Scientific Publications

## Chapter 34

Gawkrodger, D. J. 1997. *Dermatology: An Illustrated Colour Text*, 2nd edn. London: Churchill Livingstone

## Chapter 35

Grattan, C., Powell, S. & Humphreys, F. 2001. Management and diagnostic guidelines for urticaria and angio-odema. *British Journal of Dermatology* **144**:708–714

Rook, A., Wilkinson, D. S., Ebling, F. J. S., Champion, R. H. & Burton, J. L. (eds). 1998. *Textbook of Dermatology*, 6th edn. Oxford: Blackwell Scientific Publications

## Chapter 36

Graham-Brown, R. & Burns, T. 2002. *Lecture Notes on Dermatology*, 8th edn. London: Blackwell Science

MacKie, R. M. 2003. *Clinical Dermatology*, 5th edn. London: Oxford University Press

## Chapter 37

www.prodigy.nhs.uk/guidance acne vulgaris (accessed 15/Apr/2004)

Gollnick, H. P. M. & Krautheim, A. 2003. Topical treatment in acne: current status and future aspects. *Dermatology* **206**:29–36

Gawkrodger, D. J. 1997. *Dermatology: An Illustrated Colour Text*, 2nd edn. London: Churchill Livingstone

## Chapter 38

MacDonald Hull, S. P., Wood, M. L., Hutchinson, P. E., Sladden, M. & Messenger, A. G. Guidelines for the management of alopecia areata. *British Journal of Dermatology* **147**:692–699

Gawkrodger, D. J. 1997. *Dermatology: An Illustrated Colour Text*, 2nd edn. London: Churchill Livingstone

## Chapter 39

Simon, D. A., Dix, F. P. & McCollum, C. N. 2004. Management of venous leg ulcers. *British Medical Journal* **328**:1358–1362

Mekkes, J. R., Loots, M. A. M., Van Der Wal, A. C. & Bos, J. D. 2003. Causes, investigation and treatment of leg ulceration. *British Journal of Dermatology* **148**:388–401

Douglas, W. S. & Simpson, N. B. 1995. Guidelines for the management of chronic venous leg ulceration. Report of a multidisciplinary workshop. *British Journal of Dermatology* **132**:446–452

## Chapter 40, 41 and 42

MacKie, R. M. 2003. *Clinical Dermatology*, 5th edn. London: Oxford University Press

Buxton, P. K. 2003. *ABC of Dermatology*, 4th edn. London: BMJ Publishing

Gawkrodger, D. J. 1997. *Dermatology: An Illustrated Colour Text*, 2nd edn. London: Churchill Livingstone

# Index

Note: Page numbers in **bold** refer to figures and tables.